Study Guide for

Abrams' Clinical Drug Therapy
Rationales for Nursing Practice

TENTH EDITION

Wolters Kluwer | Lippincott Williams & Wilkins
Health

Philadelphia · Baltimore · New York · London
Buenos Aires · Hong Kong · Sydney · Tokyo

Acquisitions Editor: Matt Kane
Product Manager: John Larkin
Editorial Assistant: Dan Reilly
Production Project Manager: Cynthia Rudy
Design Coordinator: Joan Wendt
Illustration Coordinator: Brett MacNaughton
Manufacturing Coordinator: Karin Duffield
Prepress Vendor: SPi Global

Tenth edition

9 8 7 6 5 4 3 2 1

Printed in the United States of America

ISBN: 978-1-4511-8238-5

Care has been taken to confirm the accuracy of the information presented and to describe generally accepted practices. However, the authors, editors, and publisher are not responsible for errors or omissions or for any consequences from application of the information in this book and make no warranty, expressed or implied, with respect to the currency, completeness, or accuracy of the contents of the publication. Application of this information in a particular situation remains the professional responsibility of the practitioner; the clinical treatments described and recommended may not be considered absolute and universal recommendations.

The authors, editors, and publisher have exerted every effort to ensure that drug selection and dosage set forth in this text are in accordance with the current recommendations and practice at the time of publication. However, in view of ongoing research, changes in government regulations, and the constant flow of information relating to drug therapy and drug reactions, the reader is urged to check the package insert for each drug for any change in indications and dosage and for added warnings and precautions. This is particularly important when the recommended agent is a new or infrequently employed drug.

Some drugs and medical devices presented in this publication have Food and Drug Administration (FDA) clearance for limited use in restricted research settings. It is the responsibility of the health care provider to ascertain the FDA status of each drug or device planned for use in his or her clinical practice.

LWW.com

Preface

This Study Guide was developed for the 10th edition of *Abrams' Clinical Drug Therapy: Rationales for Nursing Practice* by Geralyn Frandsen and Sandra Pennington. The Study Guide is designed to help you practice and retain the knowledge you've gained from the textbook, and it is structured to integrate that knowledge and give you a basis for applying it in your nursing practice. The following types of exercises are provided in each chapter of the Study Guide.

Learning Objectives
Each Study Guide chapter lists the Learning Objectives of the textbook chapter, to remind you of the goals of the chapter as you work your way through the exercises.

Assessing Your Understanding
The first section of each Study Guide chapter concentrates on the basic information in the textbook chapter and helps you to remember key concepts, vocabulary, and principles.

- **Fill in the Blanks.** Fill in the blank exercises help you recall important chapter information by testing you on key points.

- **Matching.** Matching questions test your knowledge of the definition of key terms.

- **Sequencing.** Sequencing exercises ask you to remember particular sequences or orders, for instance testing processes and prioritizing nursing actions.

- **Short Answers.** Short answer questions cover the facts, concepts, procedures, and principles of the chapter. These questions ask you to recall information as well as demonstrate your comprehension of it.

Applying Your Knowledge
The second section of each Study Guide chapter consists of case study–based exercises that ask you to apply the knowledge you've gained from the textbook chapter, which was reinforced in the first section of the Study Guide chapter. A case study scenario based on the chapter's content is presented, and then you are asked to answer some questions, in writing, related to the case study. In addition to questions related to your knowledge of the drugs themselves, these case scenarios ask you to consider your nursing role in areas such as patient education and communication with physicians.

Practicing for NCLEX
The final section of each Study Guide chapter helps you practice answering NCLEX-style questions based on the content of the textbook chapter. The questions are scenario-based, asking you to reflect, consider, and apply what you know and to choose the best answer out of those posited. Some questions in the alternate format NCLEX styles are also included.

Answer Key
So that you can assess your own learning as you complete each chapter, the answers for all of the exercises in the Study Guide are provided at the back of the book.

We hope you will find this Study Guide to be helpful and enjoyable, and we wish you success in your goal of becoming a nurse.

The Publisher

Contents

CHAPTER 1

Introduction to Pharmacology

Learning Objectives

- Define a prototype drug.
- Distinguish between generic and trade names of drugs.
- Describe the main categories of controlled substances in relation to therapeutic use, potential for abuse, and regulatory requirements.
- Identify the multiple safeguards that are in place to promote drug safety in packaging, drug laws, and approval processes.
- Recognize initiatives designated to enhance safe drug administration.
- Develop personal techniques for learning about drugs and using drug knowledge in patient care.
- Identify authoritative sources of drug information.

SECTION I: ASSESSING YOUR UNDERSTANDING

Activity A FILL IN THE BLANKS

1. _____ is the study of drugs (chemicals) that alter functions of living organisms.

2. _____, also called pharmacotherapy, is the use of drugs to prevent, diagnose, or treat signs, symptoms, and disease processes.

3. Drugs given for therapeutic purposes are called _____.

4. Individual drugs that represent groups of drugs are called _____.

5. _____ involves the costs of drug therapy, which include the costs of purchasing, dispensing, storage, and administration; laboratory and other tests used to monitor patient responses; and losses due to expiration.

Activity B MATCHING

Match the term in Column A with the definition in Column B.

Column A	Column B
____ 1. Generic name	a. Designates drugs that must be prescribed by a licensed physician or nurse practitioner and dispensed by a pharmacist
____ 2. Trade or brand name	
____ 3. Food, Drug, and Cosmetic Act of 1938	b. Regulates the manufacture, distribution, advertising, and labeling of drugs
____ 4. Durham-Humphrey Amendment	c. Regulates the manufacture and distribution of narcotics, stimulants, depressants, hallucinogens, and anabolic steroids
____ 5. Controlled Substances Act	d. Often indicates the drug group
	e. Name designated and patented by the manufacturer

Activity C SEQUENCING

Since 1962, newly developed drugs have been extensively tested before being marketed for general use. Clinical trials are conducted in four phases, which are given below in random order. Write the correct sequence in which they are performed in the boxes provided.

A. A few doses are given to a certain number of healthy volunteers to determine safe dosages, routes of administration, absorption, metabolism, excretion, and toxicity.

B. Studies help to determine whether the potential benefits of the drug outweigh the risks.

C. A few doses are given to a certain number of subjects who have the disease or symptom for which the drug is being studied, and responses are compared with those of healthy subjects.

D. The FDA evaluates the data from the first three phases for drug safety and effectiveness, allows the drug to be marketed for general use, and requires manufacturers to continue monitoring the drug's effects.

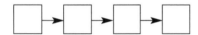

Activity D SHORT ANSWERS

Briefly answer the following questions.

1. Medications may be given for local effects. Give an example of a drug that exhibits its effects locally, and identify the action of the medication.

2. Medications may be given for systemic effects. Explain the mechanism of action for a systemic medication.

3. Identify the advantages of synthetic drugs.

4. Describe why biotechnology is an important source of drugs.

5. Describe the impact of cloning on biotechnology.

SECTION II: APPLYING YOUR KNOWLEDGE

Activity E CASE STUDIES

Consider the scenario and answer the questions.

Sally Smith, a close friend, states that she has a headache that "just won't go away." She asks if she can borrow a prescription medication that you received from your physician last year for persistent migraine headaches.

1. You want to help Sally to relieve the pain that she is experiencing. Discuss the two methods that a consumer may use to procure therapeutic medications.

2. Sally visits her doctor and is instructed to take OTC medications for her pain. Define "OTC" and the regulation of these medications.

3. Sally tells you that she borrowed a friend's prescription drug to control her headache. She states that she felt so good taking the drug that she wants to repeat the experience. Discuss the legal ramifications of self-administration of prescription drugs prescribed to another.

SECTION III: PRACTICING FOR NCLEX

Activity F

Answer the following questions.

1. The FDA approves many new drugs annually. New drugs are categorized according to their review priority and therapeutic potential. What is a new drug that is to be reviewed on a priority or accelerated basis?

   a. 1P

   b. 1D

   c. 1A

   d. 1S

2. The FDA approves drugs for OTC status, including the transfer of drugs from prescription to OTC status. What are characteristic of prescription drugs that are delegated to OTC status? (Select all that apply.)

   a. They may be administered at a higher dosage than the prescription.

   b. They may be administered at a lower dosage than the prescription.

   c. They may require additional clinical trials to determine the safety and effectiveness of the OTC use.

   d. They may be used for different indications than the original prescription medication.

   e. They shift responsibility from the consumer to the health care professional to ensure the drug may be taken safely.

3. Having drugs available OTC has potential advantages and disadvantages for consumers. What is one of the advantages?

 a. Reliable self-diagnosis

 b. Increased diagnosis of the identified illness

 c. Faster and more convenient access to effective treatment

 d. Reduction of possible drug interactions

4. When prevention or cure is not a reasonable goal, relief of symptoms can do what? (Select all that apply.)

 a. Improve a patient's quality of life

 b. Eliminate pain

 c. Improve ability to function in activities of daily living

 d. Decrease dependence on drugs

 e. Increase longevity

5. Drugs are classified according to what features?

 a. Name

 b. Therapeutic uses

 c. Side effects

 d. Actions

6. What do the names of therapeutic classifications usually reflect?

 a. Actions of the medication

 b.Conditions for which the medication is used

 c. Possible adverse reactions to the medications

 d. Possible generic names for the medication

7. How may drugs be prescribed and dispensed?

 a. By generic name only

 b. By trade name only

 c. By prescription

 d. By generic or trade name

8. Once a drug is patented, what statement is true?

 a. The drug may be manufactured by other companies.

 b. The drug may be manufactured by other companies under a generic name.

 c. The drug may not be manufactured by other companies until the patent expires.

 d. The drug may be marketed by other companies.

9. The main goal of current drug laws and standards is to ensure what?

 a. That drugs are available to all, regardless of cost

 b. That drugs marketed for therapeutic purposes are safe and effective

 c. That drugs are cost-effective

 d. That drugs are patented

10. What are the advantages of using a synthetic drug? (Select all that apply.)

 a. Increased standardized chemical characteristics

 b. Produced by cloning

 c. More consistent therapeutic effects

 d. Less allergenic

 e. Limited use for treatment of disease

11. What does the Comprehensive Drug Abuse Prevention and Control Act regulate?

 a. Classifications of narcotics

 b. Acceptable diagnoses for prescription of narcotics

 c. Manufacture and distribution of narcotics

 d. Abuse of narcotics

12. What are nurses responsible for? (Select all that apply.)

 a. Storing controlled substances in locked containers

 b. Reporting discrepancies in the narcotic inventory to the physician

 c. Recording prescribed controlled substances on medication administration records

 d. Maintaining an accurate inventory of narcotics

 e. Administering controlled substances when the prescribed analgesic is not effective.

13. People and companies that are legally empowered to handle controlled substances must do what? (Select all that apply.)

 a. Keep accurate records of all transactions

 b. Be registered with the DEA

 c. Be registered with the FDA

 d. Provide for secure storage of controlled substances

 e. Educate health care professionals about adverse effects of controlled substances

14. What does the National Institutes of Health Revitalization Act stipulate?

    a. Men must be included in drug research studies.

    b. Women and minorities must be included in drug research studies.

    c. Animal testing must be completed prior to human drug testing.

    d. Animal testing is not needed prior to human drug testing.

15. Since 1962, newly developed drugs have been extensively tested before being marketed for general use. What do drug companies do to test drugs *initially*?

    a. Test the drugs with animals.

    b. Test the drugs with humans.

    c. Test the drugs in a controlled laboratory experiment.

    d. Test the drugs on volunteers.

16. FDA approval of a drug for OTC availability includes what?

    a. Analysis of the cost of the drug to the consumer

    b. Evaluation of evidence that the consumer can use the drug safely, using information on the product label

    c. Studies involving the safe use of the medication by the consumer

    d. Analysis of the diagnoses for which the medication may be used by the consumer

17. What should the beginning student of pharmacology use as the primary source of drug data?

    a. The Internet

    b. The pharmacology text

    c. A drug book

    d. A palm pilot

18. What is the manufacturer's responsibility during Phase IV of a drug trial?

    a. Find healthy volunteers to test for adverse effects.

    b. Continue to monitor the drug's effects while the drug is in general use.

    c. Match patients with similar characteristics to test drug effectiveness.

    d. Determine if the drug is too toxic for human use.

19. What is designated by the Durham-Humphrey Amendment?

    a. Drugs that may be administered by a nurse

    b. Drugs that may be designated as OTC

    c. Drugs that must be prescribed by a licensed physician

    d. Drugs that must be given in conjunction with other drugs to be effective

20. What is a major disadvantage of using over-the-counter (OTC) medications?

    a. Causes increased visits to the health care practitioner

    b. Consumers resist the effort to learn more about their condition.

    c. People may choose an OTC that interacts with another medication.

    d. Lack of autonomy

Basic Concepts and Processes

- Discuss cellular physiology in relation to drug therapy.
- Describe the main pathways and mechanisms by which drugs cross biologic membranes and move through the body.
- Explain each process of pharmacokinetics.
- Discuss the clinical usefulness of measuring serum drug levels.
- Describe major characteristics of the receptor theory of drug action.
- Differentiate between agonist drugs and antagonist drugs.
- List drug-related and patient-related variables that affect drug actions.
- Discuss mechanisms and potential effects of drug–drug interactions.
- Identify signs and symptoms that may occur with adverse drug effects on major body systems.
- Discuss general management of drug overdose and toxicity.
- Discuss selected drug antidotes.

SECTION I: ASSESSING YOUR UNDERSTANDING

Activity A   FILL IN THE BLANKS

1. _____ are chemicals that alter basic processes in body cells.

2. Drugs must reach and interact with or cross the _____ to stimulate or inhibit cellular function.

3. _____ involves drug movement through the body (i.e., "what the body does to the drug") to reach sites of action, metabolism, and excretion.

4. _____ is the process that occurs from the time a drug enters the body to the time it enters the bloodstream to be circulated.

5. Liquid medications are absorbed _____ than tablets or capsules because they need not be dissolved.

6. _____ occur when two drugs with similar pharmacologic actions are taken.

7. _____ occurs when two drugs with different sites or mechanisms of action produce greater effects when taken together.

8. _____ by one drug with the metabolism of a second drug may result in intensified effects of the second drug.

9. _____ of one drug from plasma protein–binding sites by a second drug (i.e., a drug with a strong attraction to protein-binding sites may displace a less tightly bound drug) increases the effects of the displaced drug.

10. A/An _____ drug can be given to antagonize the toxic effects of another drug.

Activity B MATCHING

Match the term in Column A with the definition in Column B.

Column A

_____ **1.** Distribution

_____ **2.** Protein binding

_____ **3.** Metabolism

_____ **4.** Excretion

_____ **5.** A serum drug level

Column B

a. The method by which drugs are inactivated or biotransformed by the body

b. An important factor in drug distribution

c. A laboratory measurement of the amount of a drug in the blood at a particular time

d. Elimination of a drug from the body

e. Involves the transport of drug molecules within the body after a drug is injected or absorbed into the bloodstream.

Activity C SEQUENCING

Given below, in random order, are statements that refer to the movements of a drug in the body. Identify the path that the molecules of most oral drugs must take in order to be effectively absorbed and excreted by writing the correct sequence in the boxes provided.

A. Perform their action, and then return to the bloodstream

B. Circulate to their target cells

C. Cross the membranes of cells in the gastrointestinal tract, liver, and capillaries to reach the bloodstream

D. Reenter the bloodstream, circulate to the kidneys, and be excreted in urine

E. Leave the bloodstream and attach to receptors on cells

F. Circulate to the liver, and reach drug-metabolizing enzymes in liver cells

☐ → ☐ → ☐ → ☐ → ☐ → ☐

Activity D SHORT ANSWERS

Briefly answer the following questions.

1. Explain how a drug is absorbed systemically.

2. Although cells differ from one tissue to another, their common characteristics include the ability to perform what functions?

3. Identify several factors that may affect the rate and extent of drug absorption.

4. Rapid movement through the stomach and small intestine may increase drug absorption by what mechanisms or factors?

5. Why is drug distribution into the central nervous system (CNS) limited because of the blood–brain barrier?

SECTION II: APPLYING YOUR KNOWLEDGE

Activity E CASE STUDIES

Consider the scenario and answer the questions.

Stanley, age 35, is newly diagnosed with a seizure disorder. His physician arranges for blood levels to be drawn every 2 weeks during the first month that the new drug is administered.

1. Stanley asks you why he needs to have blood drawn every 2 weeks. Define serum drug levels and explain the rationale for obtaining them.

2. Stanley's physician reduces his medication dosage after the first laboratory results because the levels are near toxic. Stanley demonstrates to you that he is taking his medication correctly. He asks why his level might become toxic. Discuss conditions that may foster toxic drug levels in a compliant patient.

3. Two months later, the physician notifies Stanley that he has reached a blood therapeutic level and should continue to take the currently prescribed dosage of his medication. Explain the method by which a therapeutic range is determined by the physician.

SECTION III: PRACTICING FOR NCLEX

Activity F

Answer the following questions.

1. The nurse is explaining to the patient what bioavailability is. What statement is true of bioavailability?
   a. It is the portion of a dose that reaches the systemic circulation.
   b. It is the portion of a dose that causes toxicity.
   c. It is the portion of a dose that is absorbed by the system to achieve a therapeutic drug level.
   d. It is the portion of a dose that reaches the systemic circulation and is available to act on body cells.

2. A drug is 100% bioavailable when it is administered by what routes?
   a. Oral
   b. Parenteral
   c. Intravenous
   d. Rectal

3. Mrs. Anderson is prescribed a medication to control her hypercholesterolemia. Two years later, the physician prescribes a higher dose of her medication due to a process called *enzyme induction*. A student nurse asks the nurse to explain the change in the drug dosage. The nurse explains that with chronic administration, some drugs stimulate liver cells to produce what?
   a. Smaller amounts of drug-metabolizing enzymes
   b. Toxic amounts of drug-metabolizing enzymes
   c. Larger amounts of drug-metabolizing enzymes
   d. Therapeutic amounts of drug-metabolizing enzymes

4. Mr. Elliot is prescribed a combination of medications to treat his disease process. He is exhibiting signs of toxicity related to his new drug regimen. A possible cause of the change in the absorption of his medications may be *enzyme inhibition*. What is true of enzyme inhibition? (Select all that apply.)
   a. It may occur with concurrent administration of two or more drugs that compete for the same metabolizing enzymes.
   b. It may occur with concurrent administration of two or more drugs that compete for different metabolizing enzymes.
   c. It may necessitate the administration of larger doses of the medication.
   d. It may necessitate the administration of smaller doses of the medication.
   e. It occurs within seconds or minutes of starting an inhibiting agent.

5. In the first-pass effect or presystemic metabolism, a drug is extensively metabolized in the liver, with only part of the drug dose reaching the systemic circulation for distribution to sites of action. The first-pass effect occurs when some drugs are given by what route?
   a. Orally
   b. Parenterally
   c. Rectally
   d. Intravenously

6. Whereas some drugs or metabolites are excreted in bile and then eliminated in feces, others are excreted in bile, reabsorbed from the small intestine, and then returned to the liver. What is the name of this process?
   a. Enterohepatic recirculation
   b. Interohepatic recirculation
   c. Enterorenal recirculation
   d. Interorenal recirculation

7. For most drugs, serum levels indicate the onset, peak, and duration of drug action. After a single dose of a drug is given, onset of action occurs when the drug level reaches what?
   a. MAX
   b. MIC
   c. MEC
   d. MAC

8. In clinical practice, measurement of serum drug levels is useful in what circumstances? (Select all that apply.)

    a. When drugs with a narrow margin of safety are given, because their therapeutic doses are close to their toxic doses

    b. When the medication used is experimental

    c. To document the serum drug levels associated with particular drug dosages, therapeutic effects, or possible adverse effects

    d. To document drug interactions

    e. To monitor unexpected responses to a drug dose, such as decreased therapeutic effects or increased adverse effects

    f. When a drug overdose is suspected

9. Which skin condition would be most likely to cause increased systemic absorption of a topical medication?

    a. Multiple nevi

    b. Rosacea

    c. Port wine stain of the face

    d. Severe sunburn

10. When a drug is given at a stable dose, how many half-life periods are required to achieve steady-state concentrations and develop equilibrium between tissue and serum concentrations?

    a. 2 to 3

    b. 3 to 4

    c. 4 to 5

    d. 5 to 6

11. *Pharmacodynamics* involves drug actions on target cells and results in what?

    a. Alterations in cellular biochemical reactions and functions

    b. Alterations in cellular pharmacologic reactions

    c. Alterations in drug absorption

    d. Alterations in drug secretion

12. Relatively few drugs act by mechanisms other than combination with receptor sites on cells. Drugs that do not act on receptor sites include what? (Select all that apply.)

    a. Antacids

    b. Salicylates

    c. Osmotic diuretics

    d. Purines

    e. NSAIDs

13. Mrs. Geonity is prescribed a medication, and the physician modifies the dose on multiple occasions to achieve the maximum therapeutic effect of the drug. She asks the nurse what the rationale is for the dosage changes. How should the nurse respond?

    a. "Dosage determines whether the drug actions may be therapeutic or toxic."

    b. "Dosage varies based on the brand name."

    c. "Your generic drug does not work as efficiently, and the physician increased your dose."

    d. "Your HMO requires that we change the drug dose frequently."

14. Mr. Dow works the evening shift. The physician orders a medication that must be taken three times a day on an empty stomach. He asks the nurse if he can take his evening dose with supper for the sake of convenience. How should the nurse respond?

    a. "If it is only the one meal, the food will not make a difference."

    b. "Food may slow the absorption of the drug."

    c. "Food may increase the effectiveness of the medication."

    d. "It does not matter if the drug is taken on an empty stomach or not."

15. Mr. Ansgow is diagnosed with Parkinson's disease. His physician orders selegiline. As part of his education plan, the nurse instructs the patient to avoid what food?

    a. Grapefruit

    b. Cheese

    c. Chicken

    d. Corn

16. Mrs. Adams is diagnosed with atrial fibrillation and prescribed the drug Coumadin. The nurse would instruct her to avoid what food?

    a. Foods with vitamin B

    b. Foods with vitamin C

    c. Foods with vitamin K

    d. Foods with niacin

17. Mr. Grey is diagnosed with hypercholesterol-emia and is prescribed a statin by his physician. As part of his education plan, the nurse should teach Mr. Grey to avoid what food?

    a. Grapefruit

    b. Cheese

    c. Chicken

    d. Corn

18. Changes in aging in the geriatric patient that may affect excretion and promote accumulation of drugs in the body include what?

    a. Rigidity of the diaphragm

    b. Increased gastric motility

    c. Decreased mentation

    d. Decreased glomerular filtration rate

19. Mr. Abo, an African American male, asks the nurse why the physician orders a diuretic as part of his treatment plan for hypertension, when the physician ordered an ACE inhibitor for his friend with the same diagnosis. After consulting with the physician, how would the nurse respond?

    a. "Diuretics are more cost-effective."

    b. "Diuretics are shown to be more effective than ACE inhibitors for African American males with hypertension."

    c. "The physician ordered diuretics to reduce the stress on your heart."

    d. "You must take the drug that the doctor orders, because he knows best how to manage your hypertension."

20. Mrs. Smith has a 12-year history of ETOH abuse. She is injured in a motor vehicle accident and requires surgery with general anesthesia. What would the nurse expect for this patient?

    a. A smaller-than-normal dose of the general anesthetic

    b. A larger-than-normal dose of the general anesthetic

    c. The same dose of the general anesthetic as another female of her age and medical history

    d. No general anesthesia, because general anesthesia should not be given to a patient with her history

3 CHAPTER

Medication Administration and the Nursing Process of Drug Therapy

Learning Objectives

- Apply the rights of medication administration in the care of a patient.
- Illustrate knowledge needed to administer medications to a patient.
- Identify and interpret the drug orders for medication administration.
- Demonstrate the ability to calculate drug dosages accurately.
- Apply the steps of the nursing process in the administration of medications.
- Demonstrate safe and accurate administration of medications.
- Apply evidence-based practice research in the administration of medications.
- Identify alternative or complementary therapy that may potentiate, negate, or cause toxicity with prescribed medications.

SECTION I: ASSESSING YOUR UNDERSTANDING

Activity A FILL IN THE BLANKS

1. The _____ system is a method of drug administration in which most drugs are dispensed in single-dose containers for individual patients.

2. _____ are usually kept as a stock supply in a locked drawer or automated cabinet and replaced as needed.

3. _____ is a process designed to avoid medication errors such as omissions, duplications, dosing errors, or drug interactions that occur when a patient is admitted to a health care agency, transferred from one department or unit to another within the agency, or discharged home from the agency.

4. The nursing process involves both _____ and _____ skills.

5. _____ involves collecting data about patient characteristics known to affect drug therapy.

Activity B MATCHING

Match the term in Column A with the definition in Column B

Column A	Column B
_____ **1.** Goal	**a.** As desired
_____ **2.** Assessment	**b.** What does the patient know about current drugs? Is teaching needed?
_____ **3.** ad lib	
_____ **4.** Intervention	**c.** Experience relief of signs and symptoms
_____ **5.** mcg	**d.** Microgram
	e. Ambulating, positioning, exercising

Activity C SEQUENCING

You are administering a medication using a point-of-care bar code system. Given below, in random order, are the steps used for medication preparation and administration. Place the steps in the correct order, using the boxes provided.

A. The nurse scans the patient's ID band and the nurse's personal ID badge.

B. The nurse compares the medication with the medication ordered for the patient.

C. The nurse records the drug on the medication administration record.

D. The nurse scans the bar code on the drug label.

E. The nurse administers the medication to the patient.

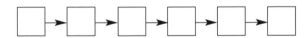

Activity D SHORT ANSWERS

Briefly answer the following questions.

1. Give three examples of commonly reported medication errors.

2. Describe the components of a medication order.

3. Describe the assessment phase of the nursing process.

4. Describe the planning/goals component of the nursing process.

5. When does evaluation occur within the nursing process?

SECTION II: APPLYING YOUR KNOWLEDGE

Activity E CASE STUDIES

Consider the scenarios and answer the questions.

Case Study 1

A physician calls you with a series of verbal orders for Ms. Walden, who is to be discharged today. You are responsible for Ms. Walden's discharge medication education.

1. Describe the parameters for a verbal order.

2. The physician gives Ms. Walden a prescription for a Schedule II controlled drug to be taken after discharge. Describe the parameters for a prescription narcotic; include the method used to refill the prescription.

3. What information would you include in the education plan regarding discharge medications for Ms. Walden?

Case Study 2

You are responsible for the initial assessment for a patient returning to the physician's office 10 days after beginning a new medication regimen to control her asthma.

1. You begin your assessment by doing which of the following?
   a. Collecting objective data
   b. Collecting both objective and subjective data
   c. Collecting subjective data only
   d. Taking the patient's vital signs

2. You interview the patient regarding the effectiveness of the medication as well as any adverse reactions. Your patient's statements are considered to be which of the following?
   a. Subjective data
   b. Objective data
   c. An icebreaker
   d. An important part of the nursing diagnosis

3. Part of your focused assessment includes taking the patient's vital signs. Vital signs are an example of which of the following?
   a. Subjective data
   b. Objective data
   c. An icebreaker
   d. An important part of the nursing diagnosis

SECTION III: PRACTICING FOR NCLEX

Answer the following questions.

1. A patient refuses a PRN medication; the nurse documents the reason for the refusal on the back of the medication administration record and disposes of the medication according to facility policy. By documenting the patient's refusal and reason for declining the medication, the nurse is adhering to which of the "rights" for medication administration?
   a. Right dose
   b. Right medication
   c. Right documentation
   d. Right patient

2. The charge nurse on the unit transcribes a physician's order onto the medication administration record. She writes, "Digoxin 0.25 mg PO qod ×3d" on the MAR. How should the order be written to prevent medication error?
   a. Digoxin 0.25 mg PO every other day ×3d
   b. Digoxin 0.25 mg PO qod for three doses
   c. Digoxin 0.25 mg by mouth every other day for three doses
   d. Digoxin 0.25 mg PO qod ×3d

3. The physician orders NPH U100 insulin 16 units SC every AM for Mrs. Styles. The nurse prepares the insulin dose, and, to ensure safety, what does the nurse do?
   a. Give the insulin to the patient.
   b. Bring the vial.
   c. Ask another nurse to double-check the measurement.
   d. Encourage the patient to administer her own insulin.

4. During a medication pass, the nurse notices that the physician ordered a dose of medication that appears to be excessive, based on the nurse's knowledge of the medication. The nurse calls the physician, and he instructs the nurse to administer the medication anyway. What should the nurse do?
   a. Administer the medication.
   b. Consult with the nursing supervisor, refuse to administer the medication, and notify the physician.
   c. Refuse to administer the medication, and notify the physician.
   d. Ask the physician on-call for a new order.

5. What specific drugs are often associated with errors and adverse drug events (ADEs)? (Select all that apply.)
   a. Insulin
   b. Acetaminophen
   c. Heparin
   d. Salicylates
   e. Warfarin

6. What is a safety feature inherent in using the bar code method to administer drugs?
   a. The bar code on the drug label contains the patient's name.
   b. When administering medications, the nurse is only required to scan the bar code on the drug label.
   c. The bar code on the patient's identification band contains the MAR.
   d. A wireless computer network processes the scanned information and gives an error message when the MAR has not been inputted onto the computer.

7. Mrs. Janis' physician orders enteric-coated aspirin 81 mg by mouth once a day. When the nurse attempts to administer the medication, the patient informs the nurse that the aspirin that she takes at home is not coated and works just fine. As part of the nurse's education plan, what does the nurse instruct the patient to do?
   a. "Enteric-coated tablets and capsules are coated with a substance that is insoluble in stomach acid. This delays dissolution until the medication reaches the intestine, usually to avoid gastric irritation or to keep the drug from being destroyed by gastric acid."
   b. "Enteric-coated tablets and capsules are coated with a substance that is soluble in stomach acid. This delays dissolution until the medication reaches the intestine, usually to avoid gastric irritation or to keep the drug from being destroyed by gastric acid."
   c. "Enteric-coated tablets and capsules are coated with a substance that is insoluble in stomach acid. This delays dissolution until

the medication reaches the intestine, usually causing gastric irritation or to keep the drug from being destroyed by gastric acid."

d. "Enteric-coated tablets and capsules are coated with a substance that is insoluble in stomach acid. This delays dissolution until the medication reaches the liver, usually to avoid gastric irritation or to keep the drug from being destroyed by gastric acid."

8. Mrs. Hone has a new order for Effexor XR. She asks the nurse why she doesn't have to take the medication as frequently as her other antidepressant. As part of the nurse's teaching plan, what does the nurse tell her?

a. "XR means that the drug is extended release, which means that there are less consistent serum drug levels and you need to take it less frequently."

b. "XR means that the drug is delayed release, which means that there are more consistent serum drug levels and you need to take it less frequently."

c. "XR means that the drug is extended release, which means that there are more consistent serum drug levels and you need to take it less frequently."

d. "XR means that the drug is extended release, which means that there are more consistent serum drug levels and you need to take it more frequently."

9. Mrs. Hone asks the nurse to open her Effexor XR capsule and mix the contents in applesauce to make it easier to swallow. How should the nurse respond?

a. "Not a problem; I will mix the medication for you."

b. "I am sorry, but opening the capsule may cause you to absorb too much medication too quickly."

c. "The physician gave you this form of your medication because it is easier to take by mouth."

d. "Effexor XR may only be mixed with food with a physician's order."

10. How many 60-mg tablets of Lasix are needed to give a dose of 120 mg? _____ Show the mathematical formula used to achieve the answer: _____.

11. The physician ordered 8 mg of morphine sulfate IM. Morphine sulfate is available as 10 mg in a 1-mL vial. How many milliliters will the nurse administer to this patient? _____ Show the mathematical formula used to achieve the answer.

_____.

12. The nurse is preparing to administer a 500-mg. dose of medication. It is available as 0.5 g per tablet. How many tablets will the nurse administer to this patient to achieve the prescribed dose?_____
Show the mathematical formula used to achieve the answer.

_____

13. Mr. Jones is self-administering garlic, St. John's wort, and echinacea. What does the anesthesiologist ask the patient to do?

a. Discontinue the herbal medications 1 week prior to surgery.

b. Maintain his current regimen regardless of the herbal supplements taken.

c. Discontinue the herbal medications 2 to 3 weeks prior to surgery.

d. Continue only the garlic and echinacea according to his current medication regimen.

14. Mrs. Abbot recently discovered that she is pregnant. She currently takes herbal medications to control her diabetes and the symptoms related to pregnancy. She asks the nurse if it is safe to take herbal medications while she is pregnant. What would the nurse tell this patient?

a. "Most herbal and dietary supplements should be avoided during pregnancy or lactation."

b. "Most herbal and dietary supplements are safe during pregnancy and are used by many cultures to control the symptoms of nausea."

c. "Dietary supplements are high in fat and protein; they are safe to take during pregnancy and help to maintain health during lactation."

d. "Herbal and dietary supplements will cause premature labor."

15. What statement would indicate that a mother is administering the *incorrect* dosage of liquid medication to her child?

 a. "I use a calibrated medication cup to administer the medication."

 b. "I use the measuring teaspoon that I cook with."

 c. "I give the medication at the times indicated on the prescription."

 d. "I use a household teaspoon to administer the medication."

16. If a dose of a medication is missed, what do most authorities recommend?

 a. Double the dose the next time that the medication is due.

 b. Take the medication if it is close to the administration time.

 c. Increase the next two doses to maintain the drug's level in the system.

 d. Take the medication as long as there are 2 hours between doses.

17. The patient requests an oral pain medication. The nurse notes that the patient is NPO in preparation for laboratory tests. What is the nurse's best response to this patient?

 a. "You are not allowed to have any medication by mouth right now. I will give you this medication in an injection."

 b. "I will check with your doctor and see if it will be all right for you to take a pain pill."

 c. "I will contact your doctor and ask for an order for a different method of drug administration."

 d. "You will have to wait for this medication until you eat and drink again."

18. The nurse is preparing to administer medications via a patient's gastrostomy tube. The physician has ordered an extended-release medication. What is the nurse's most appropriate action?

 a. The nurse should open the capsule and empty the powder into 30 mL of water.

 b. Crush the capsule and flush the medication with at least 60 mL of water.

 c. Do not administer the medication because it may clog the gastrostomy tube.

 d. Call the physician and ask for an order for a different formulation of the medication.

19. The nursing instructor is observing a nursing student give a subcutaneous injection of heparin to a patient. The nursing student would receive an unsatisfactory evaluation if the student performed what action?

 a. The student uses a 25-gauge needle to administer the medication.

 b. The student inserts the needle at a 45-degree angle.

 c. The student gently aspirates the medication before administering the medication.

 d. The student applies pressure for a few sections after removing the needle.

20. The physician has ordered IV antibiotics for a patient who has had a right mastectomy. The nurse is unable to find a suitable vein to insert the IV catheter in the left hand or arm. What is the nurse's next best action?

 a. See if there are any available veins in the patient's right hand.

 b. Call the physician and report the difficulty in starting the IV.

 c. Attempt to start the IV in the patients left foot.

 d. Administer the antibiotics as an IM injection.

4

Pharmacology and the Care of the Infant and Pediatric Patient

Learning Objectives

- Identify characteristics of pediatric pharmaco-therapy in children from birth to 18 years of age.
- Describe the evolution of pediatric pharmaco-therapy and the purpose of federal legislation in the development of current practice standards.
- Describe methods for determining accurate pediatric dosing.
- Explain differences in pharmacodynamic variables between children and adults.
- Explain pharmacokinetic differences between children and adults.
- Describe nursing interventions that include caregivers to help ensure safe and effective medication administration to children.

SECTION I: ASSESSING YOUR UNDERSTANDING

Activity A FILL IN THE BLANKS

1. Both the _____ and _____ actions of medications are influenced by physiological changes throughout development.

2. When caring for children, the nurse is aware that the _____ the patient, the greater the variation in medication action.

3. Children differ from adults in the percentages of _____, which is the total amount of water within the body.

4. The nurse should always use a _____ approach when administering medications to children.

5. When patients go through _____, they respond more like adults physiologically.

Activity B MATCHING

Match the term in Column A with the definition in Column B

Column A	Column B
_____ 1. Premature infant	a. From full-term newborn 0 to 4 weeks of age
_____ 2. Neonate	b. 13 to 18 years of age
_____ 3. Infant	c. Less than 38 weeks of gestational age
_____ 4. Child	d. From greater than 4 weeks to 1 year of age
_____ 5. Adolescent	e. From greater than 1 to 12 years of age

Activity C SHORT ANSWERS

Briefly answer the following questions.

1. Briefly discuss the way in which drug dosages are calculated for infants and children.

2. Discuss the factors that influence the drug effectiveness in the pediatric population and give an example of a drug that has different pharmacodynamics dependent upon age.

3. Identify the factors that affect drug absorption in the pediatric population.

4. How does the toddler's developmental level affect medication administration?

5. What assessments are important for the nurse to make related to adolescents and medication use?

SECTION II: APPLYING YOUR KNOWLEDGE

Activity D CASE STUDY

Consider the scenario and answer the questions.

Julie, aged 6 months, is admitted to the pediatric unit with a diagnosis of dehydration. Her mother states that she began experiencing vomiting and diarrhea approximately 24 hours ago. The physician has ordered IV fluids to be infused at a rate of 48 mL/h.

1. The mother asks you why her daughter became dehydrated so quickly. Discuss why dehydration may occur more quickly in children than in adults.

2. The mother asks why the physician didn't order a "shot" to help her daughter quit vomiting. Discuss why intramuscular injections are not as effective in infants as they are in older children.

3. What actions would you recommend that the mother do for her infant daughter after you start the infant's IV?

SECTION III: PRACTICING FOR NCLEX

Activity E

Answer the following questions.

1. At what age do children have the same pharmacokinetic response as an adult?
   a. 5 years of age
   b. 8 years of age
   c. 12 years of age
   d. 15 years of age

2. The nurse is instructing a mother in applying a topical medication to her infant's diaper area. The nurse instructs the mother to place the cream only on the affected area and use it sparingly. These instructions are necessary because of what physiologic characteristic of neonates?
   a. High blood flow to the skeletal muscles of neonates
   b. Abnormally strong muscle contractions of neonates
   c. Small percentage of total body water of neonates as compared to adults
   d. Highly permeable skin tissue of neonates

3. An infant with a seizure disorder who must take phenytoin (Dilantin) is at risk for developing toxic levels of the medication. This is because of what immature organ function?
   a. Liver
   b. Heart
   c. Brain
   d. Integument

4. Which is the best area to place oral medications in infants?
   a. Back of the tongue
   b. Between the cheek and gums
   c. Inner aspect of the cheek
   d. Under the tongue

5. The nursing student is preparing to administer an IM injection to a 7-month-old infant. What is the best site for injecting a medication into an infant?
   a. Dorsogluteal
   b. Vastus lateralis
   c. Ventrogluteal
   d. Deltoid

6. What areas are the best sites that the nurse is aware of for starting IVs in infants? (Select all that apply.)
   a. Hands
   b. Feet
   c. Antecubital fossa
   d. Jugular
   e. Scalp

7. What is the best device for administering oral medications to an infant?
   a. Plastic medicine cup
   b. Calibrated teaspoon
   c. Oral syringe
   d. Feeding nipple

8. Suppositories are a very appropriate method of medication delivery in what age group?
   a. Infant
   b. Toddler
   c. Preschooler
   d. School age

9. What topics are important for the nurse to share with an adolescent related to self-care and medication administration? (Select all that apply.)
   a. Use of acne medications
   b. Adverse effects of prescribed medications
   c. Birth control pills and other drug interactions
   d. Safe use of alcohol
   e. How to get a sun tan

10. The nurse is aware that pharmacodynamic variability in the pediatric patient is due to what factors? (Select all that apply.)
    a. Fat stores
    b. Skin permeability
    c. Gastric emptying
    d. Total body water
    e. Protein-carrying ability

11. The exact dose of a medication for a pediatric patient is based on what parameter?
    a. Total body water
    b. Weight
    c. Height
    d. Gastric acidity

12. The nurse is aware that CNS adverse effects of medications given to infants are higher because of what immature function?
    a. Liver function
    b. Renal function
    c. Blood–brain barrier
    d. Peripheral nervous system function

13. A 9-year-old child has been prescribed a medication but is not able to safely swallow pills. What type of medication formulation would work best for this child?
    a. Chewable tablets
    b. Capsules
    c. Scored tablets
    d. Extended-release tablets

14. The nurse must start an IV on a 4-year-old child. What sites would be best for IV placement in this child? (Select all that apply.)
    a. Hands
    b. Feet
    c. Antecubital fossa
    d. Scalp
    e. Wrist

15. The nurse is aware that renal function of a child reaches that of an adult at which age?
    a. 2 years
    b. 5 years
    c. 10 years
    d. 15 years

16. What is the total water body percentage in infants?
    a. 50%
    b. 60%
    c. 80%
    d. 95%

17. What factors affect drug absorption in neonates? (Select all that apply.)
    a. Increased gastric acidity
    b. Delayed gastric emptying
    c. Increased gastric pH
    d. Irregular gastric emptying
    e. Constricted pyloric sphincter

18. The nurse is aware that the use of antidepressants in adolescents is associated with what issue?

    a. Suicide

    b. Schizophrenia

    c. Bulimia

    d. Anorexia nervosa

19. The nurse knows that pharmacodynamics across the lifespan are affected by what variables? (Select all that apply.)

    a. Skin permeability

    b. Body composition

    c. Genetic makeup

    d. Route of administration

    e. Immature organ systems

20. What type of pediatric drug calculation is expressed in square meters?

    a. Weight based

    b. Body surface area

    c. Height based

    d. Age based

Pharmacology and the Care of the Adult and Geriatric Patient

Learning Objectives

- Understand pharmacodynamics and pharmacokinetic changes related to age in older adults.
- Understand the relevance of the Beers Criteria to medication administration in the aging population.
- Identify the physiological changes associated with increased age related to pharmacokinetics (absorption, distribution, metabolism, and excretion) of medications.
- Understand the effect of polypharmacy on the medication response of older adults.
- Implement patient education about medications to prevent medication-related reactions and adverse effects.

SECTION I: ASSESSING YOUR UNDERSTANDING

Activity A   FILL IN THE BLANKS

1. _____ is the relationship between negative effects and the positive effects of a medication.

2. Older patients are more _____ to the pharmacological effects of medication.

3. Older adults are prone to adverse drug reactions because of a _____ in the number of _____ needed for drug distribution.

4. _____ is the number one cause of death in adults.

5. _____ is a list of potentially inappropriate medications for use in older adults.

Activity B   MATCHING

Match the drug in Column A with the adverse effect in Column B.

Column A	Column B
___ **1.** Cimetidine (Tagamet)	**a.** Anticholinergic effects, weakness
___ **2.** Cyclobenzaprine (Flexeril)	**b.** Renal toxicity
___ **3.** Diphenhydramine hydrochloride (Benadryl)	**c.** Confusion
	d. Urinary retention
___ **4.** Ketorolac (Toradol)	**e.** Bleeding
___ **5.** Nitrofurantoin (Macrodantin)	

Activity C **SHORT ANSWERS**

Briefly answer the following questions.

1. Explain why older adults are at a greater risk for respiratory depression after receiving anesthetic agents during surgery.

2. Discuss how economic factors may influence adherence to a medication regimen in older adults.

3. What should the nurse assess in the older adult to determine this patient's ability to maintain adherence to medications?

4. Discuss what the nurse should teach adult patients and their families to help prevent adverse effects related to medications.

5. Discuss the differences in medication response related to ethnicity and race and give an example of a medication that has different responses dependent upon racial population.

SECTION II: APPLYING YOUR KNOWLEDGE

Activity D **CASE STUDY**

Edward, an 85-year-old man, is admitted to the hospital unit with a severe urinary tract infection. He has a temperature of 101°F. He is incontinent of urine and confused. The doctor orders IV fluids and IV antibiotics.

1. Explain why Edward is at risk for developing toxicity to the antibiotics.

2. Edward also has mild congestive heart failure. How could this affect his response to the antibiotic therapy?

3. What blood tests will the nurse anticipate the physician ordering for Edward to ensure that he is able to excrete the antibiotic appropriately?

SECTION III: PRACTICING FOR NCLEX

Activity E

Answer the following questions.

1. The nurse is aware that the most relevant way in which aging affects the pharmacokinetic process of drug administration is what?
   a. Decreased affinity to receptor sites for medication
   b. Decreased function of vital organs
   c. Decreased function of the beta-receptor system
   d. Decreased cellular biochemical reactions

2. What is the relation between the activity level of older adults and the response to medication?
   a. There is no relation between activity level and medication response.
   b. The more active the older adult, the greater the chance for adverse effects to prescribed drugs.
   c. The less physical activity an older adult engages in, the less chance there is for an altered response to a medication.
   d. The older adult who is more physically active is less likely to have an adverse drug effect.

3. A 92-year-old woman is beginning to take a new medication. What may affect drug absorption in this patient? (Select all that apply.)
   a. Increased gastric acidity
   b. Increased gastric pH
   c. Decreased blood flow to the stomach
   d. Increased surface area of the stomach related to weight gain
   e. Diminished gastric emptying

4. An older adult complains that it seems like it takes him forever to digest his meals. How would this affect this patient's ability to absorb medications? (Select all that apply.)
   a. Edema of the stomach lining
   b. Nausea and vomiting
   c. Dehydration
   d. Diarrhea
   e. Constipation

5. The nurse is preparing to give an older adult patient an IM injection. How will this patient's history of heart failure affect the administration of this medication? (Select all that apply.)

   a. Decreased absorption of the medication

   b. Lipodystrophy at the injection site

   c. Edema at the injection site

   d. Abnormal blood concentrations of the medication

   e. Increased incidence of pulmonary difficulties

6. What is the most consistent issue that arises in the older adult when the rate of absorption is slowed?

   a. Slower responses to the medication

   b. Increased chance of adverse effects

   c. Changes in peak serum drug levels

   d. Decreased dosages in medications

7. What physiological factors in older adults contribute to alterations in distribution of medications? (Select all that apply.)

   a. Diminished cardiac output

   b. Increased body fat

   c. Increased body mass

   d. Decreased body fluid

   e. Increased serum albumin

8. An older adult is concerned because his clothes feel tight though he hasn't gained any weight. The nurse knows that this is because of what physiologic change related to aging?

   a. It is normal for older adults to develop edema.

   b. As adults age, their limited vision distorts their ability to read the scale.

   c. Aging results in an increase in body fat and a decrease in lean body mass.

   d. Many of the medications that are taken by older adults result in truncal obesity.

9. What is the most reliable measure to evaluate renal function?

   a. Creatinine clearance

   b. Glomerular filtration rate

   c. Cockroft-Gault method

   d. Blood urea nitrogen

10. The nurse who is caring for an older patient and the latest laboratory report reveals a decreased creatinine clearance. The nurse anticipates what modification to the patient's drug regimen?

    a. A decrease in the dosage of medication

    b. An increase in the dosage of medication

    c. No change in the dosage of medication

    d. The physician will cancel all medication orders

11. How is the renal system affected by the aging process? (Select all that apply.)

    a. Decrease in blood flow to the kidneys

    b. Increased glomerular filtration rate

    c. Decrease in the number of functioning nephrons

    d. Decrease in tubular secretion

    e. Increased creatinine clearance

12. The nurse knows that the physician has ordered a creatinine clearance test for a 77-year-old patient because this test reveals what information?

    a. The best medication for the patient's illness

    b. The ability of the kidney to excrete medications

    c. The maximum amount of medication that the body can handle

    d. The best route for administration of the medication

13. What factors contribute to improper medication use in older adults? (Select all that apply.)

    a. Altered mental status

    b. Few medications to keep track of

    c. Unable to read small print well

    d. Lack of adequate income

    e. Ability to set up a medication schedule

14. What schedule of medication dosing assists older adults in adhering to a medication regimen?

    a. Begin with a high dose to relieve symptoms quickly

    b. Begin with a low dose to minimize adverse effects

    c. Begin with a high dose until the patient develops severe adverse effects

    d. Begin with a low dose and give it every 2 to 3 hours so it is the same as a large dose

15. Which condition contributes to nonadherence to the medication regimen due to its lack of identifiable symptoms?

    a. Arthritis

    b. Congestive heart failure

    c. Gout

    d. Hypertension

16. What interventions will the nurse use to improve adherence to a medication regimen for the older adult? (Select all that apply.)

    a. Use brand name drugs

    b. Plan medication administration every 2 hours

    c. Keep the cost of the medications as low as possible

    d. Provide easy-to-follow directions

    e. Educate patient and family to the medication regimen

17. What physiologic changes related to aging affect metabolism? (Select all that apply.)

    a. Increase in size of liver

    b. Decrease in circulation to the liver

    c. Increased number of hepatic enzymes

    d. Decreased ability to remove metabolic by-products

    e. Decrease in mass of liver

18. What are the most common medical problems seen in older adults? (Select all that apply.)

    a. Diabetes mellitus

    b. Arthritis

    c. Systemic lupus erythematosus

    d. Heart disease

    e. Ventral hernia

19. Older adults are susceptible to what type of infection?

    a. Antibiotic-sensitive

    b. Antibiotic-resistant

    c. Severe skin eruptions

    d. Localized to one organ

20. The nurse is aware that almost a third of all hospital admissions in older adults are as a result of what problem?

    a. Unnecessary surgery

    b. Sepsis

    c. Medication reactions

    d. Asthma

CHAPTER 6

Pharmacology and the Pregnant or Lactating Woman

Learning Objectives

- Describe the etiology of infertility.
- Describe the drugs used for infertility.
- Identify the pregnancy-associated changes that affect drug pharmacokinetics.
- Analyze the effect of teratogens on the fetus during development.
- Identify the effects of herbal and dietary supplements on the mother and fetus during pregnancy.
- Identify pharmacological strategies to manage pregnancy-associated symptoms.
- Identify the prototype drugs that alter uterine motility and describe these drugs.
- Identify the prototype drugs used during labor and delivery and describe these drugs.
- Discuss the use of drugs and herbs during lactation, including their effect on the infant.
- Implement the nursing process in the care of the women of childbearing age.

SECTION I: ASSESSING YOUR UNDERSTANDING

Activity A FILL IN THE BLANKS

1. Drugs that cause abnormal embryonic or fetal development are _____.

2. _____ (formation of fetal organs) occurs during the first 2 to 8 weeks after conception.

3. On the maternal side, _____ carries blood and drugs to the placenta.

4. Drugs used to stop preterm labor are _____.

5. Drugs ingested by a pregnant woman reach the fetus through the maternal–placental–fetal circulation, which is completed by about the _____ after conception.

Activity B MATCHING

Match the term in Column A with the definition in Column B.

Column A	Column B
____ 1. Magnesium sulfate	a. Inhibit uterine prostaglandins that help to initiate the uterine contractions of normal labor
____ 2. Nifedipine	
____ 3. NSAIDs, such as indomethacin	b. Long given IV as a first-line agent, but now considered ineffective as a tocolytic

_____ **4.** Terbutaline

_____ **5.** Erythromy-
cin ointment
0.5%

c. Applied to each eye
at delivery; effective
against both chlamyd-
ial and gonococcal
infections

d. Calcium channel
blocking drug that
decreases uterine con-
tractions

e. Beta-adrenergic agent
that inhibits uter-
ine contractions by
reducing intracellular
calcium levels

Activity C SHORT ANSWERS

Briefly answer the following questions.

1. How do the physiologic changes during
pregnancy influence drug effects on the
mother and fetus?

2. Explain how the fetus metabolizes and
excretes most drugs.

3. What impact does the fetal blood–brain
barrier have on the absorption of drugs into
the brain?

4. What role does the maternal circulation have
in the metabolism and excretion of drugs?

5. What is the impact on the fetus of drugs taken
on a regular schedule by the mother?

SECTION II: APPLYING YOUR KNOWLEDGE

Activity D CASE STUDY

Consider the scenario and answer the questions.

Mrs. Waddell, aged 33, comes with her husband
to the physician because they have been trying
to conceive for the last 18 months.

1. What are some of the possible causes for infertility in both Mrs. Waddell and her husband?

2. After laboratory testing, Mrs. Waddell is diagnosed with an ovulation disorder. The physician prescribes menotropin (Menopur). What
instructions would be given to this patient to
ensure she takes it correctly?

3. The nurse tells Mrs. Waddell that she will be
required to return to the clinic for frequent
laboratory tests. What type of tests are they
and why are they required?

4. Mrs. Waddell asks the nurse if taking this
medication increases her chances for having
twins. What is the nurse's best response?

SECTION III: PRACTICING FOR NCLEX

Activity E

Answer the following questions.

1. Mrs. Allen develops a headache and asks
the nurse if it is safe to take aspirin 1 hour
before breast-feeding. What is an appropriate
response?
   a. The aspirin will not be absorbed by the
   baby.
   b. Aspirin should be avoided during lactation;
   consult your physician.
   c. Your headache may interfere with letdown;
   take the aspirin.
   d. Aspirin is the drug of choice for pain during the lactation period.

2. Mrs. Sikes' friend offers her a herbal tea that
helps to prevent miscarriage and promote fetal
health. She asks the nurse if the drug is safe.
What would be the nurse's response?
   a. "Herbal drugs are safe during pregnancy in
   moderation."
   b. "Teas in general are safe during pregnancy."
   c. "The tea should be administered in
   moderation."
   d. "Drugs should be avoided during
   pregnancy."

3. To prevent neural tube defects, a physician may prescribe what drug during pregnancy?
   a. Folic acid
   b. Vitamin C
   c. Iron
   d. Multivitamin with minerals

4. Mrs. Smith is considering pregnancy; she is healthy and does not take prescription medications. She asks the nurse for advice. What should the nurse suggest this patient do?
   a. Avoid over-the-counter medications before pregnancy
   b. Begin fertility drugs as soon as possible
   c. Avoid multivitamins with minerals before pregnancy
   d. Double the dose of her multivitamins with minerals before pregnancy

5. Ms. Loftner is at 33 weeks' gestation. Her obstetrician orders a medication for her to take that is intended to treat a condition in her fetus. What fetal problems are treated by medicating the mother? (Select all that apply.)
   a. Fetal skeletal abnormalities
   b. Fetal chromosomal abnormalities
   c. Fetal tachycardia
   d. Fetal hypothyroidism
   e. Fetal lung immaturity

6. Ms. Bergman is diagnosed with hyperemesis, and the physician orders a home care nurse to assess her during her pregnancy. In order to care for the patient, what qualifications should the nurse have?
   a. Experience in care of obstetric patients
   b. Obstetric specialty
   c. Maternal home care nursing specialty
   d. Scheduled next as the nurse to admit new patients

7. The physician orders short-term therapy for a disease process in a patient who is breast-feeding. The medication is transferred to the baby during lactation. What should the nurse advise the patient to do?
   a. Pump and discard her milk
   b. Disregard the prescription
   c. Continue to breast-feed
   d. Stop breast-feeding until the medication regimen is complete

8. Ms. Corday delivers a healthy daughter. The patient, who is HIV positive, asks when she should begin breast-feeding. What is the appropriate response?
   a. Breast-feeding is based on your T-cell level.
   b. As soon as the breast-feeding coach arrives.
   c. You should not breast-feed.
   d. When the child is hungry.

9. Mrs. Herrera discovers she is pregnant. She asks the physician for a rubella vaccination. What does the nurse anticipate the physician will do?
   a. Decline, because the rubella vaccine is a live-virus vaccine
   b. Decline, because a titer was not drawn
   c. Administer the vaccine, because the patient is in her first trimester
   d. Administer the vaccine regardless of the trimester, because of the risk-versus-benefit ratio

10. Mrs. Dorland suffers from migraine headaches. Her friend tells her that acetaminophen is safe to take during pregnancy. She asks the nurse if it is safe to take the drug for her migraines. What statement is true?
    a. Acetaminophen is safe in this circumstance.
    b. The patient requires a stronger medication.
    c. Acetaminophen is the drug of choice for migraines.
    d. The physician should be consulted regarding diagnosis and the medication prescribed.

11. One hour after delivery, Mrs. East is concerned that her child is listless. What would the nurse evaluate?
    a. The child's ability to breast-feed
    b. Antibiotic administration to the mother before delivery
    c. Drugs received by the mother during labor and delivery
    d. Maternal nutrition

12. A mother asks why the nurse administers phytonadione to her newborn after delivery. What condition does the drug prevent?

    a. Syphilis

    b. Gonorrhea

    c. Calcium deficiency

    d. Hemorrhagic disease

13. Debby Pinkerton is 9 weeks pregnant and calls the nurse practitioner complaining of constipation. What will the nurse practitioner suggest to this patient to relieve the problem? (Select all that apply.)

    a. Psyllium (Metamucil)

    b. Castor oil

    c. Mineral oil

    d. Docusate (Colace)

    e. Saline laxative (milk of magnesia)

14. Ophthalmia neonatorum is a form of bacterial conjunctivitis that may cause ulceration and blindness. This is most commonly caused by what infectious agent?

    a. Gonorrhea

    b. *Chlamydia trachomatis*

    c. *Staphylococcus aureus*

    d. Methicillin-resistant *Staphylococcus aureus*

15. What is one of the benefits of using regional anesthesia during labor and delivery?

    a. The neonate is rarely depressed.

    b. The mother sleeps during labor and delivery.

    c. The mother is semiconscious during labor and delivery.

    d. The neonate is lethargic after delivery.

16. Ms. Penn receives Duramorph through her epidural catheter after undergoing a cesarean section. For what should the nurse observe the patient?

    a. Hypertension

    b. Urinary retention

    c. Diarrhea

    d. Dysrhythmia

17. Ms. Harbor received parenteral opioid analgesics during labor and deliver of her first child. The nurse observes that the neonate is experiencing respiratory depression. What is the drug of choice in this case?

    a. Magnesium sulfate

    b. Terbutaline

    c. Morphine sulfate

    d. Naloxone

18. Pitocin is given to prevent what condition?

    a. Letdown

    b. Postpartum bleeding

    c. Postpartum hypotension

    d. Eclampsia

19. Mrs. Hollings who is 36 weeks' gestation is admitted to the labor and delivery unit with severe preeclampsia. What drug therapies may be used to treat this patient during this crisis? (Select all that apply.)

    a. Nifedipine (Procardia)

    b. Labetalol (Normodyne)

    c. Hydralazine (Apresoline)

    d. Terbutaline (Brethine)

    e. Magnesium sulfate

20. Mrs. Olinger exhibits symptoms related to preterm labor. She is 37 weeks pregnant. The physician orders magnesium sulfate. The nurse notes symptoms of hypermagnesemia and report this to the physician. What would the nurse expect the physician to order?

    a. Calcium gluconate

    b. Calcium magnate

    c. Magnesium sulfate

    d. Narcan

Drug Therapy for Coagulation Disorders

Learning Objectives

- Describe important elements in the physiology of hemostasis and thrombosis.
- Discuss potential consequences of blood clotting disorders.
- Compare and contrast heparin and warfarin in terms of indications for use, onset and duration of action, route of administration, blood tests used to monitor effects, and nursing process implications.
- Discuss antiplatelet agents in terms of indications for use and effects on blood coagulation.
- Discuss direct thrombin inhibitors in terms of indications and contraindications for use, routes of administration, and major adverse effects.
- Describe thrombolytic agents in terms of indications and contraindications for use, routes of administration, and major adverse effects.
- Identify the prototype drug for each drug class.
- Describe systemic hemostatic agents for treating overdoses of anticoagulant and thrombolytic drugs.
- Understand how to use the nursing process in the care of patients receiving anticoagulant, antiplatelet, and thrombolytic agents.

SECTION I: ASSESSING YOUR UNDERSTANDING

Activity A FILL IN THE BLANKS

1. Thrombosis involves the formation (*thrombogenesis*) or presence of a _____ in the vascular system.

2. _____ is a normal body defense mechanism to prevent blood loss.

3. When part of a thrombus breaks off and travels to another part of the body, it is called a/an _____.

4. Atherosclerosis begins with accumulation of lipid-filled _____ on the inner lining of arteries.

5. In atherosclerosis, _____ develop in response to elevated blood lipid levels and eventually become fibrous plaques (i.e., foam cells covered by smooth muscle cells and connective tissue).

Activity B MATCHING

Match the term in Column A with the definition in Column B.

Column A

____ **1.** Heparin

____ **2.** Low molecular weight heparins (LMWHs)

____ **3.** Warfarin

____ **4.** Aspirin

____ **5.** Fondaparinux

Column B

a. The most commonly used oral anticoagulant; acts in the liver to prevent synthesis of vitamin K–dependent clotting factors

b. Analgesic–antipyretic–anti-inflammatory drug with potent antiplatelet effects

c. The first of a new class of pentasaccharide antithrombotic agents that produces anticoagulant effects by directly binding to circulating and clot-bound factor Xa, accelerating the activity of antithrombin and inhibiting thrombin production

d. A pharmaceutical preparation of the natural anticoagulant produced primarily by mast cells in pericapillary connective tissue

e. Contain the low molecular weight fraction and are as effective as IV heparin in treating thrombotic disorders

Activity C SHORT ANSWERS

Briefly answer the following questions.

1. Define hemostasis.

2. Explain the process of clot lysis.

3. Discuss the predisposing factors for arterial thrombosis.

4. Discuss the predisposing factors for venous thrombosis.

5. Discuss the two mechanisms by which venous thrombi cause disease.

SECTION II: APPLYING YOUR KNOWLEDGE

Activity D CASE STUDY

Consider the scenario and answer the questions.

Mrs. Adams is hospitalized in her fourth month of pregnancy with a pulmonary embolism. The physician prescribes heparin to be administered in the home daily until she returns to his office in 2 weeks. He also asks the nurse to schedule blood to be drawn for laboratory analysis by the home care nurse on a daily basis, with reports to him each day by 2 PM. You are the home care nurse in charge of Mrs. Adams' education and care.

1. Mrs. Adams asks you how the heparin will help to prevent a recurrence of the pulmonary embolism. What is your understanding of how heparin works?

2. The patient is concerned because she received intravenous heparin during most of her stay in the hospital. She asks if the subcutaneous drug will be just as effective. What is the difference between the intravenous and the subcutaneous administration?

3. Mrs. Adams is concerned that the drug will cause her fetus to bleed internally. What do you know about the effect of injected heparin on a fetus?

4. Mrs. Adams' condition resolves. However, she is placed on bed rest for the duration of her pregnancy. Based on Mrs. Adams' history, what would you expect the physician to order while Mrs. Adams is on bed rest?

5. After delivery of a healthy baby girl, Mrs. Adams develops DIC. What is DIC? What is the goal of treatment? What would you expect the physician to prescribe as part of the treatment?

SECTION III: PRACTICING FOR NCLEX

Activity E

Answer the following questions.

1. The physician orders thrombolytic agents when treating a patient diagnosed with acute myocardial infarction. Which drug should the nurse keep readily available when blood flow is reestablished?
   a. Anticoagulants
   b. Antidysrhythmics
   c. Antihypertensives
   d. Antianginals

2. The FDA has issued a black box warning for the use of protamine sulfate due to the risk of which conditions? (Select all that apply.)
   a. Severe hypotension
   b. Cardiovascular collapse
   c. Cardiogenic pulmonary edema
   d. Pulmonary hypertension
   e. Pulmonary vasodilation

3. A 67-year-old man enters the emergency department complaining of severe chest pain that is radiating down his left arm. He is diagnosed with a myocardial infarction. What drug does the nurse anticipate the physician ordering for this patient?
   a. Heparin
   b. Alteplase
   c. Ticlopidine
   d. Clopidogrel

4. The nurse is concerned that the physician does not order routine aPTTs when the patient is receiving LMWH for thromboembolism prophylaxis. When the nurse calls the physician with the nurse's concern, what will be the physician's response?
   a. aPTTs should be drawn daily.
   b. aPTTs should be drawn weekly.
   c. aPTTs are not needed.
   d. INRs should be drawn weekly.

5. The physician reorders dalteparin for the patient. The pharmacy states that the drug is not available. The nurse calls the physician and asks if dalteparin can be replaced with another LMWH. What does the nurse expect to be the physician's response?

   a. "I'll change the order to enoxaparin."
   b. "I'll change the drug to Lovenox."
   c. "The drugs are not interchangeable; have the pharmacy obtain the drug ordered."
   d. "The drugs are interchangeable; the pharmacy can substitute another LMWH."

6. The black box warning associated with warfarin concerns its risk of causing what condition?
   a. DIC
   b. Severe coagulopathy
   c. Hypotension
   d. Major or fatal bleeding

7. What are the difficulties encountered when the physician orders lepirudin for management of atrial fibrillation? (Select all that apply.)
   a. No antidote is available.
   b. Must be given IV
   c. Duration of action is only 4 hours.
   d. Requires frequent lab tests
   e. It is known to cause depression.

8. The patient presents to the physician's office because the physician is unable to regulate his Coumadin dosage. During the interview, the nurse finds that the patient began taking what substance, which might increase the effects of the warfarin?
   a. Ginseng to improve his energy
   b. Red meat to increase his protein intake
   c. Milk to increase his calcium level and prevent cramps
   d. Chamomile tea to help him sleep

9. The patient is prescribed warfarin. His INR is 5.2. At what level is this dose?
   a. Subtherapeutic
   b. Therapeutic
   c. Elevated
   d. Within prescribed limits

10. The patient is admitted to the hospital after a suicide attempt. The nurse discovers that the patient overdosed on aspirin. What does the nurse expect the physician to do?
   a. Prescribe the antidote.
   b. Prescribe a transfusion of platelets.
   c. Prescribe a transfusion of whole blood.
   d. Order an IV infusion of Ringer's lactate at 100 mL/h.

11. The patient is prescribed a thrombolytic agent. The nurse understands that the purpose of this order may be to achieve which effects? (Select all that apply.)

    a. Dissolve thrombi

    b. Limit tissue damage

    c. Prevent platelet aggregation

    d. Increase coagulation

    e. Reestablish blood flow

12. A 59-year-old patient with vascular disorders is prescribed cilostazol. The nurse instructs the patient that it is for the treatment of what condition?

    a. Pulmonary embolism

    b. Deep-vein thrombosis

    c. Intermittent claudication

    d. Venous stasis

13. The physician discovers a clot in the patient's left lower leg. The physician prescribes anti-coagulant drugs to prevent formation of new clots and to achieve which other effect?

    a. Increase coagulation

    b. Regulate PTT

    c. Regulate PT, INR

    d. Prevent extension of clots already present

14. The patient takes warfarin daily for DVT prevention. The patient also takes a multivitamin with minerals. What instructions should the nurse give the patient?

    a. Discontinue the multivitamin with minerals

    b. Increase the dose of the multivitamin with minerals

    c. Change his vitamins to ones that do not contain minerals

    d. Take his vitamins with minerals consistently

15. The patient is learning to self-administer his heparin daily. The home care nurse draws blood every 2 to 3 days to monitor the patient's platelet levels. What platelet count would the nurse report to the physician as a critical laboratory result?

    a. 150,000

    b. 160,000

    c. 90,000

    d. 400,000

16. The patient is diagnosed with hepatitis A, diabetes type 1, and portal hypertension. He develops a DVT, and the physician prescribes warfarin. The nurse is concerned, for what reason?

    a. The patient is more likely to experience bleeding.

    b. The patient is less likely to achieve a therapeutic dose.

    c. The patient is at risk for further liver impairment.

    d. The patient is at risk for hyperglycemic episodes.

17. The patient is diagnosed with chronic renal insufficiency. Her vascular access site becomes incompetent, and the physician orders urokinase to dissolve the clot. What should the nurse do?

    a. Administer the drug as ordered.

    b. Hold the drug until the physician can verify the order.

    c. Refuse to administer the drug.

    d. Ask the physician to administer the drug.

18. A 75-year-old patient presents to the physician's office with complaints of bleeding gums and multiple bruises. When the nurse reviews his drug history, the nurse finds that he is prescribed aspirin 81 mg/d. What drug may cause increased bleeding when used in conjunction with the aspirin?

    a. Antibiotics

    b. Antihypertensives

    c. NSAIDs

    d. Antidysrhythmics

19. A patient enters the emergency department with symptoms of an ischemic stroke. What condition would contraindicate the use of a thrombolytic in this patient?

    a. Colon resection 7 days ago

    b. Migraine headache yesterday

    c. Sprained ankle 2 weeks ago

    d. Bronchitis 1 month ago

20. A stable daily dose of warfarin is reached when which parameter is achieved?

    a. The PTT is within the therapeutic range.

    b. The PT and INR are within their therapeutic ranges, and the dose does not cause bleeding.

    c. The INR is between 4 and 5.

    d. The INR is between 1 and 2, and the dose does not cause bleeding.

Drug Therapy for Dyslipidemia

Learning Objectives

- Recognize the role of dyslipidemia in metabolic syndrome.
- Identify sources and functions of cholesterol and triglycerides.
- Educate patients about nonpharmacologic measures to prevent or reduce dyslipidemia.
- Identify the prototype drug from each drug class used to treat dyslipidemia.
- Describe the classes of dyslipidemic drugs in terms of their mechanism of action, indications for use, major adverse effects, and nursing implications.
- Apply the nursing process in the care of patients with dyslipidemia.

SECTION I: ASSESSING YOUR UNDERSTANDING

Activity A FILL IN THE BLANKS

1. _____ drugs are used in the management of elevated blood lipids, a major risk factor for atherosclerosis and vascular disorders such as coronary artery disease, strokes, and peripheral arterial insufficiency.

2. Blood lipids, which include cholesterol, phospholipids, and triglycerides, are derived from the diet or synthesized by the liver and _____.

3. Most cholesterol is found in body cells, where it is a component of _____ and performs other essential functions.

4. In cells of the adrenal glands, ovaries, and testes, cholesterol is required for the synthesis of _____ hormones.

5. In liver cells, cholesterol is used to form _____, which is conjugated with other substances to form bile salts; bile salts promote absorption and digestion of fats.

Activity B MATCHING

Match the term in Column A with the definition in Column B.

Column A	Column B
____ 1. Atorvastatin	a. Similar to endogenous fatty acids
____ 2. Cholestyramine	b. Binds bile acids in the intestinal lumen
____ 3. Gemfibrozil, fenofibrate	c. Decreases both cholesterol and triglycerides
____ 4. Niacin (nicotinic acid)	d. Acts in the small intestine to inhibit absorption of cholesterol and decrease the delivery of intestinal cholesterol to the liver
____ 5. Ezetimibe	e. Most widely used statin and one of the most widely used drugs in the United States

Activity C   SHORT ANSWERS

Briefly answer the following questions.

1. Discuss the process by which blood lipids are transported.

2. Describe how lipoprotein density is determined.

3. Identify the risk factors associated with the metabolic syndrome.

4. How do these risk factors affect the cardiovascular, cerebrovascular, and peripheral vascular systems?

5. Discuss the first line of treatment for metabolic syndrome.

SECTION II: APPLYING YOUR KNOWLEDGE

Activity D   CASE STUDY

Consider the scenario and answer the questions.

Mr. Best, aged 45, presents to the physician's office for an employment-related physical examination. His last physical was 7 years ago. He leads a sedentary lifestyle and works in a high-stress environment. He is approximately 35 pounds overweight. His medication history includes ibuprofen periodically for headaches. He does not take vitamins or herbal supplements. Before the examination, the physician ordered the following laboratory studies: CBC, electrolyte panel, lipid panel, and electrocardiogram. The physician diagnoses Mr. Best with dyslipidemia.

1. Mr. Best asks you if the doctor is sure that he has dyslipidemia; he noticed that his HDL was low, and asks, "Isn't that good?" What do you know about the major risk factors for coronary artery disease?

2. Three months later, the physician orders a lipid profile and triglycerides. What instructions should you give Mr. Best about preparing for the tests?

3. What are some recommendations for reducing Mr. Best's risk factors for cardiovascular disease?

SECTION III: PRACTICING FOR NCLEX

Activity E

Answer the following questions.

1. A male patient's triglycerides are still elevated despite lifestyle changes. What does the nurse expect the physician to order for this patient?
   a. Fenofibrate
   b. Cholestyramine
   c. Niacin
   d. Atorvastatin

2. A female patient presents to the physician's office with complaints of a recurrence of her "hot flashes." The nurse understands that the patient is taking what drug to treat her dyslipidemia?
   a. Fenofibrate
   b. Cholestyramine
   c. Niacin
   d. Atorvastatin

3. How should the nurse instruct the patient to take his lovastatin?
   a. In the morning 1 hour before breakfast
   b. At night 2 hours after a meal
   c. With food
   d. Without regard to food or time of the day

4. What should the nurse suggest to assist a patient to improve his cholesterol levels?
   a. Smoking cessation
   b. Diet high in polysaturated fats
   c. Limit exercise to the weekends
   d. Weight lifting

5. What cardiac risk factors are related to metabolic syndrome? (Select all that apply.)
   a. Central adiposity
   b. Elevated triglycerides
   c. Reduced high density lipoprotein cholesterol
   d. Postural hypotension
   e. Elevated fasting blood glucose

6. The physician orders a lipid profile without triglycerides for his patient. When the nurse phones the patient with his appointment, what would the nurse tell him?

a. Fast for 12 hours before the test.

b. Fast for 6 hours before the test.

c. Fast for 4 hours before the test.

d. Fasting is not needed.

7. What is the most common reason for an elevated cholesterol level in a patient who does not have a genetic disorder of lipid metabolism?

a. His dietary intake of saturated fat

b. His sedentary lifestyle

c. His waist size

d. His alcohol intake

8. A male patient presents to the physician's office with symptoms of hyperglycemia. He is taking his oral antidiabetic medication and has not modified his diet or exercise program in any way. When the nurse interviews the patient, he states that he now takes flax seed to reduce his cholesterol level. What may occur as a result of taking flax seed?

a. Increased absorption of his drugs

b. Decreased absorption of his drugs

c. Increased liver metabolism

d. Decreased excretion of the drug through the kidneys

9. The physician prescribes fibrate for his patient with elevated triglycerides. The patient begins to self-administer niacin approximately 3 mg daily. What would the nurse expect the physician to order?

a. LFTs

b. CBC

c. Electrolyte panel

d. Fibrate level

10. A male patient takes cholesterol absorption inhibitors as a monotherapy without statins. He develops mild hepatic insufficiency. What would the nurse expect the physician to do?

a. Increase the dosage of his medication

b. Decrease the dosage of his medication

c. Maintain the current dosage of his medication

d. Discontinue his medication

11. A male patient presents to the physician's office for his annual visit. He takes statins to control his hyperlipidemia. When the physician reviews the patient's laboratory results and notes that there is an unexplained elevation in the serum aspartate, what would the nurse expect the physician to do?

a. Increase the dose of the statin

b. Discontinue the statin

c. Decrease the dose of the statin

d. Maintain the current dose of the statin

12. The physician is caring for a patient who is a 2-year kidney transplant survivor. The nurse would expect the physician to order what drug for the patient's hyperlipidemia?

a. Atorvastatin

b. Fluvastatin

c. Lovastatin

d. Pravastatin

13. A 57-year-old female patient is postmenopausal. Lifestyle changes have not made a significant impact on her lipids. What would the nurse expect the physician to suggest?

a. Fenofibrate

b. Cholestyramine

c. Niacin

d. Estrogen replacement therapy

14. An 8-year-old male patient requires treatment for dyslipidemia. What would the nurse expect the physician to order?

a. Pravastatin

b. Fenofibrate

c. Cholestyramine

d. Niacin

15. Patients of which ethnic group may find diet and exercise more useful than lipid-lowering drugs?

a. African Americans

b. Asian Americans

c. Native Americans

d. Italian Americans

16. A male patient's laboratory results indicate that both cholesterol and triglycerides are elevated. Which medications may be ordered? (Select all that apply.)

    a. Statin (Atorvastatin)

    b. Ezetimibe

    c. Gemfibrozil

    d. Cholestyramine

    e. Colesevelam

17. A fibrate–statin combination should be avoided because of increased risks of what condition?

    a. Severe myopathy

    b. Rebound dyslipidemia

    c. Cardiac dysrhythmia

    d. Postural hypotension

18. What drug or drug class decreases the delivery of intestinal cholesterol to the liver?

    a. Statin

    b. Fibrate

    c. Cholesterol absorption inhibitor

    d. Bile acid sequestrant

19. What drug or drug class inhibits mobilization of free fatty acids from peripheral tissues?

    a. Statin

    b. Fibrate

    c. Cholesterol absorption inhibitor

    d. Niacin

20. A patient who had a total cholesterol-to-HDL cholesterol ratio of 5.3 has been losing weight and participating in an exercise program. His total cholesterol-to-HDL ratio is now 3.9. What LDL reading is also important to further decrease his risk of coronary artery disease?

    a. 140 mg/dL

    b. 120 mg/dL

    c. 105 mg/dL

    d. 95 mg/dL

Drug Therapy for Hematopoietic Disorders and to Enhance Immunity

Learning Objectives

- Briefly describe hematopoietic and immune functions.
- Identify common clinical manifestations of inadequate erythropoiesis and diminished host defense mechanisms.
- Discuss characteristics of hematopoietic drugs in terms of the prototype, mechanism of action, indications for use, adverse effects, principles of therapy, and nursing implications.
- Describe the characteristics of colony-stimulating factors in terms of the prototype, mechanism of action, indications for use, adverse effects, principles of therapy, and nursing implications.
- Discuss interferons in terms of the prototype, mechanism of action, indications for use, adverse effects, principles of therapy, and nursing implications.
- Implement the nursing process in the care of patients who take drugs to enhance hematopoietic and immune system function.

SECTION I: ASSESSING YOUR UNDERSTANDING

Activity A FILL IN THE BLANKS

1. Hematopoietic and immune blood cells originate in bone marrow in stem cells, which are often called _____ stem cells because they are capable of becoming different types of cells.

2. Hematopoietic growth factors or _____ control the reproduction, growth, and differentiation of stem cells and CFUs.

3. Adequate blood cell production and development are defined as _____.

4. _____ enhance communication between cells when antigens or tumors are identified.

5. Drugs that stimulate immune function are called _____, biologic response modifiers, and immunomodulators.

Activity B MATCHING

Match the term in Column A with the definition in Column B.

Column A

_____ 1. Darbepoetin alfa (Aranesp) and epoetin alfa (Epogen, Procrit)

_____ 2. Sargramostim (Leukine)

_____ 3. Filgrastim (Neupogen)

_____ 4. Interferon alfa-2b (Intron-A)

_____ 5. Interferon alfa-n1 and alfacon-1

Column B

a. A CSF (GM-CSF) used to promote the engraftment and function of transplanted bone marrow.

b. A recombinant DNA that has both antiviral and antineoplastic activities. It enhances the overall function of the immune system by increasing phagocytic activity, which augments cytotoxicity against cancer cells.

c. Approved for treatment of chronic hepatitis C, a condition that can lead to liver failure and liver cancer.

d. Drug formulations of *erythropoietin*, a hormone from the kidney that stimulates bone marrow production of red blood cells.

e. Prototype G-CSF used to stimulate blood cell production in the bone marrow of patients with bone marrow transplantation or chemotherapy-induced neutropenia.

Activity C SHORT ANSWERS

Briefly answer the following questions.

1. What are the symptoms of inadequate hematopoiesis?

2. Exogenous drug preparations have the same mechanisms of action as the endogenous products. Describe the mechanism of action.

3. Describe the antiproliferative and immunoregulatory activities of interferons.

4. Why are exogenous cytokines given only by a subcutaneous (Sub-Q) or intravenous (IV) injection?

5. What are immunostimulants and how are they used?

SECTION II: APPLYING YOUR KNOWLEDGE

Activity D CASE STUDY

Consider the scenario and answer the questions.

Mrs. Cantos is diagnosed with chronic renal failure. The physician orders epoetin alfa (Epogen). You are responsible for the education plan.

1. How does epoetin alfa work? How long will the patient have to take it?

2. Mrs. Cantos' insurance does not cover home care, and she will be administering her own medication. What must you teach Mrs. Cantos about administering Epogen at home?

3. Mrs. Cantos' last hemoglobin level was 14 grams per deciliter (g/dL). What might this indicate?

SECTION III: PRACTICING FOR NCLEX

Activity E

Answer the following questions.

1. All hematopoietic and immune blood cells are derived from which cells in the bone marrow?
   a. Stem cells
   b. Beta cells
   c. Alfa cells
   d. Theta cells

2. Cytokines regulate the immune response by stimulating or inhibiting the activation, proliferation, and differentiation of various cells and by what other action?
   a. Inhibiting the secretion of cytokines
   b. Inhibiting the secretion of antibodies
   c. Regulating the secretion of antibodies
   d. Regulating the secretion of M lymphocytes

3. A male patient is prescribed interferon. What is his probable diagnosis?
   a. Hypertension
   b. Viral hepatitis
   c. Sepsis
   d. Bacteremia

4. A male patient is diagnosed with severe neutropenia. The physician prescribes filgrastim. What is the desired effect?
   a. To increase white blood cells
   b. To increase red blood cells
   c. To increase electrolytes
   d. To decrease leukocytes

5. Adverse effects of epoetin and darbepoetin include increased risks of what condition?
   a. Hyperlipidemia
   b. Diabetes mellitus type 2
   c. Myocardial infarction
   d. Cirrhosis of the liver

6. A male patient is self-administering epoetin in the home. The nurse encourages him to include what supplements as part of his daily medication regimen?
   a. Iron
   b. Vitamin C
   c. Vitamin A
   d. Folic acid

7. The nurse is caring for a female patient in the home. The patient is prescribed filgrastim. What would be included in the nurse's education plan?
   a. Dietary restrictions
   b. Exercise restrictions
   c. Fall prevention
   d. Techniques to reduce exposure to infection

8. A male patient is prescribed sargramostim. He is diagnosed with liver impairment. What would the nurse expect the physician to do?
   a. Monitor LFTs every 2 weeks
   b. Monitor BUN and creatinine every week
   c. Monitor CBC every other day
   d. Monitor electrolytes weekly

9. A male patient is diagnosed with hepatitis B. The physician orders interferon alfa. What is the patient at risk of developing?

   a. Drug tolerance
   b. Chronic flank pain
   c. Drug resistance
   d. Subclinical hepatitis B

10. A male patient is diagnosed with multiple myeloma. What treatment regimen would the nurse expect the physician to order?
    a. Interferon alfa
    b. Sargramostim
    c. Filgrastim
    d. Epoetin

11. A male patient is diagnosed with hairy cell leukemia. The physician orders interferon therapy to normalize his WBC. The nurse expects the therapy to last how long with this drug?
    a. 4 to 6 weeks
    b. Indefinitely
    c. Until the WBC count is normal for 3 months
    d. 6 to 12 months

12. After the patient undergoes bone marrow transfusion, his physician administers sargramostim. When would the nurse expect the first dose to be administered?
    a. 30 minutes after the bone marrow infusion
    b. 1 hour after the bone marrow infusion
    c. Immediately after the bone marrow infusion
    d. 2 to 4 hours after the bone marrow infusion

13. A patient is beginning darbepoetin therapy. How often does the nurse expect the hemoglobin to be measured?
    a. Weekly until stabilized
    b. Twice weekly until stabilized
    c. Monthly until stabilized
    d. Every other day until stabilized

14. A patient is receiving darbepoetin. The laboratory report indicates that his hemoglobin level increased 2 g/dL in 2 weeks. What would the nurse expect the physician to do?
    a. Increase the medication
    b. Reduce the medication
    c. Maintain the current dose
    d. Discontinue the medication

15. The nurse is admitting a patient who has neutropenia. The nurse would expect to document which findings when taking the nursing history? (Select all that apply.)

    a. Shortness of breath when walking

    b. Bruising more easily

    c. Upper respiratory infection three times in last 4 months

    d. Bleeding from gums when brushing teeth

    e. Thrush infection of the mouth twice in last 4 weeks.

16. The home care nurse is caring for a patient who is self-administering epoetin. What assessment is most important for the nurse to complete during the visit?

    a. Pulse

    b. Blood pressure

    c. Temperature

    d. Respirations

17. The nurse is caring for a patient who has been receiving filgrastim. The nurse expects to perform which action concerning this drug on the day prior to the patient's chemotherapy treatment?

    a. Hold the medication

    b. Administer IV instead of SC

    c. Give the medication both morning and evening

    d. Ensure that the patient's diet has no herbs

18. The nurse would contact the prescriber immediately if interferon was prescribed for which patient?

    a. 34-year-old male with chronic hepatitis B

    b. 48-year-old female with hepatitis C

    c. 72-year-old male with AIDS-related Kaposi's sarcoma

    d. 11-month-old female with HIV acquired from her mother

19. The clinic nurse receives a call from a patient who has been taking interferon alfa for 7 days. The patient states that he has become very sad and wonders if life is worth living. What is the best response by the nurse to this patient?

    a. "Don't worry, this medication will make you well again."

    b. "Wait another 7 days and if you are still feeling sad, call back."

    c. "Come to the clinic as soon as possible."

    d. "This is an expected effect. Your depression should lift in another 2 weeks."

20. The nurse is caring for a patient with a WBC of 700 cells/mm^3. Which discharge instruction is most important for the nurse to share with this patient?

    a. "Go for a walk in the mall everyday to increase your endurance."

    b. "Eat foods rich in iron to increase your energy level."

    c. "Stay out of crowded places such as grocery stores."

    d. "Watch for signs of excessive bruising."

Drug Therapy: Immunizations

Learning Objectives

- Describe the types of immunity and the agents that produce them.
- Identify immunizations recommended for children and adolescents.
- Identify immunizations recommended for adults.
- Identify authoritative sources for immunization information.
- Be able to teach parents (and their children) about the importance of immunizations to public health.
- Be able to teach people about recommended immunizations and record keeping.

SECTION I: ASSESSING YOUR UNDERSTANDING

Activity A FILL IN THE BLANKS

1. _____ involves administration of an antigen to induce antibody formation (for active immunity) or administration of serum from immune people (for passive immunity).

2. _____ are suspensions of microorganisms or their antigenic products that have been killed or attenuated (weakened or reduced in virulence) so that they can induce antibody formation while preventing or causing very mild forms of the disease.

3. _____ live vaccines produce immunity, usually lifelong, that is similar to that produced by natural infection.

4. _____ are bacterial toxins or products that have been modified to destroy toxicity while retaining antigenic properties.

5. Immunization with toxoids is not permanent; scheduled repeat doses called _____ are required to maintain immunity.

Activity B MATCHING

Match the vaccine in Column A with its use in Column B.

Column A

_____ 1. *Haemophilus influenzae* b

_____ 2. *Haemophilus influenzae* b (Hib) with hepatitis B (Comvax)

_____ 3. Human papillomavirus (HPV) (Gardasil)

Column B

a. Prevention of diseases caused by HPV types 6, 11, 16, and 18 (cervical, vaginal, and vulvar cancer; genital warts) in girls and women aged 9 to 26 years

b. Routine immunization of children 12 months to 12 years of age

c. Prevention of infection with Hib, a common cause of serious bacterial infections, including meningitis, in children younger than 5 years of age

_____ **4.** Measles, mumps, rubella, and varicella (ProQuad)

_____ **5.** Meningitis/meningococcal disease (Menactra, Menomune)

d. Recommended for college students living in dormitories

e. Routine immunization of children 6 weeks to 15 months of age born to HB_sAg-negative mothers

Activity C   SHORT ANSWERS

Briefly answer the following questions.

1. Some vaccines may include aluminum. What method should be used to administer these medications, and what may occur if this method is not used?

2. Why are additives included in the creation of vaccines?

3. What is the impact of widespread use of vaccines on populations?

4. Why are single doses of the measles, mumps, and rubella vaccines rarely used?

5. Why is it important to immunize prepubertal girls against rubella?

SECTION II: APPLYING YOUR KNOWLEDGE

Activity D   CASE STUDY

Consider the scenario and answer the questions.

Ms. Banks, a nurse assistant, experiences a blood exposure when caring for a patient with hepatitis B. She presents to the occupational health department and explains to the nurse what happened. The physician orders immune globulin. You are responsible for the education plan for Ms. Banks.

1. The physician informs Ms. Banks that the immune globulin is given to foster passive immunity. She asks you what this means and how long it will last. How would you respond? Ms. Banks expresses concern that immune globulin may cause hepatitis B. How would you address this concern?

2. What is the goal of therapy in this case?

3. Explain why immunoglobulin fractions are preferred over serum. What type of plasma is used to prepare these products?

4. Ms. Banks asks whether there are hyperimmune serums available if she is exposed to other diseases. What other serums are available?

SECTION III: PRACTICING FOR NCLEX

Activity E

Answer the following questions.

1. What is the nurse's responsibility when obtaining a history from a new patient?

    a. Offer all available new immunizations

    b. Assess the patient's immunization status

    c. Inform the patient that immunizations will be administered

    d. Inform the patient that a new immunization schedule will begin

2. A male patient is treated for his cancer of the colon with a combination of chemotherapy and radiation therapy. During a routine physician's visit, the nurse determines that the patient is behind in his immunizations. For when should the nurse schedule immunizations?

    a. This appointment

    b. Three months after his cancer treatment is completed

    c. The next routine appointment

    d. 30 days after his cancer treatment is completed

3. For children with HIV infection, what is true about most routine immunizations?

    a. They are determined by the patient's T-cell count.

    b. They are determined by the WBC.

    c. They are recommended.

    d. They are not recommended.

4. A patient with asymptomatic HIV calls the clinic and reports that he just found out that his 2-year-old nephew has just been diagnosed with chickenpox. What therapy will be recommended for this patient?

   a. Varicella vaccine

   b. Shingles vaccine

   c. Varicella-zoster immune globulin

   d. No therapy is indicated

5. A male patient is diagnosed with HIV. He also is diagnosed with mild bladder cancer. The physician does not prescribe BCG, for what reason?

   a. It is not effective when the patient is diagnosed with HIV.

   b. It is an attenuated vaccine.

   c. It is a live vaccine.

   d. It will further impair the patient's immune system.

6. A female patient is living with HIV. She is exposed to measles. What is the treatment of choice in this case?

   a. Live vaccine

   b. No vaccine and presumptive treatment of the disease

   c. Varicella-zoster immune globulin for active immunization

   d. Immune globulin

7. The patient has been on a systemic corticosteroid for the last 3 weeks. How long should the patient wait before receiving a live virus vaccine?

   a. 6 weeks

   b. 3 months

   c. 6 months

   d. 1 year

8. A female patient presents to the physician's office with shoulder pain and is diagnosed with bursitis. The physician administers an intra-articular injection of a corticosteroid. The nurse discovers that the patient requires a tetanus booster. What would the nurse expect the physician to do?

   a. Postpone the booster for 1 week

   b. Postpone the booster until the next physician's visit

   c. State that the booster is contraindicated at this time

   d. Order the booster

9. A male patient presents to the emergency department with an asthma attack. He is treated and sent home with prednisone 10 mg on a taper and is encouraged to see his physician within 1 week. During an assessment of the chart, the nurse notices that the patient is overdue for his tetanus booster. What would the nurse expect the physician to do?

   a. Postpone the booster until the next physician's visit

   b. State that the booster is contraindicated at this time

   c. Order the booster

   d. Postpone the booster for 1 week

10. What type of vaccine is contraindicated in patients who have active malignant disease?

    a. Killed vaccines

    b. Toxoids

    c. Attenuated vaccines

    d. Live vaccines

11. A female patient is receiving chemotherapy for breast cancer. She requires a vaccine booster. For when would the physician order the administration of the vaccine?

    a. 1 year after chemotherapy is completed

    b. 3 months after chemotherapy is completed

    c. 30 days after chemotherapy is completed

    d. 6 months after chemotherapy is completed

12. Patients diagnosed with diabetes mellitus or chronic pulmonary, renal, or hepatic disorders who are not receiving immunosuppressant drugs may be given what types of vaccine? (Select all that apply.)

    a. Live attenuated vaccines

    b. Killed vaccines

    c. Toxoids

    d. Conjugated vaccines

    e. Immune serums

13. A 65-year-old male patient lives in a long-term care facility. The infection control nurse identifies a cluster of patients on the unit diagnosed with shingles. What would the nurse expect the patient's physician to order?

    a. Isolation of the patient

    b. Shingles vaccine

    c. Isolation of the patient's peers

    d. HBV vaccine

14. The nurse is aware that an 8-year-old child who had a splenectomy should receive which vaccination in addition to those recommended for his age group?

 a. Quadrivalent human papillomavirus vaccine

 b. Pneumococcal vaccine

 c. Hib vaccine

 d. Shingles vaccine

15. What type of modification may be necessary for a patient with diabetes mellitus who requires immunizations?

 a. Immunizations are contraindicated for this patient.

 b. The patient will require reduced doses of vaccines.

 c. The patient will require less frequent administration of vaccines.

 d. The patient will require increased doses of vaccines.

16. What immunizations are recommended for older adults? (Select all that apply.)

 a. A tetanus–diphtheria (Td) booster every 10 years

 b. An MMR every 7 to 10 years

 c. An annual influenza vaccine

 d. A one-time administration of pneumococcal vaccine at 65 years of age

 e. Rotavirus vaccine

17. A 60-year-old male patient received a dose of pneumococcal vaccine during a physician's visit. What would the nurse recommend?

 a. A second dose when he turns 65

 b. A second dose when he turns 70

 c. That he maintain his healthy lifestyle; a second dose is not needed

 d. That he receive a booster in 6 months

18. A 15-year-old male patient presents to the physician's office with his mother. Assuming that he received all of his primary immunizations as an infant and young child, what immunization would the nurse expect the physician to order? (Select all that apply.)

 a. A second dose of varicella vaccine

 b. A tetanus–diphtheria–pertussis booster

 c. An MMR booster

 d. A hepatitis B booster

 e. Shingles vaccine

19. What is a contraindication to an MMR booster for an adolescent female?

 a. Menses

 b. Pregnancy

 c. A positive titer

 d. History of rubeola

20. What is the best source of information for current recommendations regarding immunizations and immunization schedules?

 a. Department of public health

 b. Department of epidemiology

 c. Local physician's office

 d. Centers for Disease Control and Prevention

CHAPTER 11

Drug Therapy to Suppress Immunity

Learning Objectives

- Describe the allergic and immune disorders as well as organ transplantation in terms of etiology, pathophysiology, and clinical manifestations.
- Discuss the characteristics and uses of major immunosuppressant drugs in autoimmune disorders and organ transplantation.
- Describe the cytotoxic immunosuppressant agents in terms of prototype, action, use, adverse effects, contraindications, and nursing implications.
- Discuss the conventional antirejection agents in terms of prototype, action, use, adverse effects, contraindications, and nursing implications.
- Describe the adjuvant drugs in terms of prototypes, indications and contraindications for use, major adverse effects, and administration.
- Understand how to use the nursing process in the care of patients receiving immunosuppressant drugs.

SECTION I: ASSESSING YOUR UNDERSTANDING

Activity A FILL IN THE BLANKS

1. Immunosuppressant drugs interfere with the production or function of immune cells and _____.

2. Autoimmune disorders occur when a person's immune system loses its ability to differentiate between _____ and its own cells.

3. Autoantigens for some disorders have been identified as specific _____ and are found in affected tissues.

4. Allergic asthma, Crohn's disease, psoriasis, psoriatic arthritis, and RA are inflammatory disorders that may be treated with _____ drugs.

5. Although many factors affect graft survival, including the degree of matching between donor tissues and recipient tissues, drug-induced _____ is a major part of transplantation protocols.

Activity B MATCHING

Match the term in Column A with the definition in Column B.

Column A

____ 1. Azathioprine

____ 2. Methotrexate

____ 3. Mycophenolate

____ 4. Cyclosporine

____ 5. Sirolimus

Column B

a. Folate antagonist that inhibits dihydrofolate reductase, the enzyme that converts dihydrofolate to the tetrahydrofolate required for biosynthesis of DNA and cell reproduction

b. Used to prevent rejection reactions and prolong graft survival after solid organ transplantation (e.g., kidney, liver, heart, lung) or to treat chronic rejection in patients previously treated with other immunosuppressive agents

c. Used for prevention and treatment of rejection reactions with renal, cardiac, and hepatic transplantation

d. Antimetabolite that interferes with production of DNA and RNA and thus blocks cellular reproduction, growth, and development

e. Used to prevent renal transplant rejection; inhibits T-cell activation and is given concomitantly with a corticosteroid and cyclosporine

Activity C SHORT ANSWERS

Briefly answer the following questions.

1. How does the body react when foreign tissue is transplanted into the body?

2. What role does tumor necrosis factor (TNF)-alpha play in the response to infection?

3. Identify two factors that prevent the immune system from "turning off" an abnormal immune or inflammatory process.

4. Discuss the mechanism that causes rejection reaction.

5. What are the characteristics of acute organ reactions?

SECTION II: APPLYING YOUR KNOWLEDGE

Activity D CASE STUDY

Consider the scenario and answer the questions.

Mr. Wallace received a bone marrow transplant 6 weeks ago. He presents to the physician's office for a scheduled visit. He is in distress, and the physician requests that you initiate an education plan regarding his disease process, drugs, and symptomatology.

1. The physician diagnoses Mr. Wallace with graft versus host disease (GVHD). How would you explain this disease to the patient?

2. What symptom would you look for that indicates that Mr. Wallace has acute GVHD? If Mr. Wallace's symptoms persist for 3 months after transplantation, the physician would diagnose him with chronic GVHD. What are the characteristics of chronic GVHD?

3. After transplantation, the physician prescribed a combination of methotrexate and cyclosporine to prevent GVHD. The dose of methotrexate ordered was lower than doses you have administered for chemotherapeutic purposes. What consequence does the lower dose have? Organ damage is possible with this combination of drugs. What should you monitor?

SECTION III: PRACTICING FOR NCLEX

Activity E

Answer the following questions.

1. The physician changes a female patient's immunosuppressant to a newer drug. The patient asks the physician why this is necessary. What is true about the newer immunosuppressants?

   a. They have fewer severe adverse effects.

   b. They are less expensive.

   c. They will prolong her life.

   d. They will enhance her health and well-being.

2. A recent transplant patient is prescribed enzyme-inhibiting drugs by his physician. He is also prescribed tacrolimus. What could be the result of this drug combination?

   a. Increased blood levels

   b. Decreased blood levels

   c. Drug-induced diabetes mellitus

   d. Drug-induced liver failure

3. Six months after undergoing transplantation, a female patient asks her physician if it would be alright for her to volunteer at the local children's health clinic. She has limited adverse effects from her immunosuppressant drugs and is beginning to feel healthy again. The physician suggests alternate volunteer options; what is he most likely concerned about?

   a. She may not have the stamina to work at the clinic.

   b. It is too soon to volunteer in a clinic setting.

   c. She may develop an infectious process at the clinic.

   d. It will increase the risk of rejection.

4. A male patient received a kidney transplant 2 years ago. He asks the physician if he may begin to wean himself off of the immunosuppressive drug therapy. He is healthy and works as an engineer full time, and he finds the cost of the medication prohibitive. What would the nurse expect the physician to do?

   a. Discontinue the medication

   b. Titrate the medication and discontinue the medication

   c. Use an alternative, less expensive medication and then titrate the new medication

   d. Continue the medication, because it is lifelong therapy

5. What disorder of the immune system may affect both the skin and the joints?

   a. Rheumatoid arthritis

   b. Crohn's disease

   c. Psoriasis

   d. Graft versus host disease

6. The home care nurse is caring for a female patient who underwent renal transplantation 8 weeks ago and is self-administering immunosuppressant drugs. What situation in the patient's life is the greatest cause for concern?

   a. She runs a secretarial business from home.

   b. She runs a sick child day care.

   c. She is a vegetarian.

   d. She likes to walk ½ mile a day.

7. A female patient physician prescribes leflunomide for her rheumatoid arthritis. Six months later, the patient presents for routine laboratory testing. The physician would discontinue the medication if what laboratory test was abnormal?

   a. Serum albumin

   b. HDL

   c. LDL

   d. LFT

8. If a patient who is prescribed tacrolimus has impaired liver function, what would the nurse expect the physician to do?

   a. Increase the dose

   b. Discontinue the medication

   c. Decrease the dose

   d. Continue the current dose

9. A male patient is status post-kidney transplantation; he also has impaired liver function. What would the nurse expect the physician to do regarding the loading dose of sirolimus?

   a. Reduce it

   b. Increase it

   c. Keep it the same as for someone without liver impairment

   d. Titrate it over 48 hours

10. A male patient is prescribed cyclosporine after renal transplantation to prevent rejection. Initially, his BUN and creatine levels were elevated; they diminished with medication adjustment and 3 weeks later are elevated again. What would the nurse expect the physician to do?

    a. Evaluate the patient for transplant rejection

    b. Repeat the laboratory tests

    c. Evaluate the CBC

    d. Order an electrolyte panel

11. A 78-year-old male patient begins an immunosuppressant therapy for his rheumatoid arthritis. The nurse is concerned because this patient is at greater risk for what complication, compared with younger adults using the same treatment modality?

a. Falls

b. Infections

c. Mental status changes

d. Self-care deficit

12. A patient is recovering from a kidney transplant. The nurse educates the patient that which symptoms may signify organ rejection? (Select all that apply.)

a. Weight loss

b. Edema

c. Fever

d. Increased urine output

e. Numbness over the graft organ site

13. A female patient asks the nurse why her 4-year-old son is not receiving corticosteroids. The patient read in an article that they are more effective to prevent transplant rejection than the medication that is currently prescribed. What is the appropriate response by the nurse?

a. Corticosteroids impair the child's mental status.

b. Corticosteroids impair growth in children.

c. Corticosteroids increase the risk for childhood illness.

d. Corticosteroids increase the risk for rejection in children younger than 6 years of age.

14. A patient who must use long-term immunosuppressant agents is at risk for what complications? (Select all that apply.)

a. Lymphoma

b. Hypotension

c. Metabolic bone disease

d. Migraine headaches

e. Liver disease

15. The nurse is caring for a patient who is receiving a TNF-alpha blocking agent. The nurse understands that what condition can occur as a result of taking this medication?

a. Rheumatoid arthritis

b. Systemic lupus erythematosus

c. Psoriasis

d. *Pneumocystis* pneumonia

16. The physician is planning to prescribe mycophenolate mofetil for a 28-year-old woman. The nurse understands that the patient is required to do what before receiving this prescription?

a. Have proof of income

b. Have a head CT scan

c. Have a negative pregnancy test

d. Have a bone density test

17. A female nursing student is diagnosed with rheumatoid arthritis. What is the probable cause of her rheumatoid arthritis?

a. Injury

b. Abnormal immune response

c. Overuse of NSAIDs

d. Overuse of acetaminophen

18. Psoriatic arthritis is a type of arthritis associated with psoriasis that is similar to RA. Which TNF-alpha inhibitor is used for the treatment of psoriatic arthritis?

a. Cyclosporine

b. Methotrexate

c. Lithium

d. Etanercept

19. A male patient is diagnosed with Crohn's disease. The nurse explains that Crohn's disease is a chronic, recurrent, inflammatory bowel disorder. Which organ can it affect?

a. The large intestine

b. The small intestine

c. The duodenum

d. Any area of the GI tract

20. What is a common adverse effect that patients may experience who take methotrexate (Rheumatrex) for the treatment of rheumatoid arthritis?

a. Fever

b. Severe nausea

c. Stomatitis

d. Constipation

CHAPTER 12

Drug Therapy for the Treatment of Cancer

Learning Objectives

- Outline the etiology of cancer development.
- Describe major types of antineoplastic drugs in terms of mechanism of action, indications for use, and the nursing process.
- Discuss adverse effects of cytotoxic antineoplastic drugs and their prevention or management.
- Be able to teach patients about the administration of some anticancer drugs.
- Understand how to implement the nursing process in the care of patients undergoing drug therapy for cancer, including how to teach and promote efforts to prevent cancer.

SECTION I: ASSESSING YOUR UNDERSTANDING

Activity A FILL IN THE BLANKS

1. _____ is the study of malignant neoplasms and their treatment.

2. _____ is a major treatment modality for cancer, along with surgery and radiation therapy.

3. The term _____ is used to describe many disease processes with the common characteristics of uncontrolled cell growth, invasiveness, and metastasis, as well as numerous etiologies, clinical manifestations, and treatments.

4. _____ cells reproduce in response to a need for tissue growth or repair and stop reproduction when the need has been met.

5. The normal _____ is the interval between the "birth" of a cell and its division into two daughter cells.

Activity B MATCHING

Match the term in Column A with the definition in Column B.

Column A

_____ 1. Alkylating agents

_____ 2. Methotrexate

_____ 3. Antitumor antibiotics (e.g., doxorubicin)

_____ 4. Camptothecins (also called DNA topoisomerase inhibitors)

_____ 5. L-Asparaginase (Elspar)

Column B

a. Bind to DNA so that DNA and RNA transcription is blocked

b. Includes nitrogen mustard derivatives, nitrosoureas, and platinum compounds

c. Enzyme that inhibits protein synthesis and reproduction by depriving cells of required amino acids

d. Blocks folate and enzymes essential for cancer cell reproduction and may increase blood levels of homocysteine

e. Inhibit an enzyme required for DNA replication and repair

Activity C SHORT ANSWERS

Briefly answer the following questions.

1. Describe the mechanism used by antimetabolites to interfere with cell reproduction.

2. What does the term *cell cycle–specific* mean in relation to the action of antimetabolites on cancer cells?

3. Why are nitrosoureas used in the treatment of brain tumors?

4. Describe the toxic effects related to the use of folic acid antagonists.

5. What types of cancers are treated with folic acid antagonists, purine antagonists, and pyrimidine antagonists?

SECTION II: APPLYING YOUR KNOWLEDGE

Activity D CASE STUDY

Consider the scenario and answer the questions.

Mr. Caisse, a microbiologist, discovers a lump in the region of the clavicle. Biopsy reveals lymphoma stage IIIB, and the treatment modality chosen is surgery and cytotoxic antineoplastic drugs. You are responsible for the treatment plan.

1. Mr. Caisse states that he is having difficulty absorbing the information that he needs to cope with his diagnosis. He feels overwhelmed. He asks you to review how the drugs kill malignant cells. How can you explain to this patient how the cytotoxic antineoplastic drugs work?

2. The physician prescribes daunorubicin in a liposomal preparation. What are the advantages of liposomal preparations? What can you tell this patient about the risks for tumor lysis syndrome?

3. Mr. Caisse states that he understands that the symptoms of tumor lysis syndrome depend on the severity of metabolic imbalances. He develops a mild anemia and is concerned that he is beginning to experience the syndrome. Based on the patient's comment, would you say that he needs more teaching or not? What else might you be able to tell him?

4. What can be done to help prevent tumor lysis syndrome?

SECTION III: PRACTICING FOR NCLEX

Activity E

Answer the following questions.

1. A 75-year-old male patient is diagnosed with cancer. His current treatment modality is only minimally successful. He asks his physician to research clinical trials of drugs that may be successful for his type of cancer. The physician agrees, for what reason?

    a. Clinical trials and their subsequent costs will be covered by Medicare.

    b. The physician anticipates that no clinical trials are available for the patient's cancer.

    c. Physicians are legally permitted to present patients for clinical trials.

    d. The patient's age will no longer prevent his acceptance for a clinical trial.

2. A male patient is diagnosed with prostate cancer. The treatment modality of choice includes both surgery and chemotherapy. What does the chemotherapeutic option include?

    a. Hemoglobin replacement therapy

    b. Diuretics

    c. Hormonal therapies

    d. Antidiuretic hormone

3. The nurse is preparing a patient who will begin chemotherapy in a few days. The nurse knows that which are the most common adverse effects encountered by most patients who receive chemotherapy? (Select all that apply.)

    a. Alopecia

    b. Neutrocytosis

    c. Thrombocytopenia

    d. Anemia

    e. Stomach ulcers

4. A female patient is ending an extensive chemotherapeutic regimen that included cytotoxic antineoplastic drugs. The nurse is concerned when the patient begins to experience bone marrow toxicity, for what reason?

    a. It is a common adverse effect of her treatment.

    b. It is a rare side effect of the chemotherapy.

    c. It will cause the physician to increase the dose of chemotherapeutic medications.

    d. It will ultimately lead to death.

5. A male patient is receiving parenteral cytotoxic medications in the home. Adjunct therapy may include what substance?

   a. Erythropoietin

   b. Heparin

   c. Normal saline 0.9% intravenously

   d. Antidiuretic hormone

6. A female patient develops hepatotoxicity from the antineoplastic drugs that she is receiving. She has abnormal levels of AST, ALT, and bilirubin. The physician may not decrease the drugs, for what reason?

   a. These findings do not indicate hepatotoxicity.

   b. These findings may indicate renal dysfunction.

   c. These findings do not indicate decreased ability to metabolize drugs.

   d. These findings may indicate cardiac dysfunction.

7. A female patient is receiving L-asparaginase. She is at the end of her chemotherapeutic course and is concerned because her liver function tests are abnormal. What is an appropriate response by the nurse?

   a. "Liver damage is an outcome of chemotherapy; a transplant may be advised after you recover."

   b. "The liver damage is an acceptable consequence to chemotherapy."

   c. "Liver impairment usually subsides when chemotherapy is complete."

   d. "You are correct to worry; the chemotherapy may be canceled and your cancer will recur."

8. A male patient is informed by his physician that the latest tests indicate that his cancer has spread to his liver. The patient receives capecitabine as part of his treatment regimen. What would the nurse expect the physician to do?

   a. Increase the dose of capecitabine

   b. Discontinue the capecitabine

   c. Add routine blood transfusions to the patient's treatment regimen

   d. Monitor the patient closely and repeat LFTs routinely

9. A male patient is receiving cisplatin as part of his cancer therapy and develops renal impairment. The physician chooses to titrate the dose of the cisplatin based on what laboratory value?

   a. BUN

   b. LFTs

   c. CBC

   d. CrCl levels

10. The nurse will assess the patient receiving chemotherapy for which symptoms related to tumor lysis syndrome? (Select all that apply.)

    a. Polyuria

    b. Numbness and tingling of the extremities

    c. Nausea

    d. Confusion

    e. Hypotension

11. In addition to comorbidities, what other issues affect treatment for older adults? (Select all that apply.)

    a. Access to care

    b. Social service

    c. Financial and transportation issues

    d. Functional status

    e. Physiologic age-related changes

12. A 71-year-old male patient is receiving chemotherapy as part of the treatment regimen for his cancer. To monitor renal function, what laboratory measurements would the nurse expect the physician to order?

    a. BUN

    b. Serum creatinine

    c. Electrolytes

    d. Creatinine clearance

13. In recent years, there have been rapid advances in cancer care for children and high cure rates for many pediatric malignancies. What is the reason behind many of these advances?

    a. The sensitivity of the child's immune system to chemotherapeutic agents

    b. Prolonged radiation therapy

    c. The systematic enrollment of children in well-designed clinical trials

    d. Compliance with treatment regimens

14. The patient asks the nurse why many chemotherapy drugs must be given IV. What is the nurse's best response?

    a. Most chemotherapy drugs go directly to cancer cells if given IV.

    b. Most chemotherapy drugs are inactivated by enzymes in the stomach.

    c. Most chemotherapy drugs cause blistering of the lips if taken orally.

    d. Most chemotherapy drugs are given IV because cancer patients are too sick to take the medications orally.

15. Dosage of cytotoxic drugs for children is based on what factor?

    a. Weight

    b. Body surface area

    c. Height

    d. Disease process

16. A child is prescribed an anthracycline drug. The nurse would teach the parents to observe for signs and symptoms of what adverse effect?

    a. Cardiotoxicity

    b. Dehydration

    c. Gallbladder disease

    d. Esophageal varices

17. A male patient is prescribed cytotoxic antineo-plastic drugs as part of his cancer treatment regimen. His wife is 2 months pregnant. The nurse teaches both the patient and his wife that she should avoid contact with the drug, for which reasons? (Select all that apply.)

    a. It is carcinogenic.

    b. It is mutagenic.

    c. It is teratogenic.

    d. It is hepatogenic.

    e. It is nephrogenic.

18. The nurse is teaching the handling of cytotoxic antineoplastic drugs to the wife of a patient receiving them. What should the nurse teach her to do?

    a. Wear personal protective equipment when handling the drug.

    b. Dispose of the drug in the regular trash.

    c. Store the drug in the cellar of the home.

    d. Save the medications on the kitchen counter, so the home care nurse may dispose of them.

19. When caring for patients receiving cytotoxic antineoplastic drugs, the nurse understands that blood and body fluids are contaminated with drugs or metabolites for how long?

    a. About 72 hours after a dose

    b. About 24 hours after a dose

    c. About 12 hours after a dose

    d. About 48 hours after a dose

20. When both hormone inhibitor and cytotoxic drug therapies are needed, how are they administered?

    a. Given concurrently

    b. Not given concurrently

    c. Administered 3 hours apart

    d. Administered 2 hours apart

Inflammation, Infection, and the Use of Antimicrobial Agents

- Identify the common etiologies of inflammation.
- Discuss the pathophysiology of inflammation.
- Describe, in general, the groups of drugs used to treat inflammation.
- Identify the common pathogens and methods of infection control.
- Discuss the pathophysiology of infection.
- Discuss ways to minimize emergence of drug-resistant microorganisms.
- Discuss ways to increase the benefits and decrease the risk associated with antimicrobial drug therapy.
- Know how to apply the nursing process to the care of the patient who is receiving antimicrobial therapy.

SECTION I: ASSESSING YOUR UNDERSTANDING

Activity A FILL IN THE BLANKS

1. _____ drugs are used to prevent or treat infections caused by pathogenic (disease-producing) microorganisms.

2. In an infection, _____ initially attach to host cell receptors (i.e., proteins, carbohydrates, lipids).

3. _____ are intracellular parasites that survive only in living tissues.

4. Human pathogens include _____, herpes viruses, and retroviruses.

5. _____ are plant-like organisms that live as parasites on living tissue or as saprophytes on decaying organic matter.

Activity B MATCHING

Match the term in Column A with the definition in Column B.

Column A

____ **1.** Opportunistic microorganisms

____ **2.** Gram's stain

____ **3.** Culture

____ **4.** Detection of antigens

____ **5.** Polymerase chain reaction (PCR)

Column B

a. Involves growing a microorganism in the laboratory

b. Usually normal endogenous or environmental flora, nonpathogenic

c. Uses features of culture and serology but reduces the time required for diagnosis

d. Can detect whether DNA for a specific organism is present in a sample

e. Identifies microscopic appearance, including shape and color of the organisms

Activity C   **SHORT ANSWERS**

Briefly answer the following questions.

1. Explain how infections occur in the human body.

2. Give an example of normal flora and discuss the role of normal flora in the human body.

3. Define colonization.

4. Describe the conditions needed for opportunistic infections to invade the human body.

5. How do broad-spectrum antibiotics affect the human body?

SECTION II: APPLYING YOUR KNOWLEDGE

Activity D   **CASE STUDY**

Consider the scenario and answer the questions.

You are part of a group of nursing students who are studying the immune system. Your section to share with the group is the role of normal flora as it relates to health and illness.

1. What are the sterile areas of the body? What are some colonized areas of the body?

2. Discuss the pathogenicity of the microorganisms that are part of the normal flora. How does this normal flora protect the human host? What vitamins does the normal bowel flora synthesize?

3. What happens if the normal flora is suppressed by antimicrobial drug therapy? What happens to the normal flora when antibiotics are used? Use *Candida albicans* as an example.

SECTION III: PRACTICING FOR NCLEX

Activity E

Answer the following questions.

1. A female patient is treated with antibiotics for bacterial pneumonia. When obtaining a drug history, the nurse finds that the patient ceased her medication regimen when she no longer experienced symptoms during the first round of antibiotics. The nurse is responsible for the patient's education plan. In order to effectively treat the pneumonia, what must the patient do?

   a. Complete a full course of antibiotics as prescribed

   b. Continue the antibiotics for 1 week after cessation of symptoms

   c. Take the antibiotics at breakfast, lunch, and supper

   d. Take the antibiotics every 3 hours during the day

2. A female patient takes an antibiotic, left over from her last bout with bronchitis, when she discovers that her child has developed strep throat. She takes the antibiotic as a preventive measure. What effects might this practice have? (Select all that apply.)

   a. Increasing adverse drug effects

   b. Increasing the risk of infections with drug-resistant microorganisms

   c. Becoming a cost-effective method to manage infectious processes

   d. Reducing health care costs

   e. Increased sensitivity to antibacterials

3. The physician orders an antibiotic for a female patient, who states that she cannot take antibiotics on an empty stomach because they make her nauseous. What instructions should the nurse give her?

   a. Take the medication with food to reduce nausea.

   b. Take the medication three times a day with meals.

   c. Take the medication on an empty stomach.

   d. Take the antibiotic on an empty stomach until symptoms abate.

4. A patient has been receiving an antibiotic for the past 36 hours for treatment of a bacterial infection, and the infection has shown no signs of improving. What does the nurse suspect is the most likely reason for a lack of improvement?

   a. The patient isn't taking the medication

   b. The patient's infection is resistant to the medication

   c. The patient is allergic to this medication

   d. The patient has a viral infection, not bacterial

5. A male patient is treated for urinary tract infections several times a year, secondary to urinary retention and an enlarged prostate. He also is treated for chronic renal failure, hypertension, and type 2 diabetes. What might happen when the patient is treated with antibiotics?

   a. He may be nephrotoxic.

   b. He may be at increased risk for congestive heart failure.

   c. It may precipitate a hypertensive crisis.

   d. It may cause prostate enlargement.

6. A female patient is 48 hours post-op for a hip replacement. When the nurse assesses her incision line, the nurse finds redness, warmth, and drainage from the proximal section of the wound. What would the nurse expect the physician to order?

   a. Amoxicillin

   b. Penicillin

   c. Bactrim

   d. Cefazolin

7. The physician orders an antibiotic for a male patient three times a day for 7 days. The patient asks the nurse if this is correct, because his son took the same antibiotic for 5 days. On what factor is the amount and frequency of the antibiotic dosing based?

   a. Characteristics of the causative organism

   b. Age of the patient

   c. Sex of the patient

   d. Condition of the gastrointestinal system

8. The nurse is aware that which areas of the body are difficult to treat with antimicrobial drugs? (Select all that apply.)

   a. Bladder

   b. Prostate gland

   c. Brain

   d. Eyes

   e. Stomach

9. A male patient is diagnosed with osteomyelitis secondary to an untreated bone fracture. What type of IV therapy is required to treat this disease?

   a. Short term

   b. Long term

   c. Modified based on the patient's age

   d. Modified based on the patient's home environment

10. The nurse is discharging a patient who will be taking an antimicrobial at home. What adverse effects related to antimicrobial therapy should be reported to the physician? (Select all that apply.)

    a. Skin rash

    b. Any sign of a new infection

    c. Metallic taste in the mouth

    d. Halitosis

    e. Diarrhea

11. A male patient is diagnosed with a drug-resistant infection in his wound. What should the home care nurse teach the patient and his family?

    a. To avoid social contact while the infection is treated

    b. To avoid using the same bathroom until the infection abates

    c. To use gloves when handling drainage from the wound

    d. To use bleach when washing all laundry

12. A male patient is admitted to the critical care unit from a trauma center. He is status postsurgery after a fall from a roof in a construction site. He has multiple fractures and internal injuries. What factor will help determine the dosage of his IV antibiotic?

    a. Cardiovascular assessment of the critically ill patient

    b. Neurovascular assessment of the critically ill patient

    c. Changing physiology of the critically ill patient

    d. Altered mentation of the critically ill patient

13. On his second day in the critical care unit, a patient develops a left lower lobe infiltrate and is diagnosed with nosocomial pneumonia. What does the nurse expect is the cause of the pneumonia?

    a. *Pseudomonas*

    b. *Streptococcus*

    c. *Clostridium difficile*

    d. *Staphylococcus aureus*

14. A patient is diagnosed with bacterial pneumonia. Pending culture results, what would the nurse expect the physician to order?
    a. Broad-spectrum antibiotics
    b. Short-term oral antibiotic therapy
    c. Short-term IV antibiotic therapy
    d. Long-term oral antibiotic therapy

15. A male patient is placed on a ventilator. To reduce the rate of ventilator-associated pneumonia and mortality, what would the nurse expect the physician to order?
    a. Antibiotic rotation
    b. IV antibiotics in intervals of 4 to 6 weeks
    c. Oral antibiotics in intervals of 4 to 6 weeks
    d. An antifungal alternated with an antibiotic

16. The nurse is aware that a patient is at risk for the development of an infection because of what factors? (Select all that apply.)
    a. Patient is 35 pounds underweight
    b. Patient has diabetes mellitus
    c. Patient takes a shower every day
    d. Patient is taking chemotherapy for a malignancy
    e. Patient has a WBC of 7500

17. Which laboratory value of CrCl indicates severe renal impairment?
    a. Greater than 15 to 30 mL/min
    b. Less than 45 to 60 mL/min
    c. Less than 15 to 30 mL/min
    d. Greater than 45 to 60 mL/min

18. The nursing instructor is discussing normal body defense against infection. The nursing students answer correctly when they identify what as defense factors? (Select all that apply.)
    a. Coughing
    b. Stomach acid
    c. Impaired blood supply
    d. Use of a prosthetic device
    e. Swallowing

19. A female patient is receiving hemodialysis three times weekly. The physician orders an antibiotic. What does the nurse expect will happen with the dosage of the antibiotic related to the dialysis?
    a. The dosage may be decreased on dialysis days.
    b. An extra dose may be needed on dialysis days.
    c. A double dose may be needed on dialysis days.
    d. It is not necessary to modify the dose of the antibiotic on dialysis days.

20. Which patient is most at risk for an opportunistic infection?
    a. A 14-year-old patient with HIV infection
    b. A 25-year-old patient with asthma
    c. A 33-year-old patient with hepatitis A
    d. A 45-year-old patient with contact dermatitis

CHAPTER 14

Drug Therapy to Decrease Pain, Fever, and Inflammation

Learning Objectives

- Discuss the role of prostaglandins in the etiology of pain, fever, and inflammation.
- Identify the major manifestations of fever and inflammation.
- Understand the pathophysiology of osteoarthritis.
- Understand the pathophysiology of gout.
- Identify the prototype and describe the action, use, adverse effects, contraindications, and nursing implications for the salicylates.
- Identify the action, use, adverse effects, contraindications, and nursing implications for acetaminophen.
- Identify the prototype and describe the action, use, adverse effects, contraindications, and nursing implications for the propionic acid derivatives.
- Identify the prototype and describe the action, use, adverse effects, contraindications, and nursing implications for the oxicam derivatives.
- Identify the prototype and describe the action, use, adverse effects, contraindications, and nursing implications for the acetic acid derivatives.
- Identify the prototype and describe the action, use, adverse effects, contraindications, and nursing implications for the selective COX-2 inhibitors.

- Identify the prototype and describe the action, use, adverse effects, contraindications, and nursing implications for the mitotic agents.
- Identify the prototype and describe the action, use, adverse effects, contraindications, and nursing implications for uricosuric medications.
- Know how to implement the nursing process in the care of patients undergoing drug therapy for pain, fever, and inflammation.

SECTION I: ASSESSING YOUR UNDERSTANDING

Activity A FILL IN THE BLANKS

1. Aspirin, NSAIDs, and acetaminophen can also be called _____.

2. _____ sensitize pain receptors and increase the pain associated with other chemical mediators of inflammation and immunity.

3. Body temperature is controlled by a regulating center in the _____.

4. _____ is the normal body response to tissue damage from any source, and it may occur in any tissue or organ. It is an attempt by the body to remove the damaging agent and repair the damaged tissue.

5. Inflammation may be a component of virtually any illness. Inflammatory conditions affecting organs or systems are often named by adding the suffix _____ to the involved organ or system.

Activity B MATCHING

Match the term in Column A with the definition in Column B.

Column A

____ **1.** Acetaminophen

____ **2.** Aspirin

____ **3.** Ketorolac

____ **4.** Bursitis

____ **5.** Rheumatoid arthritis

Column B

a. Injectable NSAIDs often used for pain

b. Inflammation of the bursa

c. Nonprescription drug commonly used as an aspirin substitute because it does not cause nausea, vomiting, or GI bleeding

d. Chronic, painful, inflammatory disorder that affects the synovial tissue of hinge-like joints, tissues around these joints, and eventually other body organs

e. Prototype of the analgesic–antipyretic–anti-inflammatory drugs and the most commonly used salicylate

Activity C SEQUENCING

Because of multiple reports of liver damage from acetaminophen poisoning, the FDA has strengthened the warning on products containing acetaminophen and emphasized that the maximum adult dose of 4 g daily, from all sources, should not be exceeded. Given below, in random order, are the symptoms of acetaminophen overdosage. Write them in the correct order, from early onset to end-stage, in the boxes provided.

A. Symptoms may subside, but tests of liver function begin to show increased levels.

B. Anorexia, nausea, vomiting, and diaphoresis may occur.

C. Jaundice, vomiting, and CNS stimulation with excitement and delirium occur.

D. Vascular collapse, coma, and death occur.

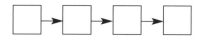

Activity D SHORT ANSWERS

Briefly answer the following questions.

1. Explain how prostaglandins are formed when cellular injury occurs.

2. Describe the role of pyrogens in the febrile process.

3. Identify the systemic manifestations that occur in the inflammatory process.

4. How do aspirin and other NSAIDs reduce inflammation and fever?

5. Aspirin and nonselective NSAIDs are also antiplatelet medications. Describe the antiplatelet process created by ingestion of these drugs.

SECTION II: APPLYING YOUR KNOWLEDGE

Activity E CASE STUDY

Consider the scenario and answer the questions.

Mrs. Anderson presents to her physician's office with long-term joint pain that is interfering with her ability to perform her activities of daily living. She is currently self-administering ibuprofen 400 mg four times a day for pain relief, but the drug is beginning to upset her stomach. The physician diagnoses the client with osteoarthritis and prescribes celecoxib for pain and inflammation. You are responsible for developing an education plan for Mrs. Anderson.

1. Mrs. Anderson asks you to explain why she is in so much pain. Using a model of a joint, explain how DJD causes the pain cycle.

2. Mrs. Anderson is concerned that the new medication will work as well as the ibuprofen. Explain the mechanism of action for COX-2 inhibitors.

SECTION III: PRACTICING FOR NCLEX

Activity F

Answer the following questions.

1. A male patient presents to the physician's office with inflammation and edema in his left great toe, lasting several days. The physician orders a uric acid level and diagnoses the patient with gout, and orders oral colchicine. The nurse is responsible for developing an education plan. The patient asks how long it will take for the pain and swelling to subside from his ankle. When colchicine is taken for acute gout, how long does it usually take until pain is relieved?

   a. 7 to 10 days

   b. 24 to 48 hours

   c. 48 to 72 hours

   d. 3 to 5 days

2. A patient with the diagnosis of chronic gout asks how long he should take his colchicine when he experiences symptoms. What are the correct instructions for this patient?

   a. Take as directed when pain begins until relief is obtained or nausea, vomiting, and diarrhea occur.

   b. Take for a minimum of 7 to 10 days.

   c. Take for a minimum of 5 to 7 days.

   d. Take as directed when you notice swelling, and continue for 7 to 10 days.

3. The patient with chronic gout asks how he can reduce the uric levels in his body when he begins to self-administer colchicine. What would be the nurse's response?

   a. "You should maintain a fluid restriction, drinking no more than 800 to 1000 mL of fluid a day."

   b. "You should increase your caffeine intake; it will help you to eliminate the uric acid crystals."

   c. "Only the medication will reduce the uric acid levels in your body; your fluid intake will not affect the levels."

   d. "Drink 2 to 3 quarts of fluid daily; this will decrease uric acid levels and help prevent formation of uric acid kidney stones."

4. A female patient complains of a mild headache. The physician orders acetaminophen 325 mg, two tablets by mouth every 4 to 6 hours. The patient states that she usually takes ibuprofen for her headaches and asks why the physician ordered acetaminophen. Which explanation would the nurse give?

   a. "Acetaminophen is more effective than ibuprofen for headaches."

   b. "Acetaminophen is less expensive and more efficient for pain relief."

   c. "Acetaminophen is often the initial drug of choice for relieving mild to moderate pain."

   d. "Acetaminophen will reduce the inflammation causing your headache."

5. A male patient's physician orders aspirin 81 mg PO each day as a treatment related to his recent myocardial infarction. The patient asks the nurse if he can take acetaminophen instead. What is the nurse's best response?

   a. "Acetaminophen is an effective aspirin substitute for pain or fever but not for prevention of heart attack or stroke."

   b. "Acetaminophen will work just as well; I will call the doctor to notify him of your drug preference."

   c. "Acetaminophen will prevent strokes but not heart attacks."

   d. "You must follow your doctor's order."

6. A 16-year-old patient asks the nurse if she can take two Tylenol every 2 hours during exams, because it helps relieve her tension headaches. What is the nurse's most appropriate response?

   a. "Why do you feel so tense regarding exams?"

   b. "Do not exceed recommended doses of acetaminophen due to the risk of life-threatening liver damage."

   c. "Consult your physician."

   d. "Acetaminophen is a benign drug and will relieve your pain."

7. A male patient is taking aspirin 81 mg by mouth each day for prevention of recurrent myocardial infarction. He makes a dentist appointment for a tooth extraction. He calls the physician's office and asks the nurse if he is at risk for bleeding. Which response is correct?

   a. "Yes, low doses of aspirin may increase your risk of bleeding; I will call you with your new physician's orders."

   b. "No, the dose of aspirin is too low to increase your risk of bleeding."

   c. "Yes, you need to stop the aspirin immediately."

   d. "Your dentist must extract the tooth in a hospital setting to reduce the risk of hemorrhage."

8. An 80-year-old male patient presents to the physician's office with complaints of fatigue and a change in the color of his stools. He self-administers ibuprofen 400 mg each night for general discomfort. The physician orders a stool test for guaiac, which yields positive results. The physician discontinues the ibuprofen. The nurse is responsible for a patient education plan. The patient should be educated regarding what as a risk with chronic use of NSAIDs?

   a. GI discomfort

   b. GI distress

   c. GI bleed

   d. GI upset

9. The nurse knows that what is the most significant risk factor in the development of osteoarthritis?

   a. Gender

   b. Ethnic background

   c. Age

   d. Occupation

10. What is the most effective treatment for a febrile episode in a child aged 6 to 36 months?

    a. Acetaminophen alone

    b. Alternating acetaminophen and ibuprofen every 4 hours over a 3-day period

    c. Ibuprofen alone

    d. Alternating acetaminophen and ibuprofen every 2 hours over a 3-day period

11. A female patient asks why she must consult with her physician when she uses cold products for her children. What is the nurse's best response?

    a. "Your health insurance requires that you notify the physician whenever you administer over-the-counter medications to your children."

    b. "Notification is just a precaution to protect you and your children."

    c. "You really aren't required to do so, it is just a precaution."

    d. "There is a risk of overdose, because acetaminophen is a very common ingredient in OTC cold, flu, fever, and pain remedies."

12. A student nurse asks the nurse why acetaminophen and NSAIDs help to reduce cancer pain. What is the nurse's most correct explanation?

    a. Cancer often produces chronic pain from tumor invasion of tissues or complications of treatment. These drugs prevent sensitization of peripheral pain receptors by inhibiting prostaglandin formation.

    b. Cancer rarely produces chronic pain from tumor invasion of tissues or complications of treatment. These drugs eliminate sensitization of peripheral pain receptors by inhibiting prostaglandin formation.

    c. Cancer often produces chronic pain from tumor invasion of tissues or complications of treatment. These drugs potentiate sensitization of peripheral pain receptors by increasing prostaglandin formation.

    d. Cancer rarely produces severe pain from tumor invasion of tissues or complications of treatment. These drugs prevent sensitization of peripheral pain receptors by inhibiting prostaglandin formation.

13. Aspirin increases the risk of bleeding and should generally be avoided for how many weeks before and after surgery?

    a. 3 to 4 weeks

    b. 1 to 2 weeks

    c. 6 to 8 weeks

    d. 2 to 3 weeks

14. A male patient is seeking an over-the-counter medication to ease both the pain and inflammation associated with his osteoarthritis of his knee. The nurse knows that which drug will only reduce pain?

    a. Acetaminophen
    b. Aspirin
    c. Naproxen sodium
    d. Ibuprofen

15. Both categories of migraine abortive drugs (ergot alkaloids and serotonin agonists) exert powerful vasoconstrictive effects and also have what potential?

    a. Lower blood pressure
    b. Manage hypertension
    c. Raise blood pressure
    d. Manage hypotension

16. A 78-year-old male patient calls the clinic and complains of severe pain and swelling in his right great toe. The patient states that the pain is worse at night and has been present for at least 2 weeks. The nurse understands that this patient has what type of inflammatory disorder?

    a. Osteoarthritis of the toe
    b. Probable fracture of the toe
    c. Gout
    d. Spondyloarthritis

17. A female patient's physician orders an ergot preparation for her migraine headaches. The nurse is responsible for the education plan. What would be the nurse's teaching regarding how the patient is to take her medication?

    a. Take it at the onset of a headache, and lie down in a quiet, darkened room.
    b. Take it when the pain becomes unbearable, so the medication will be more effective.
    c. Take it when sleep alone does not relieve the pain.
    d. Take it whenever you experience a headache.

18. What would a patient who self-administers the medication butalbital experience?

    a. Nausea and vomiting after 6 months of use
    b. Resolution of all headache types
    c. Overuse headaches and withdrawal issues
    d. Weight loss after 6 months of use

19. A 7-year-old patient is admitted to the pediatric critical care unit with a probable diagnosis of Reye's syndrome. The nurse will be assessing the child for what symptoms? (Select all that apply.)

    a. Jaundice
    b. Brain swelling
    c. Painful joints
    d. Ringing in the ears
    e. Elevated liver enzymes

20. A patient is in the surgical intensive care unit after having a coronary bypass grafting approximately 6 hours ago. What medication will the nurse be expected to administer at this time?

    a. Naproxen sodium 220 mg
    b. Aspirin 81 mg
    c. Ibuprofen 200 mg
    d. Aspirin 625 mg

Drug Therapy With Corticosteroids

Learning Objectives

- Understand the physiologic effects of endogenous corticosteroids.
- Identify the pathophysiology of adrenal cortex disorders.
- Describe the action and the clinical indications for use of exogenous corticosteroids.
- Understand the contraindications and adverse effects of corticosteroids as well as the nursing implications of their use.
- Analyze how other drugs and substances as well as other factors may affect the need for corticosteroids.
- Apply the nursing process when a patient is administered a corticosteroid.

SECTION I: ASSESSING YOUR UNDERSTANDING

Activity A FILL IN THE BLANKS

1. _____, also called *glucocorticoids* or *steroids*, are hormones produced by the adrenal cortex, part of the adrenal glands.

2. _____ corticosteroids are used as drugs in a variety of disorders.

3. When plasma corticosteroid levels rise to an adequate level, secretion of corticosteroids _____ or _____.

4. The mechanism by which the hypothalamus and anterior pituitary "learn" that no more corticosteroids are needed is called a _____ _____ _____.

5. _____ are secreted directly into the bloodstream.

Activity B MATCHING

Match the term in Column A with the definition in Column B.

Column A	Column B
____ 1. Hyperaldosteronism	a. Produced by inadequate secretion of corticotropin, most often caused by prolonged administration of corticosteroids
____ 2. Congenital adrenogenital syndromes and adrenal hyperplasia	
____ 3. Secondary adrenocortical insufficiency	b. Associated with destruction of the adrenal cortex by disease processes or hemorrhage and with atrophy of the adrenal cortex
____ 4. Primary adrenocortical insufficiency (Addison's disease)	

_____ **5.** Adrenocortical hyperfunction (Cushing's disease)

c. A rare disorder caused by adenoma or hyperplasia of the adrenal cortex cells that produce aldosterone

d. Result from deficiencies in one or more enzymes required for cortisol production

e. May result from excessive corticotropin or a primary adrenal tumor

3. Corticosteroids are effective in the treatment of neoplastic diseases. What mechanism of action do they have that makes them effective?

4. Mr. Castile received a kidney transplant 6 months ago. He is not comfortable with the changes in his body related to the corticosteroids he must take. He asks why they are necessary. How would you respond?

5. In patients with asthma, what is the effect of corticosteroids? In patients with anaphylactic shock resulting from an allergic reaction, what is the effect of corticosteroids?

Activity C **SHORT ANSWERS**

Briefly answer the following questions.

1. Discuss the process by which corticosteroid secretion is controlled.

2. How does the stress response affect the sympathetic nervous system?

3. What are glucocorticoids, and how do they affect the body's processes?

4. What are mineralocorticoids, and how do they affect the body's processes?

5. What are adrenal sex hormones, and how do they affect the body's processes?

SECTION II: APPLYING YOUR KNOWLEDGE

Activity D **CASE STUDY**

Consider the scenario and answer the questions.

You are participating in a study group of nursing students studying the indications for the various uses of corticosteroids.

1. Mr. Janis is diagnosed with systemic lupus erythematosus. Where would you expect to find inflammation in this patient?

2. Name some skin disorders that may be treated with corticosteroids.

SECTION III: PRACTICING FOR NCLEX

Activity E

Answer the following questions.

1. A female patient's physician discontinues her systemic corticosteroid using a sliding scale and orders an inhaler. The patient asks if she can begin flunisolide; her friend uses it and suggested it as the patient's next option. How should the nurse respond?

a. "I will ask the physician to change his original prescription."

b. "Flunisolide is a safe option."

c. "Flunisolide is not the primary medication to treat her disease process."

d. "The physician did not order flunisolide because it may cause death."

2. Systemic corticosteroids may cause which side effects? (Select all that apply.)

a. Hirsutism

b. Hypertension

c. Glucose intolerance

d. Premature puberty in children

e. Fat pad on the buttocks (Buffalo hump)

3. What is a strategy to minimize HPA suppression and risks of acute adrenal insufficiency?

a. Reducing the dose of systemic corticosteroids when the patient on long-term therapy experiences high-stress situations

b. Administering a systemic corticosteroid during high-stress situations in patients on long-term systemic therapy

c. Concurrent use of oral contraceptives and corticosteroids in women to reduce the stress on the adrenal gland

d. Drug holidays for patients with long-term corticosteroid use

4. A male patient experiences an acute exacerbation of his asthma secondary to an allergic reaction. The physician orders what type of therapy to minimize HPA suppression and risks of acute adrenal insufficiency?

a. A short course of systemic therapy

b. Long-term systemic therapy to prevent future exacerbations of his asthma

c. Long-term systemic therapy with drug holidays every 6 months

d. A short course of systemic therapy with a prn prescription of corticosteroids

5. A female patient experiences weight gain secondary to her systemic steroid therapy for temporal arteritis. She calls the physician's office to ask if she can discontinue the medication for 1 week, to fit into her dress for her class reunion. Which response is appropriate?

a. "A temporary discontinuance will not adversely affect your health."

b. "I will ask the physician for a change in your prescription."

c. "Your prescription must be tapered gradually with the physician's order."

d. "Your prescription must be tapered for 2 days only with the physician's order."

6. A male patient develops a mild rash secondary to sensitivity to a new laundry detergent. The physician orders a topical corticosteroid. The patient states that this medication will take too long to work and asks whether he can just take a steroid by mouth. What is the most appropriate response?

a. "Oral corticosteroids will not reduce the inflammation of contact dermatitis."

b. "Oral corticosteroids are contraindicated for cases of contact dermatitis."

c. "Local therapy will resolve the symptoms of the dermatitis quicker than the use of oral corticosteroids."

d. "Using local rather than systemic corticosteroids reduces adrenal insufficiency."

7. The mother of a child who has just been diagnosed with asthma is receiving medication teaching about the prednisone (Deltasone)

that the child will be taking for the next 2 weeks. Which statement by the mother indicates the need for further instruction?

a. "I will make sure and give him the medication around the same time every day."

b. "I will watch for other signs of illness other than fever while he takes this medicine."

c. "I am so glad that this medication will cure his asthma."

d. "I will contact the physician if I am unable to give him the medication one day."

8. A male patient is diagnosed with Addison's disease. What daily medication would the nurse expect to be administered?

a. Warfarin

b. Hydrochlorothiazide

c. Apresoline

d. Prednisone

9. A 65-year-old patient who has been on long-term corticosteroid therapy is admitted to the hospital and will need an IV inserted. What adverse effect of corticosteroid may negatively affect this procedure?

a. Truncal obesity

b. Insomnia

c. Thinning of the skin

d. Moon face

10. What are the most frequently desired pharmacologic effects of exogenous corticosteroids? (Select all that apply.)

a. Anti-inflammatory

b. Immunosuppressive

c. Anticoagulant

d. Antianxiety

e. Analgesic

11. The nurse is working in a home care setting. A female patient is prescribed oral corticosteroids by her physician secondary to a diagnosis of Addison's disease. What is the nurse's responsibility in this situation?

a. Supervising and monitoring the administration of the drug

b. Administering all doses of the oral medication

c. Administering all doses of the oral medication for the first month of use

d. Teaching all family members to administer the medication

12. A male patient is diagnosed with pneumocystosis, and his physician orders corticosteroids. What is an accurate statement to include in the teaching plan for the patient?
   a. Corticosteroids may reduce his survival rate but improve his quality of life.
   b. Corticosteroids decrease risks of respiratory failure.
   c. Corticosteroids decrease cerebral edema associated with pneumocystosis.
   d. Corticosteroids decrease the white blood cell count related to pneumocystosis.

13. A female patient is diagnosed with septic shock. What would the nurse expect a long course of low-dose corticosteroids to do?
   a. Diminish her survival secondary to impaired immunity
   b. Improve her survival without causing harm
   c. Improve her survival with long-term adrenal insufficiency
   d. Diminish her survival secondary to superinfection

14. A male patient is diagnosed with adult respiratory distress syndrome. His family asks whether corticosteroids may help him to breathe easier. Which statement about corticosteroids is accurate?
   a. They are successfully used for the long-term treatment of ARDS.
   b. They are successful for the short-term treatment of ARDS.
   c. They are not used when the patient is at risk for *Pneumocystis* pneumonia.
   d. They are not a beneficial treatment for ARDS.

15. A male patient receives IV methylprednisolone to treat status asthmaticus. Corticosteroid use may increase the risk of what condition for the patient?
   a. Pulmonary infection
   b. Bronchospasm
   c. Pulmonary edema
   d. Bronchoconstriction

16. A female patient is diagnosed with adrenal insufficiency. She presents to the emergency department with hypotension. What would the nurse expect the physician to prescribe?
   a. Vasopressors
   b. Corticosteroids
   c. ACE inhibitors
   d. Beta-blockers

17. A patient who receives long-term corticosteroid therapy is at risk for the development of which conditions? (Select all that apply.)
   a. Diabetes mellitus
   b. Rheumatoid arthritis
   c. Peptic ulcer disease
   d. Tuberculosis
   e. COPD

18. A 45-year-old woman has been taking a corticosteroid and calls the clinic complaining of the development of acne-like lesion on her face as well as facial hair. What is the nurse's best response?
   a. "Stop taking the drug immediately."
   b. "If you shave it regularly, no one will notice."
   c. "Sadly, this is an adverse effect seen in women. It should improve when you finish the medication."
   d. "This is a permanent problem. You will need to schedule electrolysis treatments."

19. The use of corticosteroids in older adults may aggravate which conditions? (Select all that apply.)
   a. Congestive heart failure
   b. Gout
   c. Diabetes mellitus
   d. Arthritis
   e. Contact dermatitis

20. The nurse is caring for a patient who has just returned to the unit after having a craniotomy. What drug does the nurse anticipate that the physician will order for this patient?
   a. IV dexamethasone
   b. IM dexamethasone
   c. PO prednisone
   d. IV hydrocortisone

16

CHAPTER

Drug Therapy With Beta-Lactam Antibacterial Agents

Learning Objectives

- Describe the general characteristics of beta-lactam antibiotics.
- Discuss penicillins in relation to effectiveness, safety, spectrum of antibacterial activity, mechanism of action, indications for use, administration, observation of patient response, and teaching of patients.
- Recognize the importance of questioning patients about allergies before the initial dose of all drugs, especially penicillins.
- Describe characteristics of beta-lactamase inhibitor drugs.
- Give the rationale for combining a penicillin and a beta-lactamase inhibitor drug.
- Discuss the cephalosporins in relation to effectiveness, safety, spectrum of antibacterial activity, mechanism of action, indications for use, administration, observation of patient response, and teaching of patients.
- Discuss the carbapenems in relation to effectiveness, safety, spectrum of antibacterial activity, mechanism of action, indications for use, administration, observation of patient response, and teaching of patients.
- Discuss the one monobactam drug in relation to effectiveness, safety, spectrum of antibacterial activity, mechanism of action, indications

for use, administration, observation of patient response, and teaching of patients.
- Use the nursing process in the care of patients receiving beta-lactam antibacterials.

SECTION I: ASSESSING YOUR UNDERSTANDING

Activity A   FILL IN THE BLANKS

1. When _____ was introduced, it was effective against many organisms; it had to be given parenterally because it was destroyed by gastric acid; and injections were painful.

2. As a class, _____ usually are more effective in infections caused by gram-positive bacteria than in those caused by gram-negative bacteria.

3. Allergy to a drug of another class with similar chemical structure is called _____.

4. _____, _____, and _____ are the drugs of choice for methicillin-susceptible *Staphylococcus aureus*.

5. _____, _____, and _____ have a broad spectrum of antimicrobial activity, especially against gram-negative organisms such as *Pseudomonas* and *Proteus* species and *Escherichia coli*.

64

Activity B MATCHING

Match the term in Column A with the definition in Column B.

Column A	Column B
___ **1.** Augmentin	**a.** Combination of ampicillin and sulbactam
___ **2.** Unasyn	
___ **3.** Carbapenems	**b.** Broad-spectrum, bactericidal, beta-lactam antimicrobials
___ **4.** Cephalosporins	
___ **5.** Meropenem (Merrem)	**c.** Widely used group of drugs that are derived from a fungus
	d. Contains amoxicillin and clavulanate
	e. Has a broad spectrum of antibacterial activity and may be used as a single drug for empiric therapy before causative microorganisms are identified

Activity C SHORT ANSWERS

Briefly answer the following questions.

1. How should the dose of penicillins be modified if a patient is on hemodialysis?

2. What impact does Augmentin have on the liver? Should it be used in patients with hepatic disease?

3. What is the role of the home care nurse when the patient receives beta-lactam antibiotics?

4. What metabolic and electrolyte imbalances may occur in patients receiving penicillins who have renal impairment or congestive heart failure?

5. When are beta-lactam antimicrobials commonly used?

SECTION II: APPLYING YOUR KNOWLEDGE

Activity D CASE STUDIES

Consider the scenarios and answer the questions.

Case Study 1

Mrs. Spades developed an intra-abdominal infection after hernia surgery. She presents to the physician's office with a temperature of 102.4 orally, BP 180/78, AP 97 regular, and respirations 32. Her skin is cold and clammy, and pallor of the skin is evident. The physician orders hospitalization to manage the infectious process. Initial orders include a course of ertapenem IM.

1. After collecting the patient's history, you discover that the patient's current medical diagnoses include asthma and a seizure disorder; her allergies include prednisone and sulfonamides. Why would you need to call the physician prior to medication administration?

2. The physician confirms the order for ertapenem. What kind of preparation does this medication need before administration? If Mrs. Spade's culture results include the bacteria *Pseudomonas aeruginosa*, what would you expect the physician to do with the ertapenem order?

Case Study 2

Mrs. Spade is now going home. You are responsible for her discharge teaching. One of her discharge medications is aztreonam.

1. Mrs. Spade asks you if she might take the penicillin that she has instead of the aztreonam, because it is cheaper. What is an appropriate response?

2. Mrs. Spade's daughter is a nurse and states that in her experience aminoglycosides are just as effective for her mother's infectious processes. How would you respond?

SECTION III: PRACTICING FOR NCLEX

Activity E

Answer the following questions.

1. Which medication blocks renal excretion of the penicillins and can be given concurrently with penicillins to increase serum drug levels?

   a. Probenecid (Benemid)

   b. Piperacillin–tazobactam

   c. Augmentin

   d. Gentamicin

2. In the rare instance in which penicillin is considered essential, which procedure may be helpful in assessing hypersensitivity?

   a. Administering the medication in a controlled environment

   b. Administering a loading dose of the medication

   c. Administering a skin test

   d. Administering the medication by the intravenous route only

3. As a class, penicillins usually are more effective in infections caused by which type of bacteria?

   a. Gram-negative

   b. Gram-positive

   c. Anaerobic

   d. Aerobic

4. Choice of a beta-lactam antibacterial depends on which factors? (Select all that apply.)

   a. The organism causing the infection

   b. Severity of the infection

   c. Age of the patient

   d. Sex of the patient

   e. Other coexisting illnesses

5. Which classifications of antibacterials are considered beta-lactam antibiotics? (Select all that apply.)

   a. Penicillins

   b. Cephalosporins

   c. Monobactams

   d. Sulfonamides

   e. Fluoroquinolones

6. A female patient is admitted to the critical care unit with sepsis related to a contaminated central line. The physician orders intravenous beta-lactam antimicrobials. The patient's current laboratory report reflects renal impairment. What would the nurse expect the physician to do?

   a. Maintain the drug dose

   b. Increase the drug dose

   c. Decrease the drug dose

   d. Administer the drug via an intramuscular route

7. Why are the beta-lactam drugs frequently given concomitantly with other antimicrobial drugs in critically ill patients.

   a. They often have drug-resistant organisms.

   b. Their immune systems are impaired.

   c. They are susceptible to drug-resistant organisms.

   d. They often have multiorganism or nosocomial infections.

8. A male patient is placed on an IV regimen of aztreonam. The nurse would expect the physician to order which laboratory test?

   a. CBC

   b. Hematocrit

   c. Serum albumin

   d. Liver function

9. A female patient is hospitalized for sepsis. She also receives hemodialysis three times a week. How much of the initial dose of monobactam should be administered after each hemodialysis session, in addition to the maintenance doses?

   a. 12.5%

   b. 25%

   c. 10%

   d. 50%

10. A male patient received the initial loading dose of aztreonam this morning. The nurse receives his laboratory results, and his CrCl is 28 mL/min. The nurse calls the physician regarding the laboratory results. What would the nurse expect the physician to order?

    a. Increase the dose of aztreonam

    b. Decrease the dose of aztreonam by 50%

    c. Maintain the current dose of aztreonam

    d. Discontinue the aztreonam

11. Unless hemodialysis is started within 48 hours, imipenem is contraindicated for patients with severe renal impairment. What laboratory measurement would indicate renal impairment?

    a. Hematocrit

    b. White blood count

    c. Serum albumin

    d. Creatinine clearance

12. Penicillins and cephalosporins are used cautiously in neonates due to what factor?

    a. Immature liver function

    b. Immature immune function

    c. Immature kidney function

    d. Immature pancreatic function

13. A male patient is admitted to the unit for a total hip replacement. The surgeon orders a first-generation cephalosporin as a surgical prophylaxis because of what type of bacteria commonly associated with this type of procedure?

    a. Gram-negative

    b. Anaerobic

    c. Gram-positive

    d. Aerobic

14. A male patient is admitted to the unit with *Pseudomonas aeruginosa* sepsis. The physician orders aminoglycoside to be given concomitantly with penicillin intravenously. How would the nurse administer these drugs?

    a. By mixing both drugs in normal saline solution

    b. By administering the drug in separate IV bags

    c. By administering the drugs dextrose 5% and 0.9% normal saline

    d. By administering the drugs every other day

15. Prior to administration of the first dose of ampicillin, the nurse questions the patient about her drug history. What condition that developed with a previous dose of this medication would contraindicate the use of it again?

    a. Vaginal yeast infection

    b. Cholestatic jaundice

    c. Nausea

    d. Diarrhea

16. A female patient demonstrates symptoms of shock after a single intravenous dose of penicillin. What interventions are most necessary at this time? (Select all that apply.)

    a. Epinephrine

    b. A tongue blade

    c. Oxygen

    d. Tracheostomy

    e. Nasogastric tube

17. The nurse is observing a graduate nurse administering medications. The other nurse would intervene if the graduate nurse attempted to give what medication intravenously?

    a. Ampicillin

    b. Oxacillin

    c. Penicillin G benzathine

    d. Ampicillin–sulbactam

18. The nurse would prepare for what type of adverse effect in a patient receiving imipenem–cilastatin who has a creatinine clearance ≤20 mL/min?

    a. Elevated liver function tests

    b. Seizure activity

    c. Rash

    d. Respiratory distress

19. The nurse is administering cefazolin to a patient. What adverse effects are most important in providing care for this patient? (Select all that apply.)

    a. Diarrhea

    b. Vomiting

    c. Vaginal yeast infection

    d. Gastritis

    e. Rash and facial edema

20. A patient with sepsis is reading material given to him on the drug imipenem. He asks the nurse why it is formulated with cilastatin and cannot be taken alone. What is the nurse's most appropriate response?

    a. "Cilastatin prevents destruction of imipenem by an enzyme created by the renal tubules."

    b. "Cilastatin is a preservative and prevents the destruction of the imipenem in the gastrointestinal tract."

    c. "Cilastatin helps the imipenem to cross the blood–brain barrier."

    d. "Cilastatin prevents the destruction of the imipenem in the liver."

17 CHAPTER

Drug Therapy With Aminoglycosides and Fluoroquinolones

Learning Objectives

- State the rationale for the increasing use of single daily doses of aminoglycosides.
- Discuss the importance of measuring serum drug levels during aminoglycoside therapy.
- Describe measures to decrease nephrotoxicity and ototoxicity with aminoglycosides.
- Identify characteristics of aminoglycosides and fluoroquinolones in relation to effectiveness, safety, spectrum of antimicrobial activity, indications for use, administration, and observation of patient responses.
- Recognize factors influencing selection and dosage of aminoglycosides and fluoroquinolones.
- Describe the characteristics, uses, adverse effects, and nursing process implications of fluoroquinolones.
- Discuss principles of using aminoglycosides and fluoroquinolones in renal impairment and critical illness.

SECTION I: ASSESSING YOUR UNDERSTANDING

Activity A FILL IN THE BLANKS

1. The _____ have been widely used to treat serious gram-negative infections for many years.

2. The _____ are older drugs originally used only for treatment of urinary tract infections.

3. The _____ are synthesized by adding a fluorine molecule to the quinolone structure.

4. Aminoglycosides are _____ agents with similar pharmacologic, antimicrobial, and toxicologic characteristics.

5. After _____ administration, aminoglycosides are widely distributed in extracellular fluid and reach therapeutic levels in blood, urine, bone, inflamed joints, and pleural and ascitic fluids.

Activity B MATCHING

Match the term in Column A with the definition in Column B.

Column A	Column B
___ **1.** Neomycin and kanamycin	**a.** Has been associated with hypoglycemic and hyperglycemic events more commonly than other fluoroquinolones
___ **2.** Gatifloxacin	
___ **3.** Moxifloxacin	**b.** May be given to suppress intestinal bacteria before bowel surgery and to treat hepatic coma

68

_____ **4.** Kanamycin

_____ **5.** Neomycin

    c. Is not recommended for urinary tract infections

    d. Is not recommended for use in infants and children

    e. Is associated with increased risk for ototoxicity in older adults

Activity C SHORT ANSWERS

Briefly answer the following questions.

1. The fluoroquinolones are synthesized by adding a fluorine molecule to the quinolone structure. Explain how this addition changes the drug activity of this antibiotic.

2. Give examples of the microorganisms that aminoglycosides are used to treat.

3. Explain how aminoglycosides are absorbed, including IV peaks.

4. After parenteral administration, aminoglycosides are widely distributed throughout the body. Discuss the areas in the body where aminoglycosides are accumulated and the impact on body systems.

5. Where are aminoglycosides excreted in the body?

SECTION II: APPLYING YOUR KNOWLEDGE

Activity D CASE STUDY

Consider the scenario and answer the questions.

While hospitalized for multiple trauma associated with a motor vehicle accident, Ms. Blanchard develops nosocomial pneumonia. She required surgery for fractures and serious internal injuries. You are the primary nurse assigned to Ms. Blanchard's case.

1. What is the cause of most nosocomial respiratory infections?

2. What part of Ms. Blanchard's current condition or situation puts her at risk for nosocomial infection?

3. Based on a sputum culture positive for *Pseudomonas*, the physician orders an aminoglycoside concurrently with piperacillin. Why do you think the physician ordered this combination of medications? What therapeutic effect does the combination have, and what is its target?

4. Ms. Blanchard fears that the pneumonia will cause her death because her body's reserves are limited. What effect is this combination antibiotic therapy expected to have on the patient's prognosis? If Ms. Blanchard's infection was not related to *Pseudomonas*, but to another gram-negative infection, what effect might this combination therapy have?

SECTION III: PRACTICING FOR NCLEX

Activity E

Answer the following questions.

1. A 75-year-old male patient is diagnosed with an infection. He is currently being treated for type 2 diabetes, hypertension, benign prostatic hypertrophy, and chronic congestive heart failure. If the physician orders a fluoroquinolone to treat the infection, the nurse understands that what adverse effects can occur in this patient?

    a. Hypoglycemia and hyperglycemia

    b. Atrial fibrillation

    c. Exacerbation of congestive heart failure

    d. Hypertensive crisis

2. A male patient is prescribed aminoglycosides for a bladder infection secondary to benign prostatic hypertrophy. The nurse understands that these drugs reach higher concentrations in which areas of the body? (Select all that apply.)

    a. Kidneys

    b. Inner ears

    c. Pericardium

    d. Peritoneum

    e. Central nervous system

3. A male patient develops a wound infection, and the physician orders once-daily intravenous multiple-dose regimens of aminoglycosides. What kinds of monitoring does the nurse expect the physician to order?

a. Peak and trough serum levels

b. A complete blood count every 48 hours

c. A serum albumin determination every 48 hours

d. Measurement of electrolytes every 48 hours

4. A patient with a severe infection has an order for IV gentamicin and IV penicillin. How will the nurse administer these medications?

a. Mix the two antibiotics in one syringe and push it slowly over 5 minutes.

b. Mix both antibiotics in an IV piggyback and administer over 1 hour.

c. Administer the gentamicin IV and wait 1 hour and administer the penicillin.

d. Administer the penicillin and immediately administer the gentamicin.

5. What symptom should the nurse expect to find if the patient begins to exhibit signs of ototoxicity?

a. Fatigue

b. Anorexia

c. Tinnitus

d. Rash

6. Before the selection of an aminoglycoside to treat a patient's wound infection, what would the nurse expect the physician to order?

a. White blood count

b. Electrolyte panel

c. Complete blood count

d. Culture and sensitivity

7. A male patient is concerned that he cannot afford to have his wife's community-acquired pneumonia (CAP) treated in the hospital. He has limited health insurance, and the cost of intravenous antibiotic therapy is prohibitive. According to the American College of Chest Physicians' position statement, where will the patient's wife be treated?

a. In the hospital using intravenous therapy

b. In the home using oral drugs

c. In the hospital using oral medications

d. In the home using intravenous therapy

8. An 80-year-old patient is a type 2 diabetic whose condition is controlled by glyburide. The patient develops an infection, and the physician orders fluoroquinolones as a treatment. With this combination of medications, the nurse understands that what adverse effect may occur with the patient?

a. Hyperglycemia

b. Diabetic ketoacidosis

c. Severe hypoglycemia

d. Diabetic shock

9. The physician orders gatifloxacin for a patient with type 2 diabetes mellitus. The nurse understands that this drug may cause which adverse effect in this patient?

a. Hyperglycemia

b. Diabetic ketoacidosis

c. Severe hypoglycemia

d. Diabetic shock

10. A male patient is NPO as a consequence of a cerebrovascular accident sustained 3 years ago. His care is managed at home by his wife, and he receives all medications via gastrostomy tube. The physician orders a fluoroquinolone for the patient to treat an infection. The nurse would instruct the patient's wife to administer the medication in what way?

a. With the enteral feeding

b. On a full stomach

c. With antacids

d. On an empty stomach

11. A patient in the critical care unit is receiving aminoglycosides for an infectious process. What does the nurse need to monitor?

a. Complete blood count

b. Liver function tests

c. Serum albumin concentration

d. White blood count

12. The nurse would contact the physician if ciprofloxacin was prescribed for which patient diagnosed with a urinary tract infection?

a. A 13-year-old patient

b. A 25-year-old patient

c. A 44-year-old patient

d. A 65-year-old patient

13. A 72-year-old patient has been prescribed ciprofloxacin. What instruction for home care has the highest priority?
    a. Take this medication with food.
    b. Take this medication on an empty stomach.
    c. Take this medication with an antacid.
    d. Take this medication with extra fluid.

14. The physician orders an aminoglycoside for a ventilator-dependent patient who is admitted to the critical care unit. His current diagnoses include respiratory arrest, type 2 diabetes, hepatitis C, and chronic obstructive pulmonary disease. Which statement indicates the risk of using this class of medication in this patient?
    a. Risk for hepatic impairment is significant, because the drug is metabolized in the liver.
    b. Risk for hepatic impairment is significant because of a higher risk for toxicity.
    c. Risk for hepatic impairment is not significant, because the drug is excreted through the kidneys.
    d. Risk for hypertensive crisis is increased.

15. What renal effects may occur in patients treated with fluoroquinolones? (Select all that apply.)
    a. Glycosuria
    b. Azotemia
    c. Crystalluria
    d. Hematuria
    e. Pyuria

16. The patient is receiving IV gentamicin for an infection. The physician orders a peak and trough level. When should the nurse order the trough level to be drawn?
    a. 1 hour before the 8 AM dose of medication is infused
    b. Immediately before the 8 AM dose of medication is infused
    c. Immediately after the 8 AM dose of medication is infused
    d. 1 hour after the 8 AM dose of medication is infused

17. Aminoglycosides must be used cautiously in children as in adults. Dosage must be accurately calculated according to which factors?
    a. Weight and renal function
    b. Height and weight
    c. Age and weight
    d. Weight and leukocytosis

18. Why must a patient who is receiving aminoglycosides be kept well hydrated?
    a. Hydration increases drug concentration in serum and body tissues.
    b. Hydration decreases drug concentration in serum and body tissues.
    c. Hydration stabilizes peak serum levels.
    d. Hydration stabilizes trough serum levels.

19. The nurse is caring for a patient who is receiving IV gentamicin and knows that the patient should not receive what medication at the same time because it may mask symptoms of ototoxicity?
    a. Penicillin
    b. Morphine sulfate
    c. Diphenhydramine
    d. Diazepam

20. The nurse instructs the patient who is taking oral ciprofloxacin to avoid which food while taking this medication?
    a. Hamburger
    b. Chicken
    c. Cheese
    d. Tuna

18

Drug Therapy With Tetracyclines, Sulfonamides, and Urinary Antiseptics

Learning Objectives

- Identify the prototype and describe the characteristics, action, use, adverse effects, contraindications, and nursing implications of the tetracyclines.
- Identify the prototype and describe the characteristics, action, use, adverse effects, contraindications, and nursing implications of the sulfonamides.
- Identify the prototype and describe the action, use, adverse effects, contraindications, and nursing implications for the adjuvant urinary antiseptic agents used in the treatment of urinary tract infections.
- Implement the nursing process in the care of patients being treated with tetracyclines, sulfonamides, or urinary antiseptics.

SECTION I: ASSESSING YOUR UNDERSTANDING

Activity A   FILL IN THE BLANKS

1. Urinary _____ are used only in urinary tract infections (UTI).

2. Urinary antiseptics may be bactericidal for sensitive organisms in the urinary tract because these drugs are concentrated in _____ and reach high levels in urine.

3. Tetracyclines penetrate microbial cells by _____ diffusion and an active transport system.

4. All tetracyclines (except doxycycline) and sulfonamides are contraindicated in patients with _____.

5. Tetracyclines decompose with _____ , exposure to light, and extreme heat and humidity.

Activity B   MATCHING

Match the term in Column A with the definition in Column B.

Column A	Column B
____ 1. Tetracyclines and sulfonamides	a. Older, broad-spectrum, bacteriostatic drugs; rarely used for systemic infections because of microbial resistance and development of more effective or less toxic drugs
____ 2. Tetracyclines	
____ 3. Doxycycline (Vibramycin)	
	b. Useful in the treatment of bronchitis

Column A	Column B
____ **4.** Trimethoprim–sulfamethoxazole (Bactrim, Septra)	**c.** Still used to treat bacterial infections caused by *Brucella* and *Vibrio cholerae*
____ **5.** Phenazopyridine (Pyridium)	**d.** One of the drugs of choice for *Bacillus anthracis* (anthrax) and *Chlamydia trachomatis*
	e. Given to relieve pain associated with UTI

Activity C SHORT ANSWERS

Briefly answer the following questions.

1. Name two organisms/disease processes that are still treated with tetracyclines.

2. Explain how tetracyclines are excreted.

3. Name two organisms or disease processes in which sulfonamides may be an effective treatment.

4. Describe the mechanism of action used by tetracyclines.

5. For what types of UTIs are sulfonamides prescribed?

SECTION II: APPLYING YOUR KNOWLEDGE

Activity D CASE STUDY

Consider the scenario and answer the questions.

Mrs. Banks calls the physician's office with symptoms of burning on urination, left flank pain, and urinary frequency. The physician asks you to make an appointment for Mrs. Banks for an assessment. You are responsible for Mrs. Banks' medication education and treatment plan.

1. Mrs. Banks asks if the physician can just call in a prescription for her. How would you respond? Why are urine cultures and susceptibility tests needed?

2. Mrs. Banks is diagnosed with a urinary tract infection that is susceptible to sulfonamides. The physician prescribes a loading dose before the maintenance dose. What can you tell the patient about a loading dose?

3. Why is the urine pH important in drug therapy? Is alkalinization needed for this patient?

SECTION III: PRACTICING FOR NCLEX

Activity E

Answer the following questions.

1. Urinary antiseptics may be bactericidal for sensitive organisms in the urinary tract because these drugs are concentrated in what structure?

   a. Renal tubules

   b. Bladder

   c. Nephrons

   d. Renal calculi

2. Urinary antiseptics are not used in systemic infections, for what reason?

   a. They do not sustain therapeutic plasma levels.

   b. They do not attain therapeutic plasma levels.

   c. They are not effective against systemic infections in general.

   d. They attain therapeutic blood levels rapidly.

3. Sulfasalazine (Azulfidine) is contraindicated in people who are allergic to what?

   a. Salicylates

   b. Diuretics

   c. Nonopioid analgesics

   d. NSAIDs

4. Sulfonamides are bacteriostatic against a wide range of gram-positive and gram-negative bacteria, but they are becoming less useful, for what reason?

   a. Decreased resistance

   b. Increased susceptibility

   c. Intermittent resistance

   d. Increasing resistance

5. The tetracyclines are effective against a wide range of which type of organisms?

   a. Gram-positive organisms

   b. Gram-negative organisms

   c. Gram-positive and gram-negative organisms

   d. Beta-lactamase–positive organisms

6. A male patient presents to the emergency department in pain. He is diagnosed with mild to moderate burns on his forearms secondary to exposure to hot pipes in his home. The nurse expects the physician to order what topical medication?

   a. Penicillin

   b. Amoxicillin

   c. Tetracycline

   d. Sulfadiazine

7. What is the recommended medication for the treatment of choice for *Pneumocystis jiroveci* pneumonia?

   a. Trimethoprim–sulfamethoxazole

   b. Tetracycline

   c. Amoxicillin

   d. Sulfadiazine

8. The nurse is giving discharge instructions to a woman who has been prescribed tetracycline and also uses oral contraceptives. What is the most important instruction the nurse will give to this patient?

   a. "Your period will be heavier while you are taking tetracycline."

   b. "You should use alternative means of contraception while you are taking tetracycline."

   c. "You will need to take your oral contraceptive in the morning while taking tetracycline."

   d. "You must take an antacid to prevent gastric erosion from the combination of the two medications."

9. Tetracyclines are generally contraindicated in pregnant women because of what effects? (Select all that apply.)

   a. Cause fatal hepatic necrosis in the mother

   b. Cause renal impairment in the mother

   c. Cause renal impairment in the fetus

   d. Interfere with bone and tooth development in the fetus

   e. Decrease brain development in the fetus

10. A female patient is diagnosed with hepatitis C as well as a urinary tract infection. The organism is sensitive to tetracycline. Why is the physician reluctant to order tetracycline in a patient with hepatic impairment?

   a. It slows drug elimination.

   b. It increases drug elimination.

   c. It causes intermittent drug elimination.

   d. It eliminates absorption of the medication.

11. In patients with renal impairment, which IV dose of tetracycline has been associated with death from liver failure?

   a. Greater than 1.5 g/d

   b. Greater than 2 g/d

   c. Greater than 3 g/d

   d. Less than 5 g/d

12. The nurse is aware that a patient with renal failure should not be prescribed tetracycline for which reasons? (Select all that apply.)

   a. Development of azotemia

   b. Decreased blood urea nitrogen (BUN)

   c. Hypophosphatemia

   d. Hyperkalemia

   e. Acidosis

13. The nurse would recommend that a patient who is taking tetracycline should have fluid intake of how many liters of fluid?

   a. 1 L

   b. 2 L

   c. 3 L

   d. 4 L

14. The nurse is preparing to administer an infusion of trimethoprim–sulfamethoxazole. The nurse understands that this medication must be mixed with what IV fluid?

   a. 0.9% saline

   b. 5% dextrose and lactated Ringer's

   c. 5% dextrose and 0.9% saline

   d. 5% dextrose and water

15. The nurse is caring for a patient who has an indwelling Foley catheter. What nursing interventions will help prevent a urinary tract infection in this patient? (Select all that apply.)
    a. Disconnect the catheter system to drain the urine from the drainage bag.
    b. Keep the urinary drainage bag below the level of the patient's bladder.
    c. Perform perineal care frequently.
    d. Irrigate the Foley catheter three times a day.
    e. Leave the catheter in for at least 3 weeks.

16. Tetracyclines should not be used in children younger than 8 years of age because of their effects on what?
    a. Teeth and bones
    b. Kidneys
    c. Blood
    d. Liver

17. If a fetus or young infant receives a sulfonamide by placental transfer, in breast milk, or by direct administration, the drug displaces bilirubin from binding sites on albumin. As a result, what may the fetus experience?
    a. Hyperbilirubinemia
    b. Hyperkalemia
    c. Hypernatremia
    d. Kernicterus

18. The nurse is caring for a patient with ulcerative colitis who is taking sulfasalazine. What instruction will the nurse give this patient?
    a. "Expect burning during urination."
    b. "Expect your urine to turn yellow-orange."
    c. "Expect to be constipated."
    d. "Expect to have insomnia."

19. Sulfonamides are often used to treat UTI in children older than what age?
    a. 6 months
    b. 4 months
    c. 2 months
    d. 12 months

20. Tetracyclines must be used cautiously in the presence of what condition?
    a. Cerebral vascular accident
    b. Liver impairment
    c. Cardiovascular disease
    d. Kidney impairment

19

Drug Therapy With Macrolides, Ketolides, and Miscellaneous Anti-Infective Agents

Learning Objectives

- Describe the characteristics and specific uses of macrolide and ketolide anti-infective agents.
- Identify the prototype and describe the action, use, adverse effects, contraindications, and nursing implications of macrolides.
- Identify the prototype and describe the action, use, adverse effects, contraindications, and nursing implications of ketolides.
- Describe the action, use, adverse effects, contraindications, and nursing implications of miscellaneous anti-infective agents.
- Implement the nursing process in the care of patients being treated with macrolides, ketolides, and other miscellaneous anti-infective agents.

SECTION I: ASSESSING YOUR UNDERSTANDING

Activity A FILL IN THE BLANKS

1. Macrolides are widely distributed into body tissues and fluids and may be _____ or bactericidal, depending on drug concentration in infected tissues.

2. *Mycobacterium avium* complex (MAC) disease is an opportunistic infection that occurs mainly in people with advanced _____ _____ _____ infection.

3. *Helicobacter pylori*, a pathogen implicated in peptic ulcer disease, is treated by _____ or clarithromycin as part of a combination regimen.

4. Telithromycin is excreted by the _____ and kidneys.

5. The macrolides and ketolides enter microbial cells and reversibly bind to the 50S subunits of _____, thereby inhibiting microbial protein synthesis.

Activity B MATCHING

Match the term in Column A with the definition in Column B.

Column A

_____ **1.** Telithromycin (Ketek)

_____ **2.** Chloramphenicol (Chloromycetin)

_____ **3.** Clindamycin (Cleocin)

_____ **4.** Daptomycin (Cubicin)

_____ **5.** Tigecycline (Tygacil)

Column B

a. Broad-spectrum, bacteriostatic antibiotic, active against most gram-positive and gram-negative bacteria, rickettsiae, chlamydiae, and treponemes

b. A lincosamide, similar to the macrolides in its mechanism of action and antimicrobial spectrum

c. The first member of the ketolide class

d. A member of the glycylcycline class, currently the only member in its class

e. Belongs to the lipopeptide class, a new class of antibiotics

Activity C SHORT ANSWERS

Briefly answer the following questions.

1. Discuss how erythromycin is metabolized and excreted in the body. Does food have an effect on the absorption of erythromycin?

2. What is the mechanism of action of macrolides and ketolides?

3. Identify two contraindications related to the administration of macrolides and ketolides.

4. What are the clinical indications for the use of metronidazole?

5. Name two categories of drugs that should not be administered with quinupristin–dalfopristin. Explain how quinupristin–dalfopristin interferes with the identified medication's absorption.

SECTION II: APPLYING YOUR KNOWLEDGE

Activity D CASE STUDY

Consider the scenario and answer the questions.

Mr. Gresham presents to physician's office with chest pain and shortness of breath. He is taking his second course of antibiotics for pneumonia. The physician orders sputum for culture and sensitivity. The sputum culture results indicate that Mr. Gresham has methicillin-resistant *Staphylococcus aureus* pneumonia. Mr. Gresham is hospitalized and IV vancomycin is ordered.

1. Vancomycin is effective against MRSA. What is the mechanism of action of the drug?

2. Mr. Gresham develops antibiotic-induced diarrhea (*Clostridium difficile*) secondary to the use of the antibiotics prior to his diagnosis of MRSA pneumonia. He states that the vancomycin he is receiving should also treat the *C. difficile*. What information can you give Mr. Gresham? What medication would you expect the physician to order for the initial treatment of Mr. Gresham's *C. difficile*?

3. Discuss the limitations to the use of vancomycin.

4. During the second dose of parenteral vancomycin, Mr. Gresham develops "red man syndrome." What is the syndrome attributed to?

5. If Mr. Gresham were to develop kidney impairment during his hospitalization, what do you expect would happen to his vancomycin dose?

SECTION III: PRACTICING FOR NCLEX

Activity E

Answer the following questions.

1. A male patient presents to the emergency department with an abdominal dehiscence. He states he had a hernia repair 18 days earlier, and the physician removed his wound staples 5 days ago. The patient states that the dehiscence occurred when he lifted a box this morning for his wife. The wound is red, and there is evidence of foul-smelling drainage.

The wound is cultured, and an anaerobic bacterium is identified. The nurse understands that the physician orders metronidazole because it is effective against which type of organism?

a. All gram-positive bacteria

b. All gram-negative bacteria

c. *Staphylococcus*

d. Anaerobic bacteria

2. A female patient is noncompliant with the medication treatment plan for her gonococcal infection. She failed to complete the second course of antibiotics because she felt better after 5 days and states that she experienced unpleasant side effects. The nurse would expect the physician to order medication education and which drug?

a. Spectinomycin

b. Streptomycin

c. Erythromycin

d. Zithromax

3. A patient returns from a vacation with traveler's diarrhea. The nurse understands that what is the treatment of choice?

a. Robaxin

b. Rifaximin

c. Rifampin

d. Relafen

4. A patient has been prescribed metronidazole for treatment of *Giardia*. What instruction is most important for the nurse to give to this patient?

a. Do not smoke while taking this medication.

b. Do not drink alcohol while taking this medication.

c. Do not use sun screen products while taking this medication.

d. Do not eat sugary foods while taking this medication.

5. A patient who underwent abdominal surgery 6 weeks ago is diagnosed with VREF. The nurse expects the physician to order which medication?

a. Vancomycin

b. Rifampin

c. Quinupristin–dalfopristin

d. Rifaximin

6. A patient presents to the physician's office with a skin infection on her forearm. The infection is resistant to over-the-counter antibiotics. After receiving the culture and sensitivity results, the physician orders tigecycline. The nurse knows that this patient has what illness?

a. *Clostridium difficile*

b. VRE

c. MRSA

d. VREF

7. Daptomycin belongs to the lipopeptide class of antibiotics that kills gram-positive bacteria. What is the mechanism of action for this antibiotic?

a. Inhibition of synthesis of bacterial proteins

b. Inhibition of synthesis of DNA only

c. Inhibition of mitochondrial reproduction

d. Inhibition of cell wall osmosis

8. A patient is taking clindamycin for an infectious process and presents to the physician's office with symptoms of dehydration. The nurse understands that the patient is experiencing what adverse reaction from the administration of clindamycin?

a. Diuresis

b. Diaphoresis

c. Dysphasia

d. Diarrhea

9. A patient is diagnosed with VRE, and the physician orders chloramphenicol. The nurse should monitor the patient for the development of which side effect?

a. Dizziness

b. Blood dyscrasias

c. Nausea

d. Vomiting

10. A patient is diagnosed with myasthenia gravis and develops an infectious process that is sensitive to telithromycin. Telithromycin is contraindicated for the patient because of the risk of which condition?

a. Respiratory failure

b. Congestive heart failure

c. Myocardial infarct

d. Renal failure

11. A patient has been prescribed daptomycin for treatment of an infection. What instruction is most important for the nurse to tell this patient?

a. "Tell the physician immediately if you develop any muscle pain."

b. "Expect that this medication may cause bloody diarrhea."

c. "Take a laxative everyday to prevent becoming constipated."

d. "Maintain a clear liquid diet while on the medication to prevent nausea."

12. A patient is diagnosed with community-acquired pneumonia, and the physician orders telithromycin. What is the mechanism of action for this antibiotic?

a. Inhibition of microbial cell wall synthesis

b. Destruction of the microbial cell wall

c. Prevention of osmosis within the microbial cell

d. Inhibition of microbial protein synthesis

13. A patient is diagnosed with an infectious process that is sensitive to penicillin. The patient is allergic to penicillin, so the physician orders a drug with a similar antibacterial spectrum. The nurse anticipates that the physician will order what antibiotic?

a. Streptomycin

b. Erythromycin

c. Vancomycin

d. Dicloxacillin

14. A patient is diagnosed with acute bacterial sinusitis, and the physician orders azithromycin. How long a course of this drug does the nurse expect the physician to order?

a. 5 days

b. 10 days

c. 7 days

d. 3 days

15. A patient is given linezolid for a diagnosis of VREF. The drug will be administered for a period that extends beyond 2 weeks. Which laboratory test would the nurse expect the physician to order on a regular basis because of the length of administration of the drug?

a. Electrolytes

b. Complete blood count

c. Potassium

d. Serum albumin

16. A male patient is taking digoxin, SSRIs, and aspirin as part of his daily drug regimen. A patient with this drug history who is also receiving linezolid would be at risk for what serious complication?

a. Serotonin syndrome

b. Diabetes type 2

c. Congestive heart failure

d. Renal failure

17. Because linezolid is a weak monoamine oxidase (MAO) inhibitor, patients should avoid foods high in tyramine content, such as what foods? (Select all that apply.)

a. Aged cheeses

b. Milk

c. Red wine

d. Tap beers

e. Chicken

18. A female patient's medical history includes type 2 diabetes, CVA, dysphasia, and chronic renal failure. She develops an infectious process. The physician orders erythromycin. Based on the patient's medical history, why is erythromycin the drug of choice?

a. It is metabolized in the liver.

b. It is metabolized in the kidneys.

c. It is excreted into the bloodstream.

d. It is excreted into the GI tract.

19. The nurse is caring for a patient who is receiving IV vancomycin. The nurse infuses the medication at the prescribed rate to prevent what from occurring?

a. Gray syndrome

b. Red man syndrome

c. Serotonin syndrome

d. Cushing's syndrome

20. The nurse is caring for a patient who is receiving chloramphenicol. The nurse will assess this patient for what potential adverse effect?

a. Ototoxicity

b. Neurotoxicity

c. Blood dyscrasia

d. Hepatic dysfunctions

20

Drug Therapy for Tuberculosis and *Mycobacterium avium* Complex Disease

Learning Objectives

■ Describe the etiology and pathophysiology of tuberculosis and *Mycobacterium avium* complex.

■ Describe the characteristics of latent, active, and drug-resistant tuberculosis infections.

■ Describe drug therapy for tuberculosis, including the rationale for multiple-drug therapy.

■ List the action, uses, adverse effects, and nursing implications of first-line antitubercular drugs.

■ Describe how second-line antitubercular drugs are added to drug regimens to treat multidrug-resistant tuberculosis.

■ Describe the drugs used to prevent or treat *Mycobacterium avium* complex.

■ Discuss ways to increase adherence to antitubercular drug therapy regimens.

■ Understand how to implement the nursing process in the care of patients undergoing drug therapy for tuberculosis.

SECTION I: ASSESSING YOUR UNDERSTANDING

Activity A   FILL IN THE BLANKS

1. Tuberculosis (TB) is an infectious disease that usually affects the lungs but may affect lymph nodes, pleurae, bones, joints, _____, and the gastrointestinal tract.

2. Tuberculosis is caused by _____ _____, the tubercle bacillus.

3. In general, the tubercle bacilli multiply slowly; they may lie dormant in the body for many years; they resist _____ and survive in phagocytic cells.

4. Tubercle bacilli may develop resistance to _____ drugs.

5. Authorities estimate that _____ of the world's population is infected with tuberculosis organisms and that tuberculosis is the cause of death in almost 2 million people every year.

Activity B MATCHING

Match the term in Column A with the definition in Column B.

Column A

_____ **1.** Isoniazid (also called INH)

_____ **2.** Rifampin (Rifadin)

_____ **3.** Rifabutin (Mycobutin)

_____ **4.** Ethambutol (Myambutol)

_____ **5.** Pyrazinamide

Column B

a. A rifamycin that is bactericidal for both intracellular and extracellular TB organisms

b. A rifamycin that is active against mycobacteria

c. Used with INH and rifampin for the first 2 months of treating active TB

d. The most commonly used antitubercular drug and prototype; bactericidal, relatively inexpensive, and nontoxic; can be given orally or by injection

e. A tuberculostatic drug that inhibits synthesis of RNA and thus interferes with mycobacterial protein metabolism

Activity C SHORT ANSWERS

Briefly answer the following questions.

1. Explain how tuberculosis is transmitted.

2. What is *primary infection* as it relates to tuberculosis?

3. How does latent tuberculosis infection (LTBI) affect the diagnosed individual?

4. What are the causes of active tuberculosis?

5. What are the signs and symptoms of latent tuberculosis infection?

SECTION II: APPLYING YOUR KNOWLEDGE

Activity D CASE STUDY

Consider the scenario and answer the questions.

Mr. White is diagnosed with drug-resistant *Mycobacterium tuberculosis*. He recently completed 3 months of treatment for latent tuberculosis infection.

1. Mr. White states that he maintains strict compliance regarding his treatment regimen and asks how his disease became drug resistant. How would you respond? Why wasn't the mutant strain of the bacteria killed or weakened by his current drug regimen?

2. Mr. White asks you whether his family is safe from this strain of TB. Once a drug-resistant strain of TB develops, how is it transmitted to other people?

3. MDR-TB stands for *multidrug-resistant tuberculosis*. What are these organisms resistant to? What factors contribute to the development of drug-resistant disease?

4. Mr. White states that he wishes to delay treatment until he consults with his son who lives out of state. He informs you that his treatment will be delayed for only a few weeks while he discusses his condition with his son. Why would this be cause for concern?

SECTION III: PRACTICING FOR NCLEX

Activity E

Answer the following questions.

1. A patient is concerned because his drug regimen for drug-resistant TB is different from that of his friends. Which explanation by the nurse is accurate?

   a. "Treatment varies based on the length of time you are ill."

   b. "Treatment is based on the amount of sputum production."

   c. "Treatment is based on drug susceptibility reports."

   d. "There is a standardized treatment regimen."

2. The nurse is aware that patients with which conditions are at higher risk for developing active tuberculosis when exposed to infected air droplets? (Select all that apply.)

   a. Leukemia

   b. Diabetes mellitus

   c. Diverticulosis

   d. Pneumonia

   e. HIV

3. A patient is diagnosed with latent tuberculosis infection. The nurse expects that the treatment plan will include which drug?

   a. Ethambutol

   b. Pyrazinamide

   c. INH

   d. Cyclosporine

4. The public heath nurse is required to be present for each administered dose of antitubercular therapy administered to patients. What is the reason for this practice?

   a. It causes patients to resent and become noncompliant with therapy.

   b. It prevents inadequate drug therapy.

   c. It promotes safety within the home.

   d. It prevents adverse reactions to the drugs administered.

5. A patient is admitted to the hospital and is diagnosed with extensively drug-resistant TB (XDR-TB). This patient has been given six different drugs in an attempt to stop the progression of the disease, but they have not been effective. What therapy does the nurse expect to be prescribed for this patient?

   a. Double the usual dose of INH for 36 months.

   b. Begin again with the first treatment regimen used.

   c. Give all six previous drugs at the same time to fight the drug resistance.

   d. There is no effective treatment.

6. There are projected state budget cuts to the public health department in the coming fiscal year. Because TB is rarely diagnosed, the fiscal cutbacks will include elimination of the team responsible for diagnosing and treating tuberculosis. What can the nurse do as a taxpayer?

   a. Support the decision based on tuberculosis statistics in the state.

   b. Suggest a modified platform that will discontinue DOT.

   c. Suggest a modified platform that will limit diagnosis to private physicians.

   d. Suggest that the program be supported without change.

7. With individual patients receiving antitubercular drugs for latent or active infection, what must the home care nurse do? (Select all that apply.)

   a. Assist the patient in taking the drugs as directed.

   b. Teach about the importance of taking the drugs and the possible consequences of not taking them.

   c. Report drug resistance.

   d. Arrange and monitor compliance regarding follow-up appointments.

   e. Support the use of long-course drug regimens.

8. What are the responsibilities of the home care nurse in relation to TB within the community? (Select all that apply.)

   a. Being active in identifying cases

   b. Investigating contacts of newly diagnosed cases

   c. Suggesting isolation within the community setting

   d. Promoting efforts to manage tuberculosis effectively

   e. Providing disposable surgical masks for family members

9. A patient with alcoholism is diagnosed with tuberculosis. The nurse is responsible for the patient's education plan as well as administering the medication. Before administration of the medication regimen, which test does the nurse expect the physician to order?

   a. Serum ALT and AST

   b. CBC

   c. Electrolytes

   d. Serum albumin and potassium

10. A patient's treatment regimen includes rifampin. After a brief hospitalization, the patient is diagnosed with chronic renal insufficiency. Because the rifampin is an integral part of the patient's tuberculosis treatment regimen, what action would the nurse expect the physician to take?

    a. Increase the dose of rifampin

    b. Decrease the dose of rifampin

    c. Discontinue the rifampin

    d. Maintain the current dose of rifampin

11. An 80-year-old patient is diagnosed with latent tuberculosis infection. What is a risk for the elderly population when being treated with INH?

    a. Hypovolemia

    b. Hypoxemia

    c. Hepatotoxicity

    d. Renal failure

12. What is the recommended treatment for a patient younger than 18 years of age with LTBI?

    a. INH and rifampin for 9 months

    b. INH for 9 months

    c. INH for 12 months

    d. INH and rifabutin for 9 months

13. A patient is treated for HIV with NNRTIs. The patient develops tuberculosis, and the physician includes rifampin in the treatment regimen. Why would this be cause for concern?

    a. Rifampin decreases blood levels of anti-HIV drugs.

    b. Rifampin increases adverse side effects of anti-HIV drugs.

    c. Rifampin causes exacerbation of HIV infections.

    d. Rifampin causes critical anemias in patients with HIV.

14. A patient who is HIV positive develops tuberculosis. Which treatment regimen does the nurse expect the physician to order for this patient?

    a. Longer than a patient who does not have HIV

    b. Similar to a patient who does not have HIV

    c. Of shorter duration than a patient who does not have HIV

    d. Contraindicated due to his HIV status

15. A patient whose treatment regimen includes pyrazinamide develops gout. The nurse will assess what effect if the physician adds allopurinol to the treatment plan?

    a. It may cause allopurinol toxicity.

    b. It does not affect therapeutic levels of allopurinol.

    c. It is contraindicated for use concomitantly with allopurinol.

    d. It may decrease the effects of allopurinol.

16. A female patient is prescribed rifampin as part of her antitubercular regimen. She also takes oral contraceptives. The nurse is aware that this combination of medications can produce what effect?

    a. Blood clots

    b. Stroke

    c. Pregnancy

    d. DVT

17. A patient takes phenytoin for a seizure disorder. Before prescribing isoniazid for the patient's tuberculosis, what would the nurse expect the physician to do?

    a. Decrease the dose of phenytoin and monitor drug levels closely.

    b. Increase the dose of INH secondary to phenytoin administration.

    c. Increase the dose of phenytoin and add Tegretol to the drug regimen.

    d. Increase the dose of phenytoin and monitor drug levels closely.

18. The nurse is caring for a 79-year-old patient with suspected tuberculosis. What assessments does the nurse expect to make in this patient? (Select all that apply.)

    a. Afebrile

    b. Hemoptysis

    c. Night sweats

    d. Decreased sputum production

    e. Mental status changes

19. What therapeutic drug regimen will ensure patient compliance?

    a. Prescribe the medications Monday through Friday, with weekends off.

    b. Prescribe the medications, alternating the regimen weekly.

    c. Prescribe fixed-dose combinations of drugs.

    d. Prescribe medications for longer durations with fewer drugs to be administered.

20. The nurse is caring for a patient who is taking INH for tuberculosis. What adverse effect is this patient most at risk for?

    a. Renal dysfunction

    b. Central nervous system dysfunction

    c. Liver dysfunction

    d. Gastric dysfunction

CHAPTER 21

Drug Therapy for Viral Infections

Learning Objectives

- Identify the characteristics of viruses and common viral infections.
- Identify the major clinical manifestations of common viral infections.
- Identify the prototype and describe the action, use, adverse effects, contraindications, and nursing implications for antiviral agents administered for herpes simplex and varicella-zoster viruses.
- Identify the prototype and describe the action, use, adverse effects, contraindications, and nursing implications for antiviral agents administered for cytomegalovirus.
- Identify the prototype and describe the action, use, adverse effects, contraindications, and nursing implications of drugs administered for respiratory syncytial virus.
- Identify the prototypes and describe their action, use, adverse effects, contraindications, and nursing implications for administration in influenza.
- Identify the prototype and describe the action, use, adverse effects, contraindications, and nursing implications for the nucleoside analog antiviral agents administered for hepatitis.
- Identify the prototype and describe the action, use, adverse effects, contraindications, and nursing implications for the nucleoside reverse transcriptase inhibitors administered for human immunodeficiency virus (HIV).
- Identify the prototype and describe the action, use, adverse effects, contraindications, and nursing implications for the nonnucleoside reverse transcriptase inhibitors administered for HIV.
- Identify the prototype and describe the action, use, adverse effects, contraindications, and nursing implications for the protease inhibitors administered for HIV.
- Identify the prototype and describe the action, use, adverse effects, contraindications, and nursing implications for the integrase strand transfer inhibitors administered for HIV.
- Identify the prototype and describe the action, use, adverse effects, contraindications, and nursing implications for fusion protein inhibitors administered for HIV.
- Identify the prototype and describe the action, use, adverse effects, contraindications, and nursing implications for CCR5 antagonists administered for HIV.
- Implement the nursing process in the care of the patient undergoing drug therapy for viral infections.

SECTION I: ASSESSING YOUR UNDERSTANDING

Activity A FILL IN THE BLANKS

1. Viruses cause acquired immunodeficiency syndrome (AIDS), hepatitis, _____, and other disorders that affect almost every body system.

2. Viruses can be spread by secretions from infected people, ingestion of contaminated food or water, _____ in skin or mucous membrane, sexual contact, pregnancy, breast-feeding, and organ transplantation.

3. Viruses are _____ parasites that gain entry to human host cells by binding to receptors on cell membranes.

4. The locations and _____ of the receptors determine which host cells can be infected by a virus.

5. The mucous membranes lining the tracheo-bronchial tree have receptors for the influenza A virus; helper T lymphocytes and other white blood cells have CD4 molecules, which are the receptors for the _____.

Activity B MATCHING

Match the term in Column A with the definition in Column B.

Column A

_____ 1. Acyclovir, famciclovir, and valacyclovir

_____ 2. Foscarnet, ganciclovir, and valganciclovir

_____ 3. Trifluridine

_____ 4. Tenofovir (Viread)

_____ 5. Indinavir, ritonavir, and saquinavir

Column B

a. Applied topically to treat keratoconjunctivitis and corneal ulcers caused by the herpes simplex virus (herpetic keratitis)

b. Similar to the NRTIs in that it inhibits the reverse transcriptase enzyme

c. Inhibit viral reproduction after the drugs are activated by a viral enzyme found in virus-infected cells

d. The oldest PIs

e. Penetrate virus-infected cells, become activated by an enzyme, and inhibit viral DNA reproduction

Activity C SHORT ANSWERS

Briefly answer the following.

1. Describe how viruses use cellular metabolic activities for their own survival and replication.

2. How do viruses transmit their infection to other host cells?

3. Describe symptoms usually associated with acute viral infections.

4. How do herpesviruses differ from other viruses?

5. Describe how viruses induce antibodies and immunity.

SECTION II: APPLYING YOUR KNOWLEDGE

Activity D CASE STUDY

Consider the scenario and answer the questions.

Mr. Grant presents to the physician's office with complaints of a recurrent rash in his genital area. He is diagnosed with genital herpes. The physician prescribes acyclovir. You are responsible for the education plan.

1. Mr. Grant asks you how acyclovir works and whether it will treat his genital herpes. How do you respond? What effect does acyclovir have? What may prolonged or repeated courses of acyclovir result in?

2. Mr. Grant returns for a physician visit 1 year later. He is compliant with the prescribed acyclovir regimen and experiences few outbreaks. He asks if he can discontinue the medication regimen for a while. What will happen if drug therapy is discontinued?

3. Mr. Grant asks you how long will it take for the acyclovir to remove the virus from his body. What can you tell him?

4. Mr. Grant asks if there is an ointment that may be applied to the lesions during outbreaks in addition to taking his oral acyclovir. What do you think the physician will order?

SECTION III: PRACTICING FOR NCLEX

Activity E

Answer the following questions.

1. A female patient's physician orders a combination of antiretroviral drugs to treat her illness. The patient states that she is concerned because she fears increased adverse effects. What is the reason for using combination antiretroviral medications?

   a. To increase effectiveness

   b. To prevent the emergence of drug-resistant viruses

   c. To decrease adverse effects

   d. To cure the virus in less than 6 weeks

2. A male patient is concerned about how the antiviral drugs he is taking will affect his cells. Viruses are intracellular parasites and have what effect on human cells?

   a. They travel from cell to cell without causing damage.

   b. They do not affect the human cell.

   c. They incapacitate the cell for a short time before moving on.

   d. They are relatively toxic to human cells.

3. For which viral infection is drug therapy available? (Select all that apply.)

   a. Asthmatic bronchitis

   b. Hepatitis B and C

   c. HIV infection

   d. Influenza

   e. Cytomegalovirus

4. To prevent viral infections, what precaution should the general public take?

   a. Use intermittent hand hygiene

   b. Become vaccinated against prevalent virus infections

   c. Wear masks

   d. Wear personal protective equipment

5. Viral infections commonly occur in what age group?

   a. Young children

   b. Older adults

   c. All age groups

   d. Infants

6. The nurse is caring for a patient who is HIV positive. What laboratory test is used to determine this patient's ability to fight against viral infections?

   a. BUN

   b. CD4

   c. AST

   d. RBCs

7. A female patient is diagnosed with HIV and hepatitis C, and the physician orders antiviral therapy. The nurse would expect the physician to order monitoring of which laboratory value?

   a. CBC

   b. Electrolytes

   c. LFTs

   d. Serum albumin

8. The physician prescribes nevirapine for the treatment of a patient's HIV infection. Based on moderately abnormal LFTs 3 months later, what would the nurse expect the physician to do?

   a. Discontinue the drug until LFTs return to baseline

   b. Reduce the amount of drug prescribed

   c. Recheck the laboratory values

   d. Increase the amount of drug prescribed

9. A female patient is diagnosed with HIV and hepatitis B. The physician prescribes zidovudine. When the patient's LFTs become moderately elevated, the nurse expects the physician to reduce the dose of zidovudine by how much?

   a. 20%

   b. 25%

   c. 40%

   d. 50%

10. A male patient is prescribed amantadine as part of the treatment regimen for his Parkinson's disease. Because the patient also is diagnosed with renal disease, the physician titrates the dose of amantadine based on what factor?

    a. White blood cell count

    b. Potassium

    c. Creatinine clearance

    d. Calcium

11. A patient is diagnosed with CMV retinitis. The physician orders foscarnet. Renal impairment is most likely to occur within which period of time?

   a. First 72 hours of therapy

   b. First week of therapy

   c. Second week of therapy

   d. First month of therapy

12. How is the risk of renal impairment best minimized when foscarnet is administered?

   a. Monitoring renal function two or three times weekly during induction

   b. Monitoring renal function at least every 2 to 3 months during maintenance therapy

   c. Stopping the drug if creatinine clearance drops to less than 0.2 mL/min/kg

   d. Placing the patient on fluid restriction

13. A female patient is prescribed indinavir for her HIV infection. The nurse would encourage the patient to do what to avoid nephrolithiasis?

   a. Maintain a fluid restriction of 800 mL daily

   b. Maintain a fluid restriction of 1000 mL daily

   c. Consume 48 to 64 ounces of fluid a day

   d. Consume 64 to 82 ounces of fluid a day

14. A patient is prescribed amantadine to prevent influenza A. The nurse should monitor the patient for which adverse effects? (Select all that apply.)

   a. Dizziness

   b. Gastrointestinal bleeding

   c. Peripheral edema

   d. Hypertension

   e. Nasal congestion

15. A 10-year-old patient is prescribed oseltamivir to treat influenza A. The nurse understands that what is an adverse effect of this drug?

   a. Dizziness

   b. Hallucinations

   c. Difficulty breathing

   d. Diarrhea

16. A female patient is HIV positive and is pregnant with her first child. At 14 to 34 weeks of gestation, the physician orders zidovudine. Which dosage is correct?

   a. 75 mg PO five times a day

   b. 50 mg PO five times a day

   c. 25 mg PO five times a day

   d. 100 mg PO five times a day

17. What constitutes viral load?

   a. Viral levels in the tissues

   b. HIV DNA particles within the blood

   c. HIV RNA particles within the blood

   d. All sites of viral reproduction

18. The nurse is caring for a patient with AIDS who has developed cytomegalovirus (CMV). The nurse anticipates the physician will order which drug to treat this patient?

   a. Ribavirin

   b. Ganciclovir

   c. Amantadine hydrochloride

   d. Oseltamivir

19. The nurse is giving discharge instruction to a patient who has been prescribed efavirenz as treatment for HIV. Which instruction is most important for the nurse to give this patient to minimize the CNS adverse effects of this medication?

   a. "Take the medication at bedtime."

   b. "Take the medication with a high-fat meal."

   c. "Take the medication with orange juice."

   d. "Take the medication with herbal tea."

20. The nurse instructs a group of young adults about what method that is least likely to prevent sexually transmitted viral infections such as genital herpes?

   a. Complete abstinence

   b. Avoiding sex when skin lesions are present

   c. Use of a diaphragm when lesions are present

   d. Using condoms

22

Drug Therapy for Fungal Infections

Learning Objectives

- Describe the characteristics of fungi and fungal infections.
- Discuss antibacterial drug therapy and immunosuppression as risk factors for development of fungal infections.
- Identify the prototype and describe the action, use, adverse effects, contraindications, and nursing implications for polyenes.
- Identify the prototype and describe the action, use, adverse effects, contraindications, and nursing implications for azoles.
- Identify the prototype and describe the action, use, adverse effects, contraindications, and nursing implications for echinocandins.
- Identify the prototype and describe the action, use, adverse effects, contraindications, and nursing implications for the pyrimidine analog.
- Identify the prototype and describe the action, use, adverse effects, contraindications, and nursing implications for the miscellaneous antifungal agents.
- Understand how to implement the nursing process in the care of patients undergoing drug therapy for fungal infections.

SECTION I: ASSESSING YOUR UNDERSTANDING

Activity A FILL IN THE BLANKS

1. _____ are molds and yeasts that are widely dispersed in the environment and are either saprophytic or parasitic.

2. Molds are _____ organisms composed of colonies of tangled strands.

3. Some fungi, called _____, can grow only at the cooler temperatures of body surfaces.

4. _____ fungi can grow as molds outside the body and as yeasts in the warm temperatures of the body.

5. Dimorphic fungi include a number of human pathogens such as those that cause blastomycosis, histoplasmosis, and _____.

Activity B MATCHING

Match the term in Column A with the definition in Column B.

Column A	Column B
____ **1.** Amphotericin B	**a.** Has the same mechanism of action as amphotericin B; used only for topical therapy of oral, intestinal, and vaginal candidiasis because it is too toxic for systemic use
____ **2.** Nystatin	
____ **3.** Fluconazole (Diflucan)	

____ **4.** Posaconazole (Noxafil)

____ **5.** Caspofungin

b. A second-generation azole with activity against *Candida* and *Aspergillus* species

c. Is active against most types of pathogenic fungi and is fungicidal or fungistatic, depending on the concentration in body fluids and the susceptibility of the causative fungus

d. Is often the drug of choice for localized candidal infections (e.g., urinary tract infections, thrush) and is useful for systemic candidiasis

e. Is used for systemic *Candida* and *Aspergillus* infections. It is highly bound to plasma albumin, metabolized slowly, and excreted in feces and urine

Activity C SHORT ANSWERS

Briefly answer the following.

1. Identify the areas of the body in which *Candida albicans* is part of the normal flora.

2. What conditions alter the body's natural restraining forces and cause fungal overgrowth and opportunistic infections?

3. Identify the enzyme produced by *Aspergillus* organisms that allows them to destroy structural proteins and penetrate body tissues.

4. How do *Cryptococcus neoformans* organisms invade the normal defense mechanism of phagocytosis?

SECTION II: APPLYING YOUR KNOWLEDGE

Activity D CASE STUDY

Consider the scenario and answer the questions.

Mrs. Franks is diagnosed with a systemic fungal infection. She is hospitalized for management of her infection and will eventually be discharged to continue treatment at home. The physician orders IV amphotericin B.

1. Amphotericin B is only used for serious fungal infections. Why?

2. Mrs. Franks has a preexisting renal impairment. Which formulation of amphotericin B would you expect the physician to prescribe?

3. Mrs. Franks is concerned because her HMO will not cover the formulation that the physician ordered, and she asks whether another form of amphotericin B may be used. The HMO suggested an alternative. How should you respond?

4. Mrs. Franks asks how the drug will help her if the particular site of her infection is unknown. What explanation can you give?

5. Discuss two of the tactics used to decrease nephrotoxicity when amphotericin B is prescribed.

6. Mrs. Franks is concerned when her peripheral IV is discontinued and the physician orders the insertion of a central line. She asks if this is really necessary. What can you tell her about peripheral sites?

SECTION III: PRACTICING FOR NCLEX

Activity E

Answer the following questions.

1. Laboratory monitoring for patients on all systemic antifungal drugs should include what test?

   a. CBC

   b. BUN and creatinine

   c. Electrolytes

   d. LFTs (liver function tests)

2. What serious adverse effect is most associated with amphotericin B?

   a. Nephrotoxicity

   b. Hypovolemia

   c. Cardiogenic shock

   d. Septic shock

3. A male patient presents to the physician's office with complaints of a fungal infection on his foot. He informs the nurse that when the itching gets too bad, he applies fungal foot powder. Which statement is true about this patient's approach to self-care?

   a. "Intermittent treatment will eventually cure the fungal infection."

   b. "Fungal infections such as the one you have require lifelong treatment."

   c. "Fungal infections often require long-term drug therapy."

   d. "Fungal infections may be healed with a short course of antibiotics and antifungals."

4. A patient who is HIV positive is being treated for recurrent fungal infections. Patients whose immune systems are suppressed are at risk for what complication?

   a. Failure to thrive and therefore increased fungal infections

   b. Recurrent bacterial infections

   c. Impaired healing

   d. Development of serious fungal infections

5. The nurse is caring for a patient who has a severe fungal infection. The physician has prescribed a lipid formulation of amphotericin B. The nurse is aware that this form of medication is given for what reason?

   a. It is less hepatotoxic.

   b. It is less neurotoxic.

   c. It is less nephrotoxic.

   d. It is less gastrotoxic.

6. The patient is going home and will receive amphotericin B with the aid of a home care nurse. What should the nurse teach the family to ensure that the patient's immune system is not compromised while on this medication? (Select all that apply.)

   a. Keep fresh flowers in the patient's room.

   b. Clean the bathroom daily with bleach.

   c. Ensure that the air conditioning filters are clean.

   d. Remove all rugs and curtains from the house.

   e. Remove all potted plants.

7. A male patient is receiving intravenous antifungal therapy at home to treat his pneumonia. Five weeks ago, he completed a 6-week course of therapy. He feels fine and asks if he can begin woodworking projects around the home to keep himself busy. What is the most appropriate response by the nurse?

   a. "Yes, as long as you don't overexert yourself."

   b. "No, because of risk for infection."

   c. "I will have to consult the physician."

   d. "Yes, as long as you complete most of the project outdoors."

8. When itraconazole is used in critically ill patients, a loading dose of 200 mg three times daily may be given for what period of time?

   a. 3 days

   b. 48 hours

   c. 2 days

   d. 5 days

9. A female patient receives hemodialysis three times a week. She is diagnosed with a severe fungal infection, but the physician is reluctant to order amphotericin B. The patient asks if the hemodialysis could be used to remove any excess drug. What is the most appropriate response?

   a. Blood levels cannot be maintained if the patient is receiving hemodialysis.

   b. Hemodialysis should not be used to manage blood levels.

   c. Hemodialysis will not remove the drug.

   d. Hemodialysis is an effective method to manage blood levels in this case.

10. A patient's fungal infection extends to his cerebral spinal fluid. What medication does the nurse expect the physician to order?

   a. Amphotericin B

   b. Fluconazole

   c. Nystatin

   d. Itraconazole

11. The azole antifungals are contraindicated in patients with what condition?

   a. Hypovolemia

   b. Pancreatitis

   c. HIV

   d. Increased liver enzymes or active liver disease

12. The nurse is caring for a patient with a suspected fungal infection who is neutropenic after chemotherapy. The nurse anticipates that the physician will most likely prescribe which drug?

   a. Fluconazole

   b. Caspofungin

   c. Griseofulvin

   d. Flucytosine

13. The nurse is caring for a patient who will be receiving amphotericin B. The nurse will notify the physician immediately if the patient normally takes which daily medications? (Select all that apply.)

   a. Digoxin

   b. Ampicillin

   c. Diazepam

   d. Prednisone

   e. HCTZ

14. What antifungal medication has the same mechanism of action as amphotericin B but is used only in the topical treatment of candidiasis?

   a. Nystatin

   b. Terbinafine

   c. Fluconazole

   d. Griseofulvin

15. To reduce fever and chills related to the administration of amphotericin IV, the patient may be premedicated with a combination of which medications?

   a. An NSAID and diphenhydramine

   b. An NSAID and a corticosteroid

   c. Acetaminophen, diphenhydramine, and a corticosteroid

   d. Acetaminophen, antifungal, and an NSAID

16. To reduce phlebitis caused by the administration of amphotericin IV, the nurse may implement which prevention techniques? (Select all that apply.)

   a. Administer medication on alternate days

   b. Add 500 to 2000 units of heparin to the infusion

   c. Administer via heparin lock

   d. Removing the needle after infusion

   e. Administer through a separate IV line

17. A male patient is prescribed Fungizone. His physician informs him that his maintenance dose may be doubled and infused on alternate days and establishes the medication protocol. The nurse should be concerned when a single dose exceeds which amount?

   a. 1.5 mg/kg

   b. 2.0 mg/kg

   c. 1.0 mg/kg

   d. 3.0 mg/kg

18. A male patient is diagnosed with localized lymphocutaneous infection. What is the drug of choice for this infection?

   a. Fluconazole

   b. Nystatin

   c. Amphotericin B

   d. Itraconazole

19. Predisposing factors for fungal infections include what type of medications?

   a. Antihistamines

   b. Anticoagulants

   c. Antibacterials

   d. Antihypertensives

20. The nurse is caring for an obese female patient who is also HIV positive. The nurse takes special care to dry all skin folds in the patient after her bath to prevent which fungal infection?

   a. Histoplasmosis

   b. Cryptococcosis

   c. Sporotrichosis

   d. Candidiasis

CHAPTER 23

Drug Therapy for Parasitic Infections

Learning Objectives

- Describe the etiology, pathophysiology, and clinical manifestations of parasitic infections.
- Identify the prototype and describe the action, use, adverse effects, contraindications, and nursing implications for the amebicides.
- Identify the prototype and describe the action, use, adverse effects, contraindications, and nursing implications for the antimalarial drugs.
- Identify the prototype and describe the action, use, adverse effects, contraindications, and nursing implications for the anthelmintic drugs.
- Identify the prototype and describe the action, use, adverse effects, contraindications, and nursing implications for the scabicides and pediculicides.
- Implement the nursing process in the care of the patient being treated with antiparasitic agents.

SECTION I: ASSESSING YOUR UNDERSTANDING

Activity A FILL IN THE BLANKS

1. A _____ is a living organism that survives at the expense of another organism, called the host.

2. Amebiasis is caused by the pathogenic protozoan, _____.

3. Amebiasis is transmitted by ingestion of food or water contaminated with human feces containing _____.

4. _____ are active amebae that feed, multiply, move about, and produce clinical manifestations of amebiasis.

5. Trophozoites produce a/an _____ that allows them to invade body tissues.

Activity B MATCHING

Match the term in Column A with the definition in Column B.

Column A	Column B
____ 1. Chloroquine (Aralen)	a. An iodine compound that acts against active amebae (trophozoites) in the intestinal lumen
____ 2. Iodoquinol (Yodoxin)	b. Effective against protozoa that cause amebiasis, giardiasis, and trichomoniasis and against anaerobic bacilli
____ 3. Metronidazole (Flagyl)	c. Used to prevent *Plasmodium falciparum* malaria, including chloroquine-resistant strains, and to treat acute malaria caused by *P. falciparum* or *Plasmodium vivax*

_____ **4.** Tinidazole (Tindamax)

    d. Used mainly for its antimalarial effects

_____ **5.** Mefloquine (Lariam)

    e. A chemical relative of metronidazole approved for the treatment of amebiasis, giardiasis, and trichomoniasis

Activity C SHORT ANSWERS

Briefly answer the following questions.

1. Identify the populations that are most likely to contract amebiasis.

2. Describe how toxoplasmosis is transmitted.

3. Describe how trichomoniasis is transmitted.

4. Describe how scabies is transmitted.

5. How is pediculosis capitis diagnosed?

SECTION II: APPLYING YOUR KNOWLEDGE

Activity D CASE STUDY

Consider the scenario and answer the questions.

Mr. and Mrs. Bean returned from a trip to Central America about 1 week ago. They present to the physician's office with symptoms consistent with giardiasis. You are responsible for the patients' education plan.

1. Mr. Bean states that he didn't drink the water while on vacation. Which method or action on the Beans' part may have caused transmission of the disease?

2. Mrs. Bean asks why they didn't get sick while on vacation. What explanation can you give them? How does giardial infection manifest?

3. Mrs. Bean is embarrassed to pick up the prescription at the pharmacy for her treatment. She states, "What if people find out what we have?" What kind of education can you give these patients concerning their treatment? What symptoms may develop later, and what is the cause of these later symptoms?

4. The Beans' son, aged 9, presents to the pediatrician's office with symptoms of giardiasis. What would you expect the physician to order for this patient, given his age?

SECTION III: PRACTICING FOR NCLEX

Activity E

Answer the following questions.

1. The physician orders an antiparasitic drug for the patient. The drug is prescribed for treatment of local effects in the skin and which other area?
   a. GI tract
   b. Lungs
   c. Oral mucosa
   d. Ocular cavity

2. What is one method that the nurse can teach community members to prevent many parasitic infections?
   a. Avoidance of campgrounds
   b. Personal and public hygiene practices
   c. Avoidance of specific vacation spots
   d. Avoidance of nonbottled water

3. A male patient is traveling to a country where malaria is endemic. The nurse suggests that he visit his physician and receive a prescription for what medication?
   a. Tinidazole
   b. Metronidazole
   c. Iodoquinol
   d. Chloroquine

4. The student nurse is spending the day with the school nurse and will be assisting the nurse with head checks for the presence of head lice. The nurse tells the student to observe for what in the school children's hair?
   a. Patches of hair loss
   b. Ova (nits) sticking to hair shafts
   c. Scabs and open sores at the collar line
   d. Thin, red, pruritic lines

5. The home care nurse visits a female patient for a wound treatment. While the nurse is preparing to leave, the patient's child comes home from school with complaints related to a parasitic infection. What is one of the responsibilities of the nurse in this situation?

   a. Suggest a treatment modality to the mother

   b. Collaborate with the school to prevent or control outbreaks

   c. Tell the mother that her child's poor hygiene is the cause of the infection

   d. Tell the child not to return to school for 48 to 72 hours

6. A treatment is ordered for a child with a parasitic infection. What are the responsibilities of the home care nurse? (Select all that apply.)

   a. Examine close contacts of the child and assess their need for treatment

   b. Assist the parents so that drugs are used appropriately

   c. Provide treatments for the parasitic illness

   d. Teach personal and environmental hygiene measures to prevent reinfection

   e. Ensure follow-up measures

7. A female patient calls the physician's office and asks how to treat her three children for head lice after they come home from school with a note from the school nurse. She complains that she has treated them three times this month. What is an appropriate action for the nurse in the physician's office to take?

   a. Review the directions for the product ordered by the physician

   b. Inform her that some children are carriers of the parasite

   c. Inform her that sometimes treatment must be done several times before it is effective

   d. Tell the patient that she is "doing it all wrong"

8. Which medication used to treat malaria should not be given to children younger than 8 years of age?

   a. Tetracycline

   b. Mefloquine

   c. Primaquine

   d. Quinine

9. The mother of a 4-year-old child tells the nurse that her child has been sleeping very poorly. The child has also been scratching in her rectal or perineal area. The nurse suspects that this child has what parasitic infection?

   a. Pinworms

   b. Hookworms

   c. Whipworms

   d. Roundworms

10. The physician orders a pyrethrin preparation for the patient's children, who came home from school with head lice. The nurse tells the patient that the medication is available over the counter and that the initial treatment should be repeated in what period of time?

    a. In 5 days

    b. In 10 days

    c. In 48 hours

    d. In 72 hours

11. The physician has ordered mebendazole for a patient with a parasitic infection. It is important for the nurse to know that the medication must be administered in what way?

    a. IM in a large muscle

    b. Chewed and swallowed or crushed in food

    c. IV in a large vein

    d. Swallowed whole

12. The patient needs treatment for both pediculosis and scabies. The nurse expects the physician to order which drug?

    a. Metronidazole

    b. Malathion

    c. Spinosad

    d. Permethrin

13. The patient has just begun taking metronidazole and calls the clinic to report that her urine has turned very dark. What is the nurse's best response to this patient?

    a. "Please come to the clinic as soon as possible for a urinalysis."

    b. "This is an expected side effect. Your urine color will return to normal after you stop taking this drug."

    c. "Go immediately to the emergency department because the medication is causing bleeding from your bladder."

    d. "If you drink more fluid, your urine will get light in color again."

14. A female patient's son is diagnosed with cryptosporidiosis. She is concerned because he is also being treated for HIV. Which drug would the nurse expect the physician to order?

    a. Nitazoxanide (Alinia)

    b. Ivermectin (Stromectol)

    c. Mebendazole (Vermox)

    d. Pyrantel (Pin-Rid)

15. In addition to its use as an antimalarial, quinine may also be used to treat which condition?

    a. Amebiasis

    b. Pinworms

    c. CNS symptoms

    d. Cramped skeletal muscles

16. The physician orders primaquine to prevent an initial occurrence of malaria. After the patient returns from the malarious area, what would the nurse expect the physician to order?

    a. A repetition of the current order

    b. A proliferative agent

    c. A suppressive agent

    d. A causal prophylaxis

17. Chloroquine acts against erythrocytic forms of plasmodial parasites to prevent or treat what condition?

    a. Pinworm infestation

    b. Helminth infestation

    c. Pediculosis

    d. Malaria

18. What antibiotics act against amebae in the intestinal lumen by altering the bacterial flora required for amebic viability? (Select all that apply.)

    a. Tetracycline

    b. Penicillin

    c. Doxycycline

    d. Rifampin

    e. Ampicillin

19. Metronidazole should be used with caution in what type of patients?

    a. Those with central nervous system disorders

    b. Those with diabetes type 1

    c. Those with cardiac dysrhythmia

    d. Those with a history of myocardial infarction

20. The physician has ordered hydroxychloroquine as prophylaxis for malaria. The patient notifies the nurse that he already takes this medication. The nurse is aware that this patient takes this medication for treatment of which disorder?

    a. Diabetes mellitus type 2

    b. Renal failure

    c. Peptic ulcer disease

    d. Rheumatoid arthritis

CHAPTER 24

Drug Therapy for Heart Failure

Learning Objectives

- Understand the pathophysiology of right-sided and left-sided heart failure.
- Identify the major manifestations of heart failure.
- Identify the prototype and describe the action, use, adverse effects, contraindications, and nursing implications for the inotrope (cardiac glycoside) drug class.
- Identify the prototype and describe the action, use, adverse effects, contraindications, and nursing implications for the phosphodiesterase inhibitors (cardiotonic–inotropic agents).
- Identify the prototype and describe the action, use, adverse effects, contraindications, and nursing implications for human B-type natriuretic peptide.
- Identify the prototype and describe the action, use, adverse effects, contraindications, and nursing implications for adjuvant drugs used in the treatment of heart failure.
- Implement the nursing process in the care of patients undergoing drug therapy for heart failure.

SECTION I: ASSESSING YOUR UNDERSTANDING

Activity A FILL IN THE BLANKS

1. _____ is a complex clinical condition that occurs when the heart cannot pump enough blood to meet tissue needs for oxygen and nutrients.

2. Impaired myocardial contraction during systole is called _____.

3. Impaired relaxation and filling of ventricles during diastole is called _____.

4. HF has also been referred to as congestive heart failure (CHF), because frequently there are congestion and _____ in the lungs and peripheral tissues.

5. At the cellular level, _____ stems from dysfunction of contractile myocardial cells and the endothelial cells that line the heart and blood vessels.

Activity B MATCHING

Match the term in Column A with the definition in Column B.

Column A

_____ 1. Digoxin (Lanoxin)

_____ 2. Milrinone IV (Primacor)

_____ 3. Nesiritide (Natrecor)

Column B

a. Most commonly used cardiotonic–inotropic agents for short-term management of acute, severe HF that is not controlled by digoxin, diuretics, and vasodilators

b. First in its class of drugs to be used in the management of acute HF

___ **4.** Digoxin immune Fab (Digibind)

___ **5.** Lidocaine

c. Antidysrhythmic local anesthetic agent used to decrease myocardial irritability

d. The only commonly used digitalis glycoside

e. Digoxin-binding antidote derived from antidigoxin antibodies produced in sheep

Activity C SHORT ANSWERS

Briefly answer the following questions.

1. Discuss the primary causes of heart failure.

2. Discuss a compensatory mechanism of heart failure involving neurohormones.

3. What are the symptoms of heart failure?

4. What impact does the renin–angiotensin–aldosterone system have on congestive heart failure?

5. Define cardiac or ventricular remodeling.

SECTION II: APPLYING YOUR KNOWLEDGE

Activity D CASE STUDY

Consider the scenario and answer the questions.

Mrs. White is diagnosed with atrial fibrillation. Her physician orders digoxin 0.125 mg daily. You are responsible for her education plan.

1. Mrs. White asks if she should administer the medication on an empty or a full stomach. How would you respond?

2. Mrs. White is stabilized on a tablet formation of digoxin. She asks if the physician can change the formulation to Lanoxicaps, which may be easier to swallow. The physician changes the formulation but orders digoxin levels to be drawn at routine intervals. Why did the physician make this order?

3. Mrs. White develops chronic renal failure. She returns to the physician's office for a routine visit. The morning before the visit, she presents to the laboratory for assessment of her digoxin level. The level is 3. Based on this laboratory result, what would you expect the physician to do?

4. Discuss the teaching you would give Mrs. White concerning her digoxin prescription, including the reason that she is taking digoxin, the onset of action and peak effect of the drug, and the difference between IV and oral digoxin.

SECTION III: PRACTICING FOR NCLEX

Activity E

Answer the following questions.

1. The patient's digoxin level is 0.125. How does the nurse interpret this level?
   a. Normal
   b. Elevated
   c. Toxic
   d. Low

2. The nurse monitors which patient for an increased risk of digoxin toxicity?
   a. The patient with liver dysfunction
   b. The patient with renal dysfunction
   c. The patient with an integumentary dysfunction
   d. The patient with a peripheral vascular dysfunction

3. A patient presents to the emergency department with signs and symptoms of acute congestive heart failure. Assessment findings and tests confirm the diagnosis. Which type of diuretic would be the drug of choice to treat the patient?
   a. Thiazide
   b. Loop
   c. Potassium sparing
   d. Calcium wasting

4. A patient is admitted to the hospital secondary to hypoxia and acute congestive heart failure. At discharge, the patient notes that the physician discontinued his beta-blockers. The nurse explains that beta-blockers may cause which effect?

   a. Cause increased shortness of breath

   b. Cause anginal episodes

   c. Decrease myocardial contractility

   d. Increase atrioventricular conductivity

5. A 65-year-old patient presents to the physician's office with complaints of shortness of breath on exertion, edema in his ankles, and waking up in the middle of the night unable to breathe. The nurse suspects that his symptoms are indicative of which condition?

   a. Asthmatic bronchitis

   b. Pulmonary edema

   c. Heart failure

   d. Myocardial infarction

6. The nurse is preparing to administer digoxin to a 9-month-old infant. What must the nurse do prior to administration of this medication?

   a. Monitor the infant's respiratory rate

   b. Monitor the infant's blood pressure

   c. Monitor the infant's temperature

   d. Monitor the infant's apical pulse

7. The nurse is aware that heart failure may result from what problems? (Select all that apply.)

   a. Impaired myocardial contraction during systole

   b. Impaired relaxation and filling of ventricles during diastole

   c. A combination of systolic and diastolic dysfunction

   d. Impaired conduction from the SA node

   e. Cardiomyopathy

8. A male patient takes natural licorice for his arthritis. The patient complains that he is more short of breath. The nurse understands that licorice blocks the effects of spironolactone by which mechanism?

   a. Sodium retention and potassium loss

   b. Increased cardiac afterload

   c. Renal insufficiency

   d. Potassium retention and dysrhythmia

9. A female patient's drugs include a furosemide, digoxin, and hydralazine. She is unable to afford all of her medications, so she takes them intermittently to make them last longer. In addition to making a referral to social service, what should the home care nurse tell this patient?

   a. "Different types of drugs have different actions and produce different responses."

   b. "Over-the-counter drugs may be viable substitutes for the more expensive medications."

   c. "Your plan is acceptable if the physician is aware and laboratory studies are done more frequently."

   d. "Changes in doses may be better than alternating medications."

10. A male patient is diagnosed with cirrhosis of the liver. He also takes digoxin for a diagnosis of atrial fibrillation. The nurse anticipates that the physician will order what in connection with the digoxin medication?

    a. Lower the digoxin dose

    b. Increase the digoxin dose

    c. Check the patient's digoxin level

    d. Maintain the current digoxin dose

11. A male patient is diagnosed with renal failure secondary to diabetes mellitus. Based on the new diagnosis, how will the physician safely adjust the patient's digoxin dose?

    a. 0.25 mg every other day

    b. 0.125 mg every day

    c. 0.125 mg three times a week

    d. 0.25 mg five times a week

12. The pediatric cardiologist orders digoxin for the patient. The nurse understands that, during the initial doses, what may occur?

    a. The patient may experience an increased heart rate initially, and then a decreased rate.

    b. The patient may be monitored by ECG.

    c. The patient may experience a hypertensive crisis.

    d. The patient may experience an exacerbation of congestive heart failure.

13. The physician asks the nurse to obtain an ECG on a patient prior to starting digoxin therapy for what reason?

    a. To make sure the patient hasn't had a heart attack

    b. To recognize early changes that indicate digoxin toxicity

    c. To best monitor heart rate

    d. To document that the patient needs digoxin

14. A female patient presents to the emergency department with nausea, vomiting, and a heart rate of 45 beats per minute. Her husband states that she takes digoxin, Lasix, and nitroglycerin for chest pain. Laboratory results confirm digoxin toxicity. The nurse would expect the physician to order what medication to treat the bradycardia?

    a. Atropine

    b. Nifedipine

    c. Nitroglycerin

    d. Nesiritide

15. A male patient is diagnosed with heart failure. The physician orders a loading dose of digoxin. Loading doses are necessary for what reason?

    a. Digoxin's short half-life increases the risk for toxicity.

    b. The patient is at risk for dysthymia with titrated doses.

    c. Digoxin's long half-life makes therapeutic serum levels difficult to obtain without loading.

    d. Oral digoxin is ineffective for the treatment of heart failure.

16. A male patient is diagnosed with chronic heart failure. He is hospitalized for the second time this year for symptoms of hypokalemia. The nurse anticipates that the physician will change his diuretic to which type?

    a. Potassium wasting

    b. Potassium sparing

    c. Sodium sparing

    d. Sodium wasting

17. The nurse in a physician's office knows that heart failure patients will need which laboratory tests to best monitor their condition? (Select all that apply.)

    a. K^+ and Na^+ levels

    b. WBCs

    c. Creatinine clearance

    d. Digoxin levels

    e. ALT and AST

18. The nurse suggests which dietary habits for the patient with heart failure? (Select all that apply.)

    a. Only salt food once with every meal.

    b. Decrease calories to lose weight if needed.

    c. Avoid unsaturated fats and include saturated fats in every meal.

    d. Try to include vegetables, protein, and carbohydrates in each meal.

    e. Use canned soups to decrease the work of cooking.

19. A male patient is diagnosed with heart failure. He is 6 feet tall and weighs 275 pounds. By losing weight, the patient will experience what effect?

    a. Increase in his cardiac contractility and myocardial oxygen demand

    b. Decrease in his systemic vascular resistance and myocardial oxygen demand

    c. Decrease in his cardiac output

    d. Reduction in his risk for hypotensive crisis

20. What will occur when oxygen is administered to a patient in heart failure? (Select all that apply.)

    a. Relieve dyspnea

    b. Decrease pulmonary oxygenation

    c. Reduce the work of breathing

    d. Decrease constriction of pulmonary blood vessels

    e. Improve oxygen delivery

Drug Therapy for Dysrhythmias

Learning Objectives

- Give an overview of the cardiac electro-physiology and an outline of specific cardiac dysrhythmias that affect rhythm, heart rate, or both.
- Describe principles of therapy in the management of dysrhythmias, including measures that do not involve antidysrhythmic drugs.
- Identify the prototype and describe the action, use, adverse effects, contraindications, and nursing implications for class I sodium channel blockers.
- Identify the prototype and outline the action, use, adverse effects, contraindications, and nursing implications for beta-adrenergic blockers.
- Identify the prototype and explain the action, use, adverse effects, contraindications, and nursing implications for potassium channel blockers.
- Identify the prototype and describe the action, use, adverse effects, contraindications, and nursing implications for calcium channel blockers.
- Describe the nursing process implications and actions related to caring for patients using selected antidysrhythmic drugs.

SECTION I: ASSESSING YOUR UNDERSTANDING

Activity A FILL IN THE BLANKS

1. _____ are abnormalities in heart rate or rhythm.

2. The mechanical or "pump" activity of the heart resides in _____ tissue.

3. _____ is the heart's ability to generate an electrical impulse.

4. Initiation of an electrical impulse depends predominately on the movement of sodium and _____ ions into a myocardial cell and movement of potassium ions out of the cell.

5. The ability of a cardiac muscle cell to respond to an electrical stimulus is called _____.

Activity B MATCHING

Match the term in Column A with the definition in Column B.

Column A	Column B
____ 1. Quinidine	a. Similar to quinidine in pharmacologic actions and may be given orally to adults with a life-threatening ventricular tachydys-rhythmias.

___ **2.** Disopyramide

___ **3.** Lidocaine

___ **4.** Dofetilide

___ **5.** Diltiazem and verapamil

b. Indicated for the maintenance of NSR in symptomatic patients who are in A-Fib of more than 1 week's duration

c. The only calcium channel blockers approved for management of dysrhythmias

d. Prototype of class IA antidysrhythmics

e. An antidysrhythmic for treating serious ventricular dysrhythmias associated with acute myocardial infarction, cardiac catheterization, cardiac surgery, and digitalis-induced ventricular dysrhythmias

Activity C SHORT ANSWERS

Briefly answer the following questions.

1. Describe how the electrophysiology of the heart causes it to beat.

2. What is automaticity, and how does it affect the heart beat?

3. What is excitability, and how does it affect the heart beat?

4. Define absolute refractory period as it relates to the electrophysiology of the heart.

5. Define conductivity as it relates to the electrophysiology of the heart.

SECTION II: APPLYING YOUR KNOWLEDGE

Activity D CASE STUDY

Consider the scenario and answer the questions.

Mr. Bennet presents to the emergency department with palpitations, dizziness, shortness of breath, and crushing chest pain. The physician diagnoses serious ventricular dysrhythmias

related to myocardial infarction and begins treatment. He orders the administration of lidocaine via an intravenous route.

1. What is the mechanism of action of lidocaine? If Mr. Bennet were to develop an atrial dysrhythmia, what would you expect the physician to do with his lidocaine prescription?

2. Initially the physician orders a bolus dose of lidocaine to treat Mr. Bennet. What effect does a bolus dose have?

3. Mr. Bennet's wife arrives and informs you that her husband is an alcoholic and is diagnosed with cirrhosis of the liver. How would treatment of this patient change based on this new information? If the patient's history revealed that he broke out in hives after receiving procaine, how would this information change the treatment approach?

4. The physician orders measurement of Mr. Bennet's lidocaine serum levels, and the laboratory indicates that the level is 0.75 mcg/ mL. What does this result tell you?

SECTION III: PRACTICING FOR NCLEX

Activity E

Answer the following questions.

1. What is a life-threatening risk associated with the use of amiodarone?

a. Decreased myocardial contractility

b. Mitral atresia

c. Ventricular irritability

d. Pulmonary toxicity

2. Amiodarone is a potassium channel blocker that prolongs conduction in all cardiac tissues. What is another effect of amiodarone? (Select all that apply.)

a. It decreases heart rate.

b. It diminishes bradydysrhythmias.

c. It increases contractility of the left ventricle.

d. It decreases contractility of the left ventricle.

e. It is vasoconstrictive.

3. The nurse is preparing to administer quinidine intravenously. At what rate will the nurse administer this medication?

a. 25 mL/min

b. 15 mL/min

c. 10 mL/min

d. 1 mL/min

4. The nurse is administering lidocaine to a patient and anticipates a reduced dosage if the patient also has which conditions? (Select all that apply.)

a. Liver disorders

b. Alzheimer's disease

c. Right-sided heart failure

d. Ventricular dysrhythmia

e. Rheumatoid arthritis

5. A patient is released from the hospital after a myocardial infarction. The physician prescribes a class II beta-adrenergic blocker drug. Why does the physician choose this drug?

a. It is effective in reducing mortality after myocardial infarction.

b. It is the drug of choice for patients who experience myocardial infarction.

c. It is the drug of choice for patients with pulmonary edema.

d. It is the drug of choice for the treatment of pneumonia.

6. Flecainide, propafenone, and moricizine are unique in that they have no effect on the repolarization phase but do have what effect?

a. They increase conduction in the ventricles.

b. They decrease conduction in the atria.

c. They increase conduction in the atria.

d. They decrease conduction in the ventricles.

7. Lidocaine is the prototype of class IB antidysrhythmics used for treating serious ventricular dysrhythmias associated with what conditions? (Select all that apply.)

a. Cardiac catheterization

b. Cardiac surgery

c. Digitalis-induced ventricular dysrhythmias

d. Atrial dysrhythmia caused by diuretics

e. Cardiac arrest

8. The physician has prescribed quinidine. The nurse knows this drug is used for what physiologic effects on the heart? (Select all that apply.)

a. It reduces automaticity.

b. It speeds conduction.

c. It prolongs the refractory period.

d. It shortens the refractory period.

e. It increases contractility.

9. The physician has ordered quinidine for a 12-year-old child. The nurse expects to administer this medication in what form?

a. Oral

b. IM

c. SC

d. IV

10. The nurse is administering quinidine to a patient who is also taking digoxin. The nurse will assess this patient for which most important adverse effect?

a. Increased anticoagulant effects

b. Increased digoxin level

c. Decreased red blood cell count

d. Decreased white blood cell count

11. The nurse is visiting the home of a patient who is prescribed antidysrhythmic medication. The nurse will teach the patient to report which possible adverse effect?

a. Increased energy

b. Improved functional status

c. Dizziness

d. Improved mentation

12. A patient is admitted to the critical care unit after experiencing a myocardial infarction and subsequent serious dysrhythmias. He is treated successfully for ventricular dysrhythmia, and the physician orders continuous IV therapy. What may cause further development of dysrhythmias?

a. Elevated LFTs

b. Hypotension

c. Electrolyte imbalances

d. Elevated blood glucose

13. A patient is prescribed digoxin. Six months later, the patient is diagnosed with impaired liver function. What would the long-term care nurse expect the physician to do?

    a. Increase the dose of digoxin

    b. Continue to monitor the patient

    c. Decrease the dosage of the digoxin

    d. Discontinue the digoxin

14. A patient is diagnosed with a ventricular dysrhythmia. The physician orders antidysrhythmic drug therapy. Three months later, the patient is diagnosed with chronic renal insufficiency. The nurse expects the physician to order what tests? (Select all that apply.)

    a. Plasma drug levels

    b. Routine ECG

    c. Monitor for symptoms of drug toxicity

    d. Routine CBC

    e. Allergy/antigen testing

15. A 75-year-old patient presents to his physician with a cardiac dysrhythmia. The physician chooses to treat the dysrhythmia because of what symptoms?

    a. Symptoms related to circulatory impairment

    b. Symptoms related to diabetic neuropathy

    c. Symptoms related to Ménière's disease

    d. Symptoms related to cardiomyopathy

16. The nurse is assessing a patient and suspects that the patient is experiencing a dysrhythmia. What patient assessments would support this condition? (Select all that apply.)

    a. Polyuria

    b. Hypotension

    c. Mental confusion

    d. Shortness of breath

    e. Leg pain

17. The nurse is caring for a 5-year-old child with a dysrhythmia. What beta-blocker does the nurse expect the physician to order for this patient?

    a. Esmolol

    b. Acebutolol

    c. Sotalol

    d. Propranolol

18. A patient is treated in the pediatric unit with adenosine. He weighs less than 50 kg. How would the nurse expect the intravenous dose to be administered?

    a. Initially, a 0.2 mg/kg IV push is given, with a maximum dose administration of 6 mg

    b. Initially, a 0.2 mg/kg IV push is given, with a maximum dose administration of 10 mg

    c. Initially, a 0.1 mg/kg IV push is given, with a maximum dose administration of 8 mg

    d. Initially, a 0.1 mg/kg IV push is given, with a maximum dose administration of 6 mg

19. A patient presents to the emergency department with dizziness, shortness of breath, and palpitations. This is the third episode of A-Fib for this patient in 1 month. A low dose of what drug is the pharmacologic choice for preventing recurrent A-Fib after electrical or pharmacologic conversion?

    a. Diltiazem

    b. Nifedipine

    c. Amiodarone

    d. Amlodipine

20. Nonpharmacologic management for PSVT with mild or moderate symptoms includes what techniques? (Select all that apply.)

    a. Valsalva's maneuver

    b. Carotid sinus massage

    c. Warm baths

    d. Brisk exercise

    e. A cup of hot decaffeinated tea

Drug Therapy for Angina

- Recognize the etiology, pathophysiology, and clinical manifestations of angina.
- Identify the prototype and describe the action, use, contraindications, adverse effects, and nursing implications for the organic nitrates.
- Identify the prototype and outline the actions, use, adverse effects, contraindications, and nursing implications for the beta-adrenergic blockers.
- Identify the prototype and describe the actions, use, adverse effects, contraindications, and nursing implications for the calcium channel blockers.
- Apply the nursing process in the care of patients with angina.

SECTION I: ASSESSING YOUR UNDERSTANDING

Activity A FILL IN THE BLANKS

1. _____ is a clinical syndrome characterized by episodes of chest pain.

2. Angina pectoris occurs when there is a deficit in _____ oxygen supply in relation to myocardial oxygen demand.

3. Angina is most often caused by atherosclerotic plaque in the coronary arteries but may also be caused by coronary _____.

4. The development and progression of atherosclerotic plaque is called _____.

5. There are three main types of angina: classic angina, _____ angina, and unstable angina.

Activity B MATCHING

Match the term in Column A with the definition in Column B.

Column A	Column B
____ **1.** Nitroglycerin (e.g., Nitro-Bid)	**a.** Used to reduce the frequency and severity of acute anginal episodes
____ **2.** Isosorbide dinitrate (Isordil)	**b.** Represents a new classification of antianginal medication, metabolic modulators, used in people with chronic angina
____ **3.** Propranolol	**c.** Beta-blocker, used to relieve acute angina pectoris, prevent exercise-induced angina, and decrease the frequency and severity of acute anginal episodes

___ **4.** Ranolazine
(Ranexa)

___ **5.** Nifedipine
(Procardia)

d. May be used in
children with
asthma who can't
tolerate beta-
adrenergic blockers

e. Used to reduce
the frequency and
severity of acute
attacks of angina

Activity C   **SHORT ANSWERS**

Briefly answer the following questions.

1. Describe typical anginal symptoms for the male.

2. Describe typical anginal symptoms for the female.

3. Describe how the elderly experience anginal symptoms.

4. Define atherosclerosis.

5. What are the causes of myocardial ischemia?

SECTION II: APPLYING YOUR KNOWLEDGE

Activity D   **CASE STUDIES**

Consider the scenarios and answer the questions.

Case Study 1

Mrs. Smith, aged 45, is diagnosed with coronary artery disease. She self-administers a calcium channel blocker, an antilipidemic, and an anti-anginal medication. You are responsible for an education plan using nonpharmacologic methods for management of her disease process.

1. Mrs. Smith has these risk factors: obesity, elevated triglycerides, reduced HDL, hypertension, and elevated fasting glucose. What are these factors indicative of?

2. Mrs. Smith asks you what nonpharmacologic management can be followed to improve her health and cardiac status. How would you respond?

Case Study 2

Mr. Newsome is diagnosed with coronary artery disease and angina. The physician orders nitrates. You are responsible for the patient's education plan.

1. Mr. Newsome is fearful that the nitrates will not control his chest pain. He asks you how they will help him when he is in pain. How would you explain the action of nitrates?

2. The physician orders sublingual nitroglycerin. What can you tell Mr. Newsome about this drug? What are some contraindications to the use of sublingual nitroglycerin?

3. During an education session, Mr. Newsome confides that he self-administers sildenafil (Viagra) periodically. What further teaching regarding nitrates is required for this patient?

SECTION III: PRACTICING FOR NCLEX

Activity E

Answer the following questions.

1. The physician prescribes a small dose of antianginal medication to a patient newly diagnosed with coronary artery disease. What is the reason for starting with a small dose?

   a. Small doses minimize angina.

   b. Small doses minimize adverse effects.

   c. Small doses minimize myocardial enervation.

   d. Small doses minimize oxygenation to the myocardium.

2. A male patient asks the nurse why the doctor has added combined aspirin, antilipemics, and antihypertensives to his medication regimen when he feels fine and hasn't experienced an anginal episode in a year. The nurse explains that this combination of drugs is given for what reason?

   a. Prevents episodic hypertensive crisis and subsequent CVA

   b. Prevents cerebral edema and subsequent CVA

   c. Prevents progression of myocardial ischemia to MI

   d. Reduces afterload that fosters an MI

3. The physician prescribes calcium channel blockers for a patient who is diagnosed with angina pectoris. What is the action of calcium channel blockers?

   a. Induce coronary artery vasospasm

   b. Increase blood pressure to increase oxygenation to the myocardium

   c. Improve blood supply to the myocardium

   d. Prevent anginal episodes

4. A male patient presents to the physician's office for a regular visit. He takes nitrates on a regular schedule for his anginal episodes and has done so for 3 years. Which statement would the nurse expect from the patient about the action of the nitrates?

   a. "They eliminate my chest pain as they always have."

   b. "They do not work as well to manage my chest pain as they used to."

   c. "They're causing dizziness, which I haven't experienced in the past."

   d. "They're causing increased chest pain and discomfort."

5. A 75-year-old patient is being treated for type 2 diabetes, hypertension, gout, angina, coronary artery disease, and peptic ulcer disease. The nurse is concerned because the patient is taking a traditional antianginal drug in combination with seven other medications. The nurse understands that what could be the consequence?

   a. A greater incidence of adverse drug effects

   b. Decreased effectiveness of the antianginal drug

   c. Decreased effectiveness of the antihypertensive

   d. A greater incidence of hyperglycemic episodes

6. A patient is at risk for silent ischemia after experiencing a transmural MI. What would the nurse expect the physician to order?

   a. Nitrates

   b. Calcium channel blockers

   c. Antilipidemics

   d. Beta-blockers

7. The nurse is aware that the use of ranolazine is contraindicated in patients who have what condition?

   a. Congestive heart failure

   b. Arterial claudication

   c. QT-interval prolongation

   d. Sinus tachycardia

8. The nurse knows that nitroglycerin can be administered in what ways? (Select all that apply.)

   a. Oral

   b. IV

   c. Transmucosal

   d. Transdermal

   e. Intrathecally

9. The nurse knows that what are the goals of antianginal drug therapy? (Select all that apply.)

   a. To relieve acute anginal pain

   b. To prevent anginal episodes

   c. To improve exercise tolerance and quality of life

   d. To prevent MI and sudden cardiac death

   e. To increase the vascularity of the heart

10. A patient is diagnosed with atherosclerosis. What would the nurse say is the most likely cause of his angina?

    a. Decreased oxygenation to the myocardium

    b. A reduction in plaque secondary to atherosclerosis

    c. Hypertension of the myocardium

    d. Decreased musculature of the myocardium related to plaque

11. What are the home care nurse's responsibilities in the care of patients who are receiving antianginal medications? (Select all that apply.)

    a. Monitoring the patient's response to antianginal medications

    b. Teaching patients and caregivers how to use, store, and replace medications to ensure a constant supply

    c. Discussing the benefits of exercise to decrease the oxygen demands of the heart

    d. Discussing circumstances for which the patient should seek emergency care

    e. Assisting patients to modify factors that contribute to angina

12. The nurse visits a patient in the home care setting. On assessment, the nurse finds that the patient has gained 6 pounds in 2 days, has 4+ pitting edema from his ankles to his patella bilaterally, and has course crackles throughout his lung fields. In the middle of the examination, the patient states that he is experiencing an anginal episode. In this case, the nurse expects what effect when the patient uses his nitroglycerin?

    a. Its effect will be impaired.

    b. It will be effective.

    c. It will cause hypertensive crisis.

    d. It will exacerbate his congestive heart failure.

13. Antianginal drugs are most often used to manage what conditions? (Select all that apply.)

    a. Severe angina

    b. Severe postural hypotension

    c. Severe hypertension

    d. Serious cardiac dysrhythmias

    e. Serious heart failure

14. A patient is prescribed sublingual nitroglycerin for treatment of angina. The nurse instructs the patient to do what if chest pain occurs?

    a. "Use the nitroglycerin if your chest pain doesn't subside on its own in 3 minutes."

    b. "If the medication burns or causes a headache, get a new prescription."

    c. "If the chest pain doesn't go away after three tablets are given 5 minutes apart, call 911."

    d. "The pills are usually good for 12 to 18 months after the prescription is filled."

15. During surgery, a child develops hypertension. The physician orders nitroglycerin IV. The initial dose will be adjusted for weight, and later doses will be adjusted to which factor?

    a. Response

    b. Weight

    c. Age

    d. Relief of chest pain

16. For relief of acute angina and for prophylaxis before events that cause acute angina, what is the primary drug of choice?

    a. Nitroglycerin

    b. Diltiazem

    c. Nifedipine

    d. Furosemide

17. A male patient does not respond to traditional treatment for his chronic angina. The physician orders ranolazine (Ranexa) and orders a baseline ECG prior to medication administration. Three months later, the physician orders a repeat ECG. For what reason is the physician monitoring the patient?

    a. Dose-dependent QT prolongation

    b. Dose-dependent ST elevation

    c. Dose-dependent ectopic beats

    d. Dose-dependent premature ventricular beats

18. A male patient presents to the physician's office for the results of his exercise-tolerance test and for modification of his medication regimen. The physician informs the patient that he experiences tachycardia that, based on his history, may precipitate anginal episodes. Based on this information, what would the nurse expect the physician to order?

    a. Nifedipine

    b. Isosorbide

    c. Propranolol

    d. Nitroglycerin

19. The nurse cautions the patient taking nitroglycerin to avoid the use of which vitamin?

    a. Vitamin A

    b. Vitamin B

    c. Vitamin D

    d. Vitamin E

20. The physician determines the maximum tolerable dose of isosorbide dinitrate (Isordil) by increasing the dose until what happens?

    a. A headache occurs.

    b. Hypertension is managed.

    c. Postural hypotension occurs.

    d. Anginal symptoms dissipate.

CHAPTER 27

Drug Therapy to Enhance the Adrenergic Response

- Identify effects produced by stimulation of alpha- and beta-adrenergic receptors.
- Discuss the use of epinephrine to treat anaphylactic shock, cardiac arrest, and bronchospasm.
- Identify patients at risk for the adverse effects associated with adrenergic drugs.
- List commonly used over-the-counter preparations and herbal preparations that contain adrenergic drugs.
- List the characteristics of adrenergic drugs in terms of etiology, pathophysiology, and clinical manifestations, along with pharmacokinetics, action, use, adverse effects, and nursing process implications in the use of adrenergic agents.
- Discuss using adrenergic drugs in special patient populations.
- Teach patients about safe, effective use of adrenergic drugs.
- Describe signs and symptoms of toxicity due to noncatecholamine adrenergic drugs and how to treat this condition.
- Understand the nursing process for using adrenergic drugs.

SECTION I: ASSESSING YOUR UNDERSTANDING

Activity A FILL IN THE BLANKS

1. _____ drugs produce effects similar to those produced by stimulation of the sympathetic nervous system and therefore have widespread effects on body tissues.

2. Adrenergic medications, such as phenylephrine, pseudoephedrine, and _____, are synthetic chemical relatives of naturally occurring neurotransmitters and hormones.

3. Specific effects of adrenergic medications depend mainly on the type of adrenergic _____ activated by the drug.

4. Some adrenergic drugs are _____ formulations of naturally occurring neurotransmitters and hormones, such as norepinephrine, epinephrine, and dopamine.

5. Major therapeutic uses and adverse effects of adrenergic medications derive from drug action on the _____, blood vessels, and lungs.

Activity B MATCHING

Match the term in Column A with the definition in Column B.

Column A

___ **1.** Epinephrine (Adrenalin)

___ **2.** Ephedrine

___ **3.** Pseudoephedrine (Sudafed)

___ **4.** Isoproterenol (Isuprel)

___ **5.** Phenylephrine (e.g., Neo-Synephrine)

Column B

a. Mixed-acting adrenergic drug that acts by stimulating alpha$_1$ and beta receptors and causing release of norepinephrine from presynaptic terminals

b. Drug stimulating alpha$_1$ and beta receptors, used as a bronchodilator and nasal decongestant

c. Synthetic catecholamine that acts on beta$_1$- and beta$_2$-adrenergic receptors

d. Synthetic drug that acts on alpha-adrenergic receptors to produce vasoconstriction

e. Prototype of the adrenergic drugs

Activity C SHORT ANSWERS

Briefly answer the following questions.

1. Identify three clinical indications for the use of adrenergic drugs.

2. What is the role of adrenergic drugs during cardiac arrest?

3. What is the role of adrenergic drugs in the treatment of asthma?

4. What is the role of adrenergic drugs in the treatment of allergic reactions?

5. Identify two miscellaneous uses of adrenergic drugs, and explain why they are used.

SECTION II: APPLYING YOUR KNOWLEDGE

Activity D CASE STUDY

Consider the scenario and answer the questions.

Mrs. Wilson, aged 35, is diagnosed with bronchial asthma. She is noncompliant with her medication regimen secondary to the cost of her prescriptions. She presents to the emergency department today with symptoms associated with respiratory distress. You note auditory expiratory wheezing, perioral cyanosis, and a pulse oximetry of 83% in room air.

1. What would you expect to be the physician's treatment of choice to reduce bronchospasm?

2. When you interview Mrs. Wilson, you learn that she uses Primatene Mist as an over-the-counter asthma treatment at home. Why might you be concerned regarding over-the-counter asthma treatments? What are possible advantages of this approach?

3. What are the established treatment guidelines for patients with asthma?

4. What is another concern about products such as Primatene Mist?

5. What is a common ingredient in OTC anti-asthma tablets (e.g., Bronkaid, Primatene)?

6. What patient populations should not take over-the-counter asthma treatments on a regular basis?

SECTION III: PRACTICING FOR NCLEX

Activity E

Answer the following questions.

1. The nurse is assessing a patient in the emergency department who has taken an overdose of phenylephrine. What symptoms should the nurse be alert for in this patient? (Select all that apply.)

a. Dizziness

b. Headache

c. Polyuria

d. Pulmonary edema

e. Seizures

2. Which of the following receptors does phenylephrine stimulate?
   a. Alpha$_2$
   b. Beta$_1$
   c. Beta$_2$
   d. Alpha$_1$

3. Contraindications to adrenergic drugs include what conditions? (Select all that apply.)
   a. Cardiac dysrhythmias
   b. Hyperthyroidism
   c. Hypersensitivity to sulfites
   d. Hypersensitivity to penicillins
   e. Hypotension

4. The nurse understands that local anesthetics containing adrenergics should not be used on which part of the body?
   a. The abdomen
   b. The chest
   c. The back
   d. The fingers

5. The nurse knows that what is an added benefit of epinephrine in cardiac arrest situations due to asystole or pulseless electrical activity?
   a. Increase oxygenation to the brain
   b. Stimulate electrical and mechanical activity
   c. Reduce seizure activity
   d. Increase oxygenation to the myocardium

6. The nurse would contact the physician before administering an adrenergic drug to a patient who is also taking which drug?
   a. Antibiotic
   b. MAO inhibitor
   c. Diuretic
   d. Analgesic

7. Use of beta-adrenergic blocking drugs (e.g., propranolol) may have what effect?
   a. Increasing the effectiveness of epinephrine in cases of anaphylaxis
   b. No change in the effectiveness of epinephrine
   c. Decreasing the effectiveness of epinephrine in cases of anaphylaxis
   d. None of the above; epinephrine is contraindicated when the patient is taking beta-adrenergic drugs

8. A female patient is taking propranolol for migraine prophylaxis. She presents to the emergency department in cardiac distress. The nurse is aware that the dosage of epinephrine prescribed for this patient may need to be altered in what way?
   a. Higher-than-usual doses of epinephrine
   b. Lower-than-usual doses of epinephrine
   c. The same dose of epinephrine as stated in the emergency department protocol
   d. Discontinuation of epinephrine

9. Prior to beginning therapy with an adrenergic agent, the nurse would expect to obtain what assessments? (Select all that apply.)
   a. Vital signs
   b. Urinalysis
   c. Hearing screen
   d. Blood glucose
   e. Arterial blood gases

10. The nurse is aware that epinephrine may be administered in what ways? (Select all that apply.)
    a. PO
    b. Topical
    c. IV
    d. Inhalation
    e. Sublingual

11. A male patient presents to the physician's office with allergic rhinitis. What would the nurse expect the physician to order?
    a. An adrenergic drug
    b. A bronchodilator
    c. An antihistamine
    d. An anticholinergic drug

12. A 75-year-old male patient is diagnosed with chronic obstructive lung disease; he also has a history of cardiac dysrhythmias, hyperlipidemia, and hypertension. His physician orders a metered-dose inhaler. The nurse will teach the patient to report which symptom to the physician?
    a. Gastrointestinal upset
    b. Skin lesions
    c. Persistent edema
    d. Palpitations

13. A male patient is diagnosed with hepatitis C. He regularly takes an adrenergic medication. Secondary to the diagnosis of hepatitis C, what would the nurse expect the physician to do?

    a. Increase the dosage of the adrenergic medication

    b. Make no change in the dosage of the adrenergic medication

    c. Discontinue the adrenergic medication

    d. Decrease the dose of the adrenergic medication

14. A male patient is diagnosed with type 2 diabetes, asthmatic bronchitis, benign prostatic hyperplasia, and hyperlipidemia. He takes an adrenergic medication as part of his daily drug regimen. As part of his education plan, which of the following signs and symptoms would the nurse teach the patient to observe for?

    a. Muscle cramping

    b. Indigestion

    c. Painful urination

    d. Constipation

15. A male patient is prescribed an adrenergic ophthalmic medication. What should the nurse include in the teaching plan?

    a. The drug is only absorbed locally.

    b. Side effects are limited to inflammation of the conjunctiva.

    c. Allergic and adverse reactions are rare.

    d. Hypertension may be a side effect of the medication.

16. The nurse encourages people to limit use of OTC epinephrine products to prevent the occurrence of what problem?

    a. Increased body temperature

    b. Pruritus

    c. Tolerance

    d. Weight gain

17. A 6-year-old patient is given parenteral epinephrine for the treatment of bronchospasm. The nurse understands that children may experience what condition secondary to parenteral epinephrine?

    a. Hypotension

    b. Rebound shortness of breath

    c. Syncope

    d. Rhinitis

18. Ephedrine and ephedra-containing herbal preparations are often abused as an alternative to amphetamines. What substances are identified as herbal preparations? (Select all that apply.)

    a. Ma huang

    b. Herbal ecstasy

    c. Crack

    d. Smack

    e. Black tar

19. A male patient takes a nasal adrenergic medication for his allergic rhinitis. Part of the nurse's education plan should include information that overuse of adrenergic drugs may cause what effect?

    a. Tolerance

    b. Addiction

    c. Increased effectiveness

    d. Decreased congestion

20. The usual goal of vasopressor drug therapy is to maintain tissue perfusion and a mean arterial pressure of at least what level?

    a. 40 to 60 mm Hg

    b. 20 to 40 mm Hg

    c. 60 to 89 mm Hg

    d. 80 to 100 mm Hg

CHAPTER 28

Drug Therapy for Hypertension

Learning Objectives

- Describe factors that control blood pressure.
- Describe how hypertension is classified.
- Discuss nonpharmacologic measures to control hypertension.
- Identify the prototype and describe the action, use, contraindications, adverse effects, and nursing implications of the angiotensin-converting enzyme inhibitors.
- Identify the prototype and describe the action, use, contraindications, adverse effects, and nursing implications of the angiotensin II receptor blockers.
- Describe the rationale for using combination drugs in the management of hypertension.
- Review the effects of alpha-adrenergic blockers, beta-adrenergic blockers, calcium channel blockers, and diuretics in the management of hypertension.
- Apply the nursing process in the care of patients with hypertension.

SECTION I: ASSESSING YOUR UNDERSTANDING

Activity A FILL IN THE BLANKS

1. _____ blood pressure reflects the force exerted on arterial walls by blood flow.

2. Blood pressure normally remains constant because of _____ mechanisms that adjust blood flow to meet tissue needs.

3. The two major determinants of arterial blood pressure are _____ (systolic pressure) and peripheral vascular resistance (diastolic pressure).

4. _____ equals the product of the heart rate and stroke volume.

5. _____ is the amount of blood ejected with each heartbeat (~60–90 mL).

Activity B MATCHING

Match the term in Column A with the definition in Column B.

Column A	Column B
____ 1. ARBs	a. Inhibit activity of the SNS
____ 2. Antiadrenergic (sympatholytic) drugs	b. Dilate peripheral arteries and decrease peripheral vascular resistance by relaxing vascular smooth muscle
____ 3. Beta-adrenergic blocking agents	c. Cause antihypertensive effects usually attributed to sodium and water depletion

____ **4.** Calcium channel blockers

____ **5.** Diuretics

d. Developed to block the strong blood pressure–raising effects of angiotensin II

e. Decrease heart rate, force of myocardial contraction, cardiac output, and renin release from the kidneys

Activity C SHORT ANSWERS

Briefly answer the following questions.

1. Define and discuss autoregulation.

2. Define and discuss the action of histamines.

3. What is the role of kinins as they relate to the vascular system?

4. What is the role of serotonin as it relates to the vascular system?

5. What is the role of prostaglandins as they relate to the vascular system?

SECTION II: APPLYING YOUR KNOWLEDGE

Activity D CASE STUDIES

Consider the scenarios and answer the questions.

Case Study 1

Mrs. Bartley has her blood pressure taken at the local elder health clinic. Her blood pressure at that time is 145/90. She is concerned because she never had an elevated blood pressure before. She calls her physician's office and asks for medication to treat her hypertension.

1. What is the definition of hypertension?

2. Mrs. Bartley is diagnosed with secondary hypertension. What are some causes of secondary hypertension?

Case Study 2

Mrs. Goodman, aged 70, is diagnosed with isolated systolic hypertension.

1. What would you expect her blood pressure to be?

2. You understand that hypertension alters cardiovascular function by increasing the workload of the heart. What does this cause?

SECTION III: PRACTICING FOR NCLEX

Activity E

Answer the following questions.

1. A male patient is diagnosed with severe hypertension. The physician prescribes minoxidil. Three months later, the patient presents to the emergency department with angina. The nurse is concerned because minoxidil can have what effect?

    a. Exacerbate angina and precipitate effusion

    b. Cause rebound hypertension when a dose is missed

    c. Precipitate cardiovascular accidents

    d. Exacerbate pancreatitis

2. A 35-year-old female patient controls the symptoms of her cardiovascular disease with ACE inhibitors. She discovers that she is pregnant and contacts her primary physician regarding her medication regimen. What would the nurse expect the physician to do?

    a. Discontinue the drug

    b. Increase the dosage of the drug

    c. Decrease the dosage of the drug

    d. Maintain the current dosage of the drug

3. A male patient's friend tells him to stop taking his metoprolol because he read that it causes cancer. The nurse encourages the patient to consult his physician, because abrupt withdrawal from the drug may cause what effect?

    a. Postural hypotension and falls

    b. Bradycardia

    c. Exacerbation of his angina

    d. Atrial dysrhythmias

4. African Americans are more likely to have severe hypertension and to require multiple drugs, for what reasons? (Select all that apply.)

   a. Low circulating renin

   b. Increased salt sensitivity

   c. A higher incidence of obesity

   d. Increased potassium sensitivity

   e. Increased level of anxiety

5. A male patient who is an Asian executive visiting the United States presents to the emergency department with a severe headache and an elevated blood pressure. He is admitted to the hospital for treatment and regulation of his medication regimen. The patient is concerned because the dosage prescribed for his antihypertensive medication is lower than what he researched on the Internet. What is an accurate response for the nurse to make?

   a. "There is an error on the prescription."

   b. "I will contact the physician immediately."

   c. "People of Asian descent excrete the drugs more rapidly, so the doses prescribed are smaller."

   d. "People of Asian descent excrete the drugs more slowly, so the doses prescribed are smaller."

6. A 45-year-old patient is diagnosed with high-renin hypertension. What type of drug would the nurse expect the physician to order?

   a. ACE inhibitors

   b. Beta-blockers

   c. Diuretics

   d. Calcium channel blockers

7. The nurse has admitted a patient with type 1 diabetes mellitus who has been prescribed captopril for treatment of hypertension. The nurse knows this medication is used in patients with diabetes for what reason?

   a. It reduces fasting blood glucose.

   b. It will prevent the development of blindness.

   c. It reduces proteinuria.

   d. It decreases peripheral tissue ischemia.

8. The nurse instructs a male patient to administer his alpha$_1$-adrenergic receptor blocking agent at night. What does this practice help to minimize?

   a. Postural hypertension

   b. First-dose phenomenon

   c. Hypoglycemic reaction

   d. Hyperglycemic reaction

9. Key behavioral determinants of blood pressure are related to what factor?

   a. Minimal body mass

   b. Dietary consumption of calories and salt

   c. Dietary consumption of sugars and fat

   d. Comorbidities

10. A 57-year-old patient presents to the physician's office for the second consecutive month with an elevated blood pressure. His hypertension has been successfully managed with his current drug regimen for 2 years. When asked about his drug history, he states that the only new drug is the herb, yohimbe. The nurse understands that yohimbe is what?

    a. An over-the-counter antihyperglycemic

    b. A central nervous system stimulant

    c. An autonomic nervous system stimulant

    d. A diuretic

11. How can the home care nurse assist the patient or the patient's family members who have hypertension? (Select all that apply.)

    a. Modification of drug dosage

    b. Monitoring for drug effects

    c. Promoting compliance with the prescribed pharmacologic modifications

    d. Promoting compliance with the prescribed lifestyle modifications

    e. Providing financial assistance with daily expenses

12. A patient presents to the emergency department in hypertensive crisis. The nurse anticipates that the physician will order medication that will lower the blood pressure yet prevent stroke, MI, and acute renal failure, within what period of time?

    a. Immediately

    b. Within 5 minutes

    c. Within 7 minutes

    d. Over several minutes to several hours

13. A male patient is admitted to the critical care unit with severe hypertension and myocardial ischemia. The nurse understands that the physician orders nitroglycerin titrated according to what factor?

    a. Amount of chest pain or pressure

    b. Weight

    c. Blood pressure response

    d. Renal function

14. A male patient presents to the emergency department with a significantly elevated blood pressure. The physician chooses oral captopril for treatment and prescribes what dosage every 1 to 2 hours?

    a. 25 to 50 mg

    b. 10 to 20 mg

    c. 5 to 10 mg

    d. 50 to 75 mg

15. A male patient presents to the physician's office for his annual visit. His prescription regimen includes ACE inhibitors. The nurse expects the physician to perform what action if this patient's liver enzymes are elevated?

    a. Increase the dosage of the drug

    b. Decrease the dosage of the drug

    c. Discontinue the drug

    d. Identify a source for the elevation other than the ACE inhibitors

16. A female patient successfully treats her heart failure with an ACE inhibitor. She does not have evidence of severe or preexisting renal impairment. Her most recent laboratory results indicate increased BUN and serum creatinine levels. What medication modification does the nurse expect that the physician will make for this patient?

    a. Increase the dosage of the drug

    b. Decrease the dosage of the drug

    c. Discontinue the drug

    d. Maintain the dosage of the drug

17. A patient has come to the clinic for the past 7 months with elevated blood pressure. The patient has now been prescribed three different antihypertensives as well as a diuretic. The nurse knows that what other factors may be contributing to the patient's consistent hypertension? (Select all that apply.)

    a. Meditation

    b. Walking program

    c. Nasal decongestant

    d. Herbal supplement

    e. OTC appetite suppressant

18. Nonpharmacologic management should be tried alone or with drug therapy. What methods of nonpharmacologic management are used in the treatment of hypertension? (Select all that apply.)

    a. Weight reduction

    b. Limited alcohol intake

    c. Moderate sodium restriction

    d. Diet including no concentrated sweets

    e. Hot tub soaks

19. The National High Blood Pressure Education Program Working Group on High Blood Pressure in Children and Adolescents states that prehypertension in children is defined as an average of systolic or diastolic pressures within what range?

    a. 85th to 90th percentiles

    b. 90th to 95th percentiles

    c. 80th to 90th percentiles

    d. 80th to 85th percentiles

20. The nurse would encourage patients with prehypertension to follow what type of diet?

    a. High-sodium diet

    b. DASH diet

    c. Restricted-calorie diet

    d. High-protein diet

CHAPTER 29

Drug Therapy for Nasal Congestion

Learning Objectives

- Describe the characteristics of selected upper respiratory disorders and symptoms.
- Identify the prototype drug for each drug class.
- Discuss nasal decongestants in terms of their action, use, contraindications, adverse effects, and nursing implications.
- Describe antitussive agents in terms of their action, use, contraindications, adverse effects, and nursing implications.
- Describe expectorants in terms of their action, use, contraindications, adverse effects, and nursing implications.
- Discuss mucolytics in terms of their action, use, contraindications, adverse effects, and nursing implications.
- Discuss the advantages and disadvantages of using combination products to treat the common cold.
- Understand how to use the nursing process in the care of patients receiving nasal decongestants, antitussives, expectorants, and mucolytic agents.

SECTION I: ASSESSING YOUR UNDERSTANDING

Activity A   FILL IN THE BLANKS

1. The _____, a viral infection of the upper respiratory tract, is the most common respiratory tract infection.

2. Colds can be caused by many types of viruses, most often the _____.

3. _____ is inflammation of the paranasal sinuses, air cells that connect with the nasal cavity and are lined by similar mucosa.

4. _____ (inflammation and congestion of nasal mucosa) and upper respiratory tract infections are the most common causes of sinusitis.

5. _____ results from dilation of the blood vessels in the nasal mucosa and engorgement of the mucous membranes with blood.

Activity B   MATCHING

Match the term in Column A with the definition in Column B.

Column A

____ 1. Nasal decongestants

____ 2. Antitussive agents

____ 3. Expectorants

Column B

a. Agents given orally to liquefy respiratory secretions and allow for their easier removal

b. Used to reduce the incidence and severity of colds and influenza

c. Administered by inhalation to liquefy mucus in the respiratory tract

____ **4.** Mucolytics

____ **5.** Vitamin C

d. Suppress a cough by depressing the cough center in the medulla oblongata or the cough receptors in the throat, trachea, or lungs

e. Used to relieve nasal obstruction and discharge

4. The ingredients in multisystem cold and allergy remedies are often difficult to identify. Why is this?

5. Mrs. Hoyer's friend received an antiviral drug from her physician for the treatment of her viral respiratory tract infection. She asks why the physician won't prescribe it for her. How would you respond?

Activity C   SHORT ANSWERS

Briefly answer the following questions.

1. How is the common cold transmitted from one person to another?

2. What is the primary cause of sinusitis?

3. Define rhinorrhea.

4. Define rhinitis.

5. What effect does a cough have on the respiratory tract?

SECTION II: APPLYING YOUR KNOWLEDGE

Activity D   CASE STUDY

Consider the scenario and answer the questions.

Mrs. Hoyer develops signs and symptoms of the common cold. The purpose of the patient's visit is to request a medication to shorten the cold and alleviate the symptoms. The physician suggests over-the-counter treatments. You are responsible for the education plan.

1. What do over-the-counter medications commonly include?

2. Mrs. Hoyer wishes to purchase antihistamines to inhibit her rhinitis. You suggest that she avoid antihistamines because, although they dry nasal secretions, they can have other effects. What are these effects? What other information can you give Mrs. Hoyer about OTC cold medications, especially those that are advertised as "maximum strength?"

3. If Mrs. Hoyer wants a product with pseudo-ephedrine in it, how would you advise her?

SECTION III: PRACTICING FOR NCLEX

Activity E

Answer the following questions.

1. A female patient calls the pediatrician's office for a suggestion regarding the best over-the-counter cough and cold medicine for her 6-month-old child. The physician advises against the medication, for what reason?

a. The medication is not effective for croup.

b. Misuse could result in overdose.

c. The medication is contraindicated for the child's symptoms.

d. The medication is contraindicated for viral infections.

2. A male patient presents to the physician's office for his annual visit. When questioned about over-the-counter medication use, he states that he uses *Echinacea* to prevent colds. What statement is true about *Echinacea*?

a. He is healthier because he uses the *Echinacea*.

b. *Echinacea* is the OTC drug of choice for prevention of viral infections.

c. To be effective, *Echinacea* must be taken daily regardless of symptoms.

d. There is limited or no support for the use of *Echinacea* to prevent or treat symptoms of the common cold.

3. First-generation antihistamines may be effective against what symptoms? (Select all that apply.)

a. Sneezing

b. Rhinorrhea

c. Cough

d. Congestion

e. Fever

4. A male patient presents to the physician's office with complaints of inability to breathe freely. When the nurse reviews his use of over-the-counter medications, it is discovered that the patient routinely uses nasal spray three times a day for 1 year. The nurse knows that what may be causing this patient's continuous nasal congestion?

   a. Chronic nasal polyps

   b. Burning of the nares secondary to chronic use of nasal sprays

   c. Rebound nasal swelling

   d. Damage of the nasal concha

5. What home remedies are effective for mouth dryness and cough? (Select all that apply.)

   a. Administration of over-the-counter antihistamine

   b. Adequate fluid intake

   c. Humidification of the environment

   d. Sucking on hard candy or throat lozenges

   e. Swishing the mouth with astringent mouthwash.

6. A male patient presents to the physician's office with a chronic cough. What condition predisposes the patient to secretion retention?

   a. Chronic lozenge use

   b. Chronic use of antihistamines

   c. Intermittent use of exercise equipment

   d. Debilitation

7. A male patient is diagnosed with chronic bronchitis. What would the nurse expect to be one of his physical complaints?

   a. Rhinitis

   b. Rhinorrhea

   c. Retention of secretions

   d. Chronic nasal swelling

8. A patient's physician will not prescribe antibiotics for the patient's upper respiratory tract infection, for what reason?

   a. Most upper respiratory tract infections are viral in origin.

   b. The infection is resistant to antibiotics.

   c. Culture of sputum is inconclusive.

   d. The infection is multibacterial.

9. A male patient presents to the physician's office with symptoms of a common cold. He asks the nurse to suggest over-the-counter drugs to alleviate his symptoms. Before recommending an over-the-counter medication, what action should the nurse take?

   a. Obtain a prescription from the physician

   b. Obtain a complete drug history

   c. Consult the pharmacist

   d. Research medications covered by the patient's HMO

10. A 75-year-old patient is self-administering an oral nasal decongestant. The nurse is concerned that the patient is at risk for what conditions? (Select all that apply.)

    a. Somnolence

    b. Hypertension

    c. Nervousness

    d. Impaired gastric motility

11. A female patient calls the pediatrician's office because her child is experiencing cold symptoms and has an oral temperature of 99.9°F. The nurse expects the physician to take what action?

    a. Treat the fever only if it exceeds 100.3

    b. Treat the fever only if it exceeds 101

    c. Treat the fever only if the child is restless

    d. Treat the fever only if the child develops nasal drainage

12. A female patient calls the pediatrician because her baby is experiencing nasal congestion and cannot nurse. The nurse would expect the physician to order what to be given just before feeding time?

    a. Saline nasal solution

    b. Diphenhydramine nasal solution

    c. Phenylephrine nasal solution

    d. Chlorpheniramine nasal solution

13. A male patient calls the physician because his baby cannot sleep. When asked what medications his baby takes, he responds that the only drug is a topical agent to prevent nasal congestion just before breast-feeding. The nurse suspects that what condition is occurring?

    a. Central nervous stimulation

    b. Insufficient breast milk intake

    c. Irritable baby syndrome

    d. Child abuse or neglect

14. A female patient calls the pediatrician's office because her child is complaining of a sore throat. The nurse anticipates the physician will take what action?

    a. Order an antibiotic

    b. Order an antitussive

    c. Request a list of drug allergies

    d. Request a throat culture

15. A female patient's four children, aged 12 through 18, have symptoms of a common cold. She calls the physician's office regarding advice for the most economical over-the-counter cold remedy. The nurse informs the mother that which product is the least expensive to purchase?

    a. Combination products

    b. Single-drug formulations

    c. Nasal formulas

    d. Cough and cold formulas

16. The nursing instructor is discussing the use of nasal decongestants and shares what reason for their effectiveness?

    a. They are absorbed systemically.

    b. They treat multiple symptoms in a cost-effective manner.

    c. They come into direct contact with nasal mucosa.

    d. Their effects last for 48 to 72 hours.

17. A patient calls the clinic and complains of symptoms of a cold. The patient is most concerned because the cold symptoms are preventing him from sleeping. The nurse would inform the patient that what medication relieves cold symptoms and aids sleep?

    a. Diphenhydramine

    b. Phenergan

    c. Epinephrine

    d. Antihistamine

18. A 79-year-old patient calls the clinic requesting advice for something that will relieve nasal congestion. The nurse is aware that oral decongestants may cause which adverse effects in older adults? (Select all that apply.)

    a. Excessive sleepiness

    b. Hypertension

    c. Heart rhythm abnormalities

    d. Bradycardia

    e. Nervousness

19. Cough syrups serve as vehicles for antitussive drugs and also may exert antitussive effects of their own by doing what?

    a. Precipitating an anticholinergic reaction

    b. Reducing the bacterial load in the respiratory tract

    c. Soothing irritated pharyngeal mucosa

    d. Thinning pharyngeal mucus

20. The nurse would caution patients with which disorders to avoid the use of over-the-counter pseudoephedrine? (Select all that apply.)

    a. Diabetes

    b. Cardiovascular disorders

    c. Chronic sinusitis

    d. Glaucoma

    e. Diverticulosis

CHAPTER 30

Drug Therapy to Decrease Histamine Effects and Allergic Response

Learning Objectives

- Delineate the effects of histamine on selected body tissues.
- Describe the types of hypersensitivity or allergic reactions.
- Identify the effects of histamine that are blocked by histamine1 (H_1) receptor antagonist drugs.
- Discuss first-generation H_1 receptor antagonists in terms of prototype, indications and contraindications, major adverse effects, interactions, and administration.
- Describe second-generation H_1 receptor antagonists in terms of prototype, indications and contraindications, major adverse effects, interactions, and administration.
- Understand how to use the nursing process in the care of patients receiving antihistamines.

SECTION I: ASSESSING YOUR UNDERSTANDING

Activity A   FILL IN THE BLANKS

1. _____ are drugs that antagonize the action of histamine.

2. _____ is the first chemical mediator to be released in immune and inflammatory responses.

3. Histamine is discharged from _____ and basophils in response to certain stimuli (e.g., allergic reactions, cellular injury, extreme cold).

4. _____ or allergic reactions are exaggerated responses by the immune system that produce tissue injury and may cause serious disease.

5. _____ receptors are located mainly on smooth muscle cells in blood vessels and the respiratory and GI tracts.

Activity B   MATCHING

Match the term in Column A with the definition in Column B.

Column A

____ 1. Diphenhydramine (Benadryl)

____ 2. Hydroxyzine (Vistaril) and promethazine (Phenergan)

Column B

a. Second-generation H_1 antagonists

b. The only OTC antihistamine formulated as a nasal spray for topical use

_____ 3. Loratadine (Claritin) and cetirizine (Zyrtec)

_____ 4. Azelastine (Astelin)

_____ 5. Desloratadine (Clarinex)

c. The prototype of first-generation antihistamines

d. An active metabolite of loratadine

e. Strong CNS depressants causing extensive drowsiness

Activity C SHORT ANSWERS

Briefly answer the following questions.

1. Where is histamine located in the human body?

2. What happens to the human body when H_2 receptors are stimulated?

3. Define hypersensitivity or allergic reactions.

4. What is the cause of type I immune response (also called immediate hypersensitivity)?

5. Give an example of a type II immune response.

SECTION II: APPLYING YOUR KNOWLEDGE

Activity D CASE STUDY

Consider the scenario and answer the questions.

Mr. Eden presents to the physician's office with complaints of epistaxis secondary to inflamed nasal mucosa. After evaluation by the physician, Mr. Eden is diagnosed with allergic rhinitis. You are responsible for his education plan.

1. Mr. Eden is upset because the physician did not prescribe antibiotics for his rhinitis. How would you respond?

2. Mr. Eden is referred to an allergist for an analysis of the causes of his symptoms. He is diagnosed with seasonal disease (hay fever). Explain the difference between seasonal disease and perennial disease that is seasonal.

3. Explain allergic rhinitis in terms of an immune response.

4. In people with allergies, mast cells and basophils are increased in both number and reactivity. What type of response would you expect to occur due to the increase?

5. Based on his diagnosis of allergic rhinitis, what other conditions is Mr. Eden at risk for?

SECTION III: PRACTICING FOR NCLEX

Activity E

Answer the following questions.

1. A male patient's son is diagnosed with an allergy to peanuts. What is the most important instruction the nurse will give to the father?

   a. Provide his son with an emergency contact in case of exposure

   b. Provide those in contact with his son with an emergency plan

   c. Avoid situations in which his son may be exposed to peanuts

   d. Give all who are in contact with his son azelastine in case of exposure

2. The nurse is aware that systemic lupus erythematosus may be induced by which less commonly used antihistamine?

   a. Loratidine (Claritin)

   b. Diphenhydramine (Benadryl)

   c. Hydralazine (Vistaril)

   d. Brompheniramine (LoHist)

3. A male patient presents to the physician's office with allergy-related symptoms that interfere with his job as a car salesman. What nasal spray does the nurse expect the physician to order?

   a. Azelastine (Astelin)

   b. Loratadine (Claritin)

   c. Cetirizine (Zyrtec)

   d. Desloratadine (Clarinex)

4. Second-generation H_1 antagonists cause less CNS depression because they are selective for peripheral H_1 receptors and because of which other property?

   a. They are excreted by the renal system.

   b. They are metabolized by the liver.

   c. They cross the blood–brain barrier.

   d. They do not cross the blood–brain barrier.

5. A female patient is prescribed a first-generation antihistamine for her allergies. The nurse would expect her to experience what adverse effect?

a. Diarrhea

b. Incontinence

c. Dry mouth

d. Slurred speech

6. A female patient administers diphenhydramine to her child, who experiences seasonal allergies, before his first baseball game. What may the child experience if he has a paradoxical effect to the medication?

a. Hyperactivity

b. Exacerbation of allergic symptoms

c. Decreased mental alertness

d. Poor reflexes

7. Which food allergens have a higher inherent risk for triggering anaphylaxis? (Select all that apply.)

a. Shellfish

b. Egg

c. Milk

d. Butter

e. Nuts

8. What causes the inflammation of nasal mucosa that is seen in allergic rhinitis?

a. Type III hypersensitivity reaction to inhaled allergens

b. Type II hypersensitivity reaction to inhaled allergens

c. Type IV hypersensitivity reaction to inhaled allergens

d. Type I hypersensitivity reaction to inhaled allergens

9. The nurse is aware that patients who use OTC fexofenadine would use which class of antibacterial that would cause an increased plasma concentration of the fexofenadine?

a. Penicillins

b. Cephalosporins

c. Macrolides

d. Tetracyclines

10. The nurse is visiting a female patient in her home for treatment of a wound. The patient is concerned that her husband, a truck driver, is bothered by his seasonal allergies. A friend suggested diphenhydramine. What is the nurse's best response?

a. "The drug may cause drowsiness and make driving unsafe."

b. "The drug is safe in small doses."

c. "The drug is safe if it is purchased over the counter."

d. "The drug may exacerbate the allergies if used routinely."

11. A male patient presents to the emergency department with symptoms of a gastrointestinal bleed. The physician orders a blood transfusion. The patient has a history of anaphylaxis. The physician orders the administration of what drug before the blood transfusion?

a. Cetirizine

b. Desloratadine

c. Azelastine

d. Diphenhydramine

12. A female patient is diagnosed with type 2 diabetes mellitus, hyperlipidemia, and mild hepatic impairment. She presents to the emergency department after taking promethazine, obtained from a friend, for motion sickness. The nurse would expect what adverse effect?

a. Hypotension

b. Cholecystitis

c. Cholestatic jaundice

d. Abnormal hemoglobin

13. A female patient is diagnosed with severe kidney failure. The nurse would expect the physician to order diphenhydramine with what dosing interval?

a. 12 to 18 hours

b. 2 to 4 hours

c. 4 to 6 hours

d. 24 to 48 hours

14. What is one of the benefits related to second-generation antihistamine administration in older adults?

a. They do not impair thinking.

b. They reduce the number of falls in patients diagnosed with osteoporosis.

c. They increase the ability of patients with dementia to perform ADLs.

d. They do not affect oxygenation.

15. A 74-year-old patient is diagnosed with hypertension, hyperlipidemia, angina, and gout. He presents to the physician's office with complaints of seasonal allergies. His daughter has diphenhydramine at home, and he asks if it is safe for him to take it. The nurse is concerned because first-generation antihistamines may cause what adverse effects in older adults? (Select all that apply.)

a. Hypotension

b. Hypertension

c. Syncope

d. Myocardial hypoxia

e. Pulmonary edema

16. A male patient presents to the emergency department with his 4-year-old child. The child self-administered diphenhydramine of an unknown quantity. In overdosage of diphenhydramine, the nurse is aware that the child may experience what problems? (Select all that apply.)

a. Hallucinations

b. Hypotension

c. Dizziness

d. Convulsions

e. Headache

17. A male patient asks the nurse whether antihistamines will help him cope with the symptoms of the common cold. What is the nurse's best response?

a. "Antihistamines are recommended."

b. "Antihistamines do not relieve symptoms."

c. "Antihistamines should be taken only before bed."

d. "Antihistamines should be taken only if you are not driving."

18. A female patient is concerned that the antihistamine ordered by the physician is not relieving her symptoms and she will not find a medication to meet her needs. What is the nurse's best response?

a. "Antihistamines may not be the answer to your allergic symptoms."

b. "A patient who doesn't respond to one antihistamine is usually resistant to others."

c. "A patient may respond better to one antihistamine than to another."

d. "I will ask the physician to order another type of drug."

19. The nurse is providing instructions to a patient who will be taking second-generation antihistamines at home. Which statement by the patient indicates a need for further instruction?

a. "If I miss a dose of medication, I will wait until the next scheduled time to take the medication."

b. "I will take this medication with apple juice."

c. "I will be careful to take the medication exactly as it comes."

d. "I will check the prescription bottle and follow the directions carefully."

20. The physician has ordered promethazine (Phenergan) for a patient who is having a severe allergic reaction. The nurse is aware that this medication is also used to treat what condition?

a. Central nervous system depression

b. Hypotension

c. Nausea and vomiting

d. Joint pain

Drug Therapy for Asthma and Bronchoconstriction

Learning Objectives

- Describe asthma and bronchoconstriction in terms of their pathophysiology.
- Compare and contrast the short-acting (rescue) and the long-term maintenance inhaled beta$_2$-adrenergic agonists.
- Identify the prototype drug from each drug class used to treat asthma and bronchoconstriction.
- Describe drugs used to treat asthma and bronchoconstriction in terms of mechanism of action, indications for use, major adverse effects, and nursing implications.
- Understand how to use the nursing process in the care of patients with asthma and broncho-constriction.

SECTION I: ASSESSING YOUR UNDERSTANDING

Activity A FILL IN THE BLANKS

1. _____ is defined as asthma resulting from repeated and prolonged exposure to industrial inhalants.

2. Asthma is an airway disorder characterized by bronchoconstriction, inflammation, and _____ to various stimuli.

3. _____ is a high-pitched, whistling sound caused by turbulent airflow through an obstructed airway.

4. Acute symptoms of asthma may be precipitated by numerous stimuli, and hyperreactivity to such stimuli may initiate both inflammation and _____.

5. Some patients are allergic to _____ and may experience life-threatening asthma attacks if they ingest foods processed with these preservatives (e.g., beer, wine, dried fruit).

Activity B MATCHING

Match the term in Column A with the definition in Column B.

Column A

___ 1. Albuterol and levalbuterol

___ 2. Formoterol and salmeterol

___ 3. Beclomethasone, budesonide, flunisolide, fluticasone, mometasone, and triamcinolone

___ 4. Leukotrienes

___ 5. Theophylline

Column B

a. Topical corticosteroids for inhalation

b. Strong chemical mediators of bronchoconstriction and inflammation

c. Short-acting beta$_2$-adrenergic agonists

d. The main xanthine used clinically

e. Used only for prophylaxis of acute bronchoconstriction

Activity C SHORT ANSWERS

Briefly answer the following questions.

1. Describe the symptoms associated with asthma.

2. Discuss the variance in incidence and severity of asthma symptoms.

3. What impact do viral infections have on the development of asthma?

4. What instructions regarding dietary restrictions should be discussed with patients diagnosed with severe asthma?

5. What symptoms related to GERD may be associated with asthma?

SECTION II: APPLYING YOUR KNOWLEDGE

Activity D CASE STUDY

Consider the scenario and answer the questions.

Mrs. Livingston presents to the emergency department with status asthmaticus. She is diagnosed with an exacerbation of serious respiratory disease, not controlled by her current treatment regimen. Once her condition has stabilized, she is sent home. In addition to the first-line anti-asthmatic, the physician orders theophylline. You are responsible for the patient's discharge teaching.

1. Discuss what you know about the mechanism of action for theophylline.

2. Mrs. Livingston is diagnosed with mild to moderate congestive heart failure in addition to her respiratory disease. What would you expect the physician to do?

3. Mrs. Livingston complains that she has a more productive cough since she began using theophylline. She finds this annoying and states that the medication is not working as it should. How would you explain this development to the patient?

4. What should you include in your teaching plan for Mrs. Livingston?

5. If you were to discover that Mrs. Livingston is an alcoholic, what concerns would you have about her drug prescription? Patients with

alcohol addiction are at risk for development of acute gastritis. How would this development affect the prescription of theophylline?

SECTION III: PRACTICING FOR NCLEX

Activity E

Answer the following questions.

1. A female patient presents to the emergency department with acutely deteriorating asthma. Her husband shows the nurse salmeterol when the nurse asks what medications his wife takes at home. He then tells the nurse that he gave her three extra puffs when she became ill. What statement is correct in this situation?

   a. The husband made the correct decision in giving the extra doses.

   b. The extra doses facilitated bronchodilation and probably saved her life.

   c. Salmeterol is contraindicated based on his wife's condition.

   d. The physician will most likely order continuation of the salmeterol with increased dosage.

2. The FDA has ordered a black box warning for the drug omalizumab. The nurse knows that what are the risks associated with this medication?

   a. Anaphylaxis

   b. Bleeding

   c. Respiratory distress

   d. Seizures

3. A male patient presents to the emergency department in bronchospasm. He has a history of smoking two packs per day for 20 years and is prescribed phenytoin to control a seizure disorder that developed after a head injury 3 years ago. Based on the patient's history, what would the nurse expect the physician to order?

   a. A modified dose of aminophylline

   b. The standard dose of aminophylline

   c. A drug other than aminophylline

   d. Phenytoin intravenously

4. A female patient's diagnoses include type 2 diabetes, atrial fibrillation, asthma, and hyperlipidemia. The nurse is concerned because the over-the-counter aerosol product the patient uses to control her asthma most likely contains what substance?

   a. Corticosteroids

   b. Aspirin

   c. A glucose base

   d. Epinephrine

5. A male patient is concerned because ever since he began his antiasthma medication, his GERD symptoms are worse. The nurse explains that his symptoms are worse because his asthma medications have what effect?

   a. They cause acid indigestion.

   b. They tighten the gastroesophageal sphincter.

   c. They relax the gastroesophageal sphincter.

   d. They stimulate peristalsis.

6. Aerosols are often the drugs of choice to treat asthma because of what characteristics? (Select all that apply.)

   a. They act directly on the airways.

   b. They can usually be given in smaller doses.

   c. They produce fewer adverse effects than oral or parenteral drugs.

   d. They may be given less frequently.

   e. They relieve symptoms quickly.

7. A male patient presents with symptoms of bronchospasm that occurred during a birthday party for his grandson. What medication would the nurse expect the physician to give him?

   a. Albuterol

   b. Asthmacort

   c. Theophylline

   d. Omalizumab

8. The nurse is caring for a patient who is receiving IV theophylline for treatment of severe bronchospasm. The nurse will ensure that which item on the patient's food tray will be held while the patient is receiving theophylline?

   a. Milk

   b. Green leafy vegetables

   c. Coffee

   d. Eggs

9. During the summer, a female patient experiences increased periods of acute symptoms of her asthma. The physician increases the dose frequency of which of her medications?

   a. Epinephrine

   b. Omalizumab

   c. Salmeterol

   d. Albuterol

10. What is the most effective method used to monitor patients with asthma that they can use at home?

    a. Incentive spirometer

    b. Manometer

    c. Peak-flow monitor

    d. Trough-flow monitor

11. With theophylline, the home care nurse needs to assess the patient and the environment for certain products that can cause what to occur? (Select all that apply.)

    a. Affect metabolism of theophylline

    b. Decrease therapeutic effects

    c. Increase therapeutic effects

    d. Increase adverse effects

    e. Affect the excretion of theophylline

12. A male patient is experiencing dysphasia secondary to a mild stroke that he had 3 weeks ago. He states that his asthma medications are not working as well or as long as they did in the past. What does the nurse suspect is the reason for this?

    a. He is crushing the medication.

    b. He is administering the wrong medication.

    c. He is experiencing confusion.

    d. He is experiencing postural hypotension.

13. In children, high doses of nebulized albuterol have been associated with what conditions? (Select all that apply.)

    a. Hyperkalemia

    b. Tachycardia

    c. Hypokalemia

    d. Hyperglycemia

    e. Hypotension

14. A male patient is prescribed montelukast and uses it successfully to manage his asthma. He develops hepatitis C. What would the nurse expect the physician to do?

    a. Lower the dose of the montelukast

    b. Discontinue the medication and prescribe another

    c. Increase the dose of the montelukast

    d. Maintain the same dose of the montelukast

15. A male patient is prescribed cromolyn and uses it successfully to manage his exercise-induced asthma. He develops chronic renal insufficiency. What would the nurse expect the physician to do?

    a. Reduce the dosage of the medication

    b. Increase the dosage of the medication

    c. Maintain the current dose of the medication

    d. Titrate the dosage of the medication upward

16. A 75-year-old patient is diagnosed with COPD. His physician orders an adrenergic bronchodilator via inhaler and a spacer. What are the main risks associated with the drug for this patient? (Select all that apply.)

    a. Excessive cardiac stimulation

    b. Bradycardia

    c. Hypotension

    d. CNS stimulation

    e. Anaphylaxis

17. A 45-year-old patient is 6 feet tall and weighs 300 pounds. He is diagnosed with asthma, and the physician orders a combination of an antiasthmatic and theophylline. The nurse understands that on which factor is the dose of theophylline based?

    a. The patient's weight

    b. The patient's ideal body weight

    c. The patient's symptomatology

    d. The patient's comorbidities

18. The nurse is aware that the physician often orders combination therapy for the treatment of asthma for what reason?

    a. To counteract the adverse effects of each different drug

    b. To allow for smaller doses of each agent to be given

    c. To provide a comprehensive cure for asthma

    d. To decrease the cost of asthma therapy

19. A female patient is prescribed systemic corticosteroids for her asthma. The nurse knows that the patient is at risk for what problem?

    a. Pituitary insufficiency

    b. Pancreatic insufficiency

    c. Adrenal insufficiency

    d. Renal insufficiency

20. A male patient is brought to the emergency department by his son with alteration in consciousness. The physician suspects theophylline overdose. What would the nurse expect the physician to order?

    a. Dextrose and water intravenously

    b. Gastric lavage

    c. Antiemetic

    d. Saline 0.9% intravenously

Drug Therapy for Fluid Volume Excess

SECTION I: ASSESSING YOUR UNDERSTANDING

Activity A   FILL IN THE BLANKS

1. Diuretics are drugs that increase renal excretion of water, sodium, and other electrolytes, thereby increasing urine formation and
_____.

2. The primary function of the kidneys is to regulate the volume, _____, and pH of body fluids.

3. Each nephron is composed of a _____ and a tubule.

4. The glomerulus is a network of _____ that receives blood from the renal artery.

5. _____ is a thin-walled structure that surrounds the glomerulus, and then narrows and continues as the tubule.

Activity B   MATCHING

Match the term in Column A with the definition in Column B.

Column A	Column B
____ 1. Thiazide diuretics	a. Act at the distal tubule to decrease sodium reabsorption and potassium excretion
____ 2. Loop diuretics	b. Produce rapid diuresis by increasing the solute load (osmotic pressure) of the glomerular filtrate
____ 3. Potassium-sparing diuretics	c. Synthetic drugs that are chemically related to the sulfonamides
____ 4. Osmotic agents	d. Used to prevent potassium imbalances
____ 5. Diuretic combinations	e. Diuretics that inhibit sodium and chloride reabsorption in the ascending limb of the loop of Henle

Activity C SHORT ANSWERS

Briefly answer the following questions.

1. Explain how convoluted tubules enhance renal function.

2. Describe the three processes by which the nephron functions.

3. Describe the process of glomerular filtration.

4. What happens to the fluid processed during glomerular filtration?

5. What happens to blood that does not become part of the glomerular filtrate?

SECTION II: APPLYING YOUR KNOWLEDGE

Activity D CASE STUDY

Consider the scenario and answer the questions.

Mr. Stevens has just been diagnosed with congestive heart failure. The physician has ordered furosemide (Lasix) 60 mg PO once a day. He does not want to take the medicine until he understands how this medicine will help him.

1. Discuss what happens in the loop of Henle.

2. Explain why furosemide is called a loop diuretic, and discuss what the therapeutic action of this drug will be for this patient.

3. What are the most common side effects for the drug furosemide?

4. What are the important teaching points that must be given to the patient who will be taking furosemide?

SECTION III: PRACTICING FOR NCLEX

Answer the following questions.

1. A 75-year-old patient is diagnosed with atrial fibrillation and chronic congestive heart failure. The physician orders a combination of digoxin and diuretics to treat the patient's diseases. Recent laboratory results indicate that the patient's potassium level is 2 mEq/L. This patient is at risk for which problem?

a. Exacerbation of the atrial fibrillation

b. Subtherapeutic levels of serum digoxin

c. Digoxin toxicity

d. Congestive heart failure

2. A male patient presents to the emergency department with shortness of breath, dizziness, and confusion. He is diagnosed with severe congestive heart failure. The physician orders high-dose furosemide continuous IV infusions. What does the nurse expect the rate of dosage to be?

a. 4 mg/min or less

b. 5 mg/min or less

c. 6 mg/min or less

d. 8 mg/min or less

3. A female patient is diagnosed with chronic congestive heart failure and hypertension. The nurse would expect the physician to order what type of diuretic?

a. Loop

b. Osmotic

c. Thiazide

d. Potassium wasting

4. A patient who is allergic to sulfonamide would use what diuretic cautiously?

a. Hydrochlorothiazide

b. Furosemide

c. Bumetanide

d. Torsemide

5. A male patient is prescribed potassium-sparing diuretics to treat his disease process. During his annual visit to the physician, he complains that he is experiencing muscle weakness and tingling in his fingers. What does the nurse suspect is wrong with this patient?

a. Hypokalemia

b. Hyperkalemia

c. Hypocalcemia

d. Hypercalcemia

6. A female patient is diagnosed with hyponatremia. What type of diuretic would most likely cause this symptom?

a. Osmotic

b. Thiazide

c. Potassium sparing

d. Loop

7. A male patient is excited because it is football season. He has season tickets and attends most games with his friends. At his latest appointment, the patient's blood pressure is elevated. What does the nurse suspect is the cause?

   a. He is anxious about his team.

   b. He is consuming excessive salty foods at the games.

   c. He is developing comorbidities.

   d. He has become a vegetarian until his team wins the championship.

8. The nurse is caring for a patient who is receiving mannitol. The nurse knows that it is used to manage oliguria or anuria. The nurse knows that it is also used for what other conditions? (Select all that apply.)

   a. Reduction of intracranial pressure

   b. Reduction of mild to moderate swelling of the extremities

   c. Reduction of intraocular pressure

   d. Urinary excretion of toxic substances

   e. Reduction of venous jugular pressure

9. A patient who takes propranolol has just been prescribed hydrochlorothiazide. The nurse would expect that this combination of drugs would cause what effect?

   a. Decrease in the effectiveness of the hydrochlorothiazide

   b. Increase in the effectiveness of the hydrochlorothiazide

   c. No change in the effectiveness of the hydrochlorothiazide

   d. Dramatic increase in the effectiveness of the propranolol

10. Diuretics are often taken in the home setting. The home care nurse may need to assist patients and caregivers by doing what tasks? (Select all that apply.)

    a. Monitoring patient responses

    b. Assessing use of over-the-counter medications that may aggravate the patient's condition

    c. Weighing the patient daily

    d. Appropriating all sodium-rich foods in the home

    e. Teaching the patient and family to administer diuretics in the evening

11. A male patient is critically ill with a diagnosis of congestive heart failure exacerbated by a myocardial infarction. The nurse understands that what fast-acting diuretics would be appropriate for the physician to order? (Select all that apply.)

    a. Furosemide

    b. Diazide

    c. Hydrochlorothiazide

    d. Bumetanide

    e. Mannitol

12. The nurse is preparing to administer a diuretic to a patient in the critical care unit. The nurse knows that what method of administration of fast-acting diuretics would be most effective and least likely to produce adverse effects in a critically ill patient with pulmonary edema?

    a. Intravenous bolus doses

    b. Continuous intravenous infusion

    c. Subcutaneous doses

    d. Intramuscular doses

13. A male patient has cirrhosis of the liver that has caused ascites. The nurse knows that what condition may occur if diuretics are used to reduce the ascites?

    a. Ammonia absorption

    b. Subtherapeutic drug levels

    c. Hepatic encephalopathy

    d. Hepatomegaly

14. A male patient has cirrhosis and is receiving diuretic therapy. The nurse knows that what drug will help prevent metabolic alkalosis or hypokalemia in this patient?

    a. Spironolactone

    b. Diazide

    c. Hydrochlorothiazide

    d. Bumetanide

15. A patient with renal impairment is in need of a diuretic. Because of the renal problem, potassium-sparing diuretics are contraindicated but may be used if there is no other option. If they are used at all, what nursing intervention would be most important for this patient?

    a. Administration of concurrent potassium

    b. Monitoring of serum electrolytes, creatinine, and BUN

    c. Administration of a thiazide diuretic

    d. Monitoring of CBC and serum albumin

16. The nurse is preparing to hang an intermittent infusion of furosemide. To prevent accelerated degradation of furosemide, the nurse knows that the medication should be mixed in what IV solution?

    a. D5W

    b. D51/2 NS

    c. Lactated Ringer's solution

    d. D51/4 NS

17. A 71-year-old patient is hospitalized with pulmonary edema; he is discharged with a prescription for a loop diuretic. He presents to the physician's office 1 week later with symptoms indicating excessive diuresis. The nurse knows that this patient is also at risk for which condition?

    a. Rebound hypertension

    b. Hypervolemia

    c. Embolism

    d. Gastric ulcer disease

18. The physician orders hydrochlorothiazide for a male patient. The patient has multiple comorbidities, and the physician chooses the smallest effective dose of the drug. The nurse expects the physician to order a daily dose in what range?

    a. 0.25 to 0.50 mg

    b. 0.50 to 0.75 mg

    c. 8 to 12 mg

    d. 12.5 to 25 mg

19. A patient with renal impairment has been receiving hydrochlorothiazide, and lately it has been less effective than usual. The nurse knows that thiazide drugs become ineffective when the GFR is less than what level?

    a. 30 mL/min

    b. 40 mL/min

    c. 50 mL/min

    d. 60 mL/min

20. The physician orders furosemide for a pediatric patient. The nurse knows that the established dose of the drug should not exceed how many milligrams per kilogram of body weight per day?

    a. 4

    b. 6

    c. 8

    d. 10

Nutritional Support Products, Vitamins, and Mineral Supplements

Learning Objectives

- Discuss the need for vitamin and mineral supplements.
- Describe the use of vitamins and minerals in specific groups of patients.
- Identify fat-soluble vitamins used to treat deficiencies, including the nursing implications associated with their administration.
- Identify water-soluble vitamins used to treat deficiencies, including the nursing implications associated with their administration.
- Identify minerals used to treat deficiencies, including the nursing implications associated with their administration.
- Discuss the chelating agents used to remove excess copper, iron, and lead from body tissues.
- Recognize the benefit of nutritional supplements, including the nursing implications associated with their administration.
- Apply nursing process skills to prevent, recognize, or treat nutritional imbalances, which may involve monitoring laboratory reports that indicate nutritional status.

SECTION I: ASSESSING YOUR UNDERSTANDING

Activity A FILL IN THE BLANKS

1. _____ are structural and functional components of all body tissues; the recommended amount for adults is 50 to 60 g daily.

2. _____ and fats mainly provide energy for cellular metabolism.

3. Energy is measured in _____ per gram of food oxidized in the body.

4. Carbohydrates and _____ supply 4 kcal/g; fats supply 9 kcal/g.

5. _____ are required for normal body metabolism, growth, and development.

Activity B MATCHING

Match the term in Column A with the definition in Column B.

Column A

____ 1. Sodium polystyrene sulfonate (Kayexalate)

Column B

a. A parenteral drug used to remove excess iron from storage sites (e.g., ferritin, hemosiderin) in the body

_____ **2.** Deferasirox (Exjade)

_____ **3.** Deferoxamine (Desferal)

_____ **4.** Penicillamine (Cuprimine)

_____ **5.** Succimer (Chemet)

b. Chelates copper, zinc, mercury, and lead to form soluble complexes that are excreted in the urine

c. Chelates lead to form water-soluble complexes that are excreted in the urine

d. Used to treat hyper-kalemia

e. An oral iron-chelating agent used to treat chronic iron overload

3. What are some adverse effects of this drug? What adjustments to the treatment might be made in reaction to some of these effects?

SECTION III: PRACTICING FOR NCLEX

Activity E

Answer the following questions.

1. A female patient presents to the physician's office for her yearly physical examination. When the nurse asks about her current drug regimen, she states that she self-administers megadoses of vitamin C to prevent cancer. Which statement is an appropriate response?

a. "You require large doses of multiple vitamins to prevent cancer."

b. "Large doses of single vitamins do not prevent cancer."

c. "Large doses of vitamin C will also prevent cardiovascular disease."

d. "Large doses of vitamin C will also prevent HIV."

2. A male patient tells the nurse that he obtains all of his nutrients from vitamins. What is the correct explanation the nurse would give this patient?

a. "The effectiveness of the vitamins depends on the brand."

b. "You cannot obtain enough vitamin B_6 from vitamins."

c. "You should consult your physician for the correct strength of the vitamins."

d. "Nutrients are best obtained from foods."

3. The nurse is assessing a patient in the clinic who admits to taking megadoses of vitamins, but he is not sure which ones he has been taking. The patient presents with hair loss, double vision, headaches, and nausea and vomiting. The nurse suspects that this patient has taken a toxic amount of which vitamin?

a. A

b. C

c. D

d. E

Activity C SHORT ANSWERS

Briefly answer the following questions.

1. Discuss how nutritional deficiency states may occur.

2. What are liquid enteral products, and why are they administered?

3. When are IV fluids used instead of liquid enteral products? What types of solutions are used?

4. Under what circumstances are pancreatic enzymes used, and what is their purpose to maintain a patient's health and well-being?

5. What is considered the best source of vitamins to maintain health? Why do patients take commercially prepared vitamins?

SECTION II: APPLYING YOUR KNOWLEDGE

Activity D CASE STUDY

Consider the scenario and answer the questions.

Mrs. Angelis presents to the physician's office with symptoms of fatigue, listlessness, and dyspnea on exertion. She is diagnosed with iron deficiency anemia. The physician orders ferrous sulfate. You are responsible for Mrs. Angelis' education care plan.

1. In addition to treating iron deficiency anemia, how are iron preparations used to prevent iron deficiency anemia?

2. Mrs. Angelis asks you how long the iron will take to work. What can you tell her about how the iron preparation works? How would you respond if she asks for an enteric-coated preparation?

4. The nurse is caring for a patient who relates in his medication history that he takes large doses of vitamin E daily to keep his heart healthy. What sign/symptom if observed by the nurse may indicate that the patient is taking too much vitamin E?

   a. Constipation

   b. Insomnia

   c. Excessive bruising

   d. Difficulty swallowing

5. What is the home care nurse's responsibility related to the patient's nutrition?

   a. Providing care to the patient with physician's orders

   b. Assessing the nutritional status of the patient that the nurse has physician's orders to visit

   c. Assessing the nutritional status of all members of the household

   d. Providing nutrition counseling to the person who is the primary cook within the family

6. The home care nurse is caring for a patient who is receiving tube feedings. What teaching topics are most important to share with this patient and his family? (Select all that apply.)

   a. The patient should be lying down while the tube feeding is administered

   b. Don't give more than 500 mL per feeding

   c. Give the feeding over 30 to 60 minutes

   d. Change the tube feeding containers every week

   e. Keep a record of how much is given each day

7. The nurse is caring for a critically ill patient in the unit who has an IV dedicated to fluid and electrolyte replacement. To prevent imbalances and adverse reactions, what should the nurse closely monitor?

   a. Hemoglobin and hematocrit levels

   b. Serum electrolyte levels

   c. Serum albumin levels

   d. BUN and creatine levels

8. The nurse is responsible for the administration of total parenteral nutrition for a patient, and the physician orders the addition of a fat emulsion. How should the nurse administer the fat emulsion?

   a. Rapidly over 30 minutes

   b. Over 1 to 2 hours

   c. Slowly over an 8-hour period

   d. Slowly over 24 hours

9. The nurse is comparing the recipe for a TPN with the physician's orders for an adult male, aged 35. How will the nurse administer vitamin K?

   a. Separately by injection

   b. Separately orally

   c. Included in the TPN order

   d. Monthly subcutaneously

10. A male patient is diagnosed with COPD. His enteral feeding formula will be individualized and will contain what combination of nutrients?

   a. More carbohydrates and less protein

   b. Less carbohydrate and more fat

   c. Less carbohydrate and more protein

   d. Less fat and more protein

11. The nurse is caring for a patient who is receiving an iron supplement for treatment of anemia. What food/liquid will the nurse offer the patient to take with the iron that will increase the iron's absorption?

   a. Water

   b. Orange juice

   c. Toast

   d. Milk

12. A male patient is admitted to the nursing unit for treatment of pneumonia. His diagnoses include cirrhosis of the liver. The nurse would expect his diet to include restriction of which element?

   a. Carbohydrate

   b. Fat

   c. Calcium

   d. Protein

13. The nurse is caring for a patient who has a potassium level of 6.3 mEq/dL. The nurse expects the physician to treat this lab value in what manner?

    a. Repeating the lab value in the morning

    b. Administering PO potassium supplements

    c. Administering IV potassium

    d. Administering insulin and glucose

14. The nurse is caring for a patient with acute renal failure who is receiving total parenteral nutrition. The nurse is aware that the physician will not prescribe IV fat emulsions if serum triglyceride levels exceed what level?

    a. 400 mg/dL

    b. 300 mg/dL

    c. 200 mg/dL

    d. 100 mg/dL

15. A 75-year-old patient is admitted to the nurse's unit. His diagnoses include type 2 diabetes mellitus, arthrosclerosis, and a past medical history of a myocardial infarction in 1989. The nurse would be most concerned if his enteral feeding contains what element?

    a. Animal fats

    b. Low amounts of glucose

    c. Potassium

    d. Calcium

16. The nurse is providing home care instruction about iron replacement therapy to a young mother who has iron deficiency anemia. She also has young children in the home. To prevent accidental ingestion of iron-containing medications by children, how must products with 30 mg or more of iron be provided?

    a. They must have childproof caps.

    b. They must be packaged as individual doses.

    c. They must be supplied by prescription only.

    d. They must be prescribed only for adults.

17. The nurse has just administered oral niacin to a patient. What is the most important instruction the nurse can give to this patient at this time?

    a. "You can expect to feel very cold for the next ten minutes. This will subside in about 10 minutes."

    b. "Lie down for about 30 minutes, and then be careful when you sit and stand up."

    c. "This medication has better absorption if you go for a brisk 10-minute walk."

    d. "If your face becomes flushed, it is important not to take any type of medication."

18. The nurse is caring for a 34-week preterm infant and knows that preterm infants need proportionately more vitamins than term infants, for what reason?

    a. They often experience electrolyte imbalances.

    b. Their growth rate is faster.

    c. Their metabolism is slower.

    d. Their growth rate is slower.

19. A female patient is diagnosed with a seizure disorder, and the physician prescribes phenytoin. She is preparing to conceive her second child and begins to self-administer folic acid. The concurrent use of these medications places the patient at risk for what adverse effect?

    a. Phenytoin toxicity

    b. Seizures

    c. Folic acid toxicity

    d. Subtherapeutic levels of folic acid

20. The nurse is caring for a child in the emergency department who ate her grandmother's iron tablets. What drug does the nurse anticipate the physician ordering for this child?

    a. Penicillamine

    b. Deferasirox

    c. Deferoxamine

    d. Sodium polystyrene sulfonate

Drug Therapy for Weight Management

Learning Objectives

- Identify the various factors associated with obesity.
- Describe the clinical manifestations of obesity.
- Identify the prototype drug from each drug class used to manage obesity.
- Describe the anorexiants used in weight management in terms of their action, use, contraindications, adverse effects, and nursing implications.
- Describe the lipase inhibitors used in weight management in terms of their action, use, contraindications, adverse effects, and nursing implications.
- Understand how to apply the nursing process in the care of patients who are overweight or obese.

SECTION I: ASSESSING YOUR UNDERSTANDING

Activity A   FILL IN THE BLANKS

1. _____ is defined as a *body mass index* (BMI) of 25 to 29.9.
2. _____ is defined as a BMI of 30 or more.
3. The _____ reflects weight in relation to height and is a better indicator than weight alone.
4. The desirable range for _____ is 18.5 to 24.9.

5. A large waist circumference (greater than 35 inches for women or 40 inches for men) is another risk factor for overweight and _____.

Activity B   MATCHING

Match the term in Column A with the definition in Column B.

Column A	Column B
____ 1. Phentermine (Adipex-P)	a. Antidiabetes drug being tested as a weight-loss agent in nondiabetic patients.
____ 2. Metformin (Glucophage)	
____ 3. Orlistat (Xenical, Alli)	b. Most frequently prescribed adrenergic anorexiant
____ 4. Glucomannan	c. Decreases absorption of dietary fat from the intestine
____ 5. Guarana	d. Major source of commercial caffeine; found in weight-loss products and many other supplements and other food products
	e. Expands on contact with body fluids

Activity C SHORT ANSWERS

Briefly answer the following questions.

1. What is the primary cause of obesity?

2. What is central or visceral obesity?

3. What is the prevalence of obesity in the United States?

4. What is the etiology of excessive weight gain?

5. Explain how energy expenditure influences weight control.

SECTION II: APPLYING YOUR KNOWLEDGE

Activity D CASE STUDY

Consider the scenario and answer the questions.

During a routine physician's appointment, Mrs. Romano requests more information about orlistat. She is concerned about her obesity and does not want to take a prescription medication. You are responsible for her education plan.

1. Mrs. Romano asks how orlistat works. How would you respond?

2. Mrs. Romano wants to know whether the drug will lower her cholesterol. What is your understanding of the relationship between weight loss and effects on cholesterol with this drug?

3. Explain the absorption of the drug. Does it cause any adverse effects? What are the disadvantages of taking orlistat?

4. Mrs. Romano asks if there are any other medications or supplements that she should take with the orlistat to remain healthy. What can you suggest?

SECTION III: PRACTICING FOR NCLEX

Activity E

Answer the following questions.

1. A male patient presents to the physician's office 1 year after losing 50 pounds. He complains that he is rapidly regaining his weight and doesn't know what to do about it. What should the nurse review with this patient? (Select all that apply.)

   a. His lifestyle habits
   b. His exercise habits
   c. His work habits
   d. His eating habits
   e. His drinking habits

2. A female patient presents to the physician's office for a routine physical examination. She is 10 pounds overweight and asks the physician for a prescription for a weight-loss drug. She is healthy and her laboratory values are within normal limits. The nurse expects the physician to do what?

   a. Order the medication with a short-term prescription
   b. Encourage the patient to increase her exercise and eat a healthy diet
   c. Refuse to order the weight-loss drugs because her HMO will not pay for them
   d. Order an open prescription of a weight-loss drug

3. A patient arrives at the emergency department with tachycardia. He states he hasn't slept in the past 3 days. He also states that he has been drinking "energy" drinks in place of meals in an effort to lose weight. The nurse suspects that the patient's symptoms are related to what ingredient in these drinks?

   a. Sugar
   b. Cola flavoring
   c. Electrolytes
   d. Caffeine

4. A male patient asks the physician how to lose weight without drugs. The physician informs the patient that if he decreases his intake by 500 calories per day, he can expect to lose how much weight?

   a. 2 pounds per week
   b. 4 pounds per week
   c. 3 pounds per week
   d. 1 pound per week

5. A patient is 50 pounds overweight and is reluctant to try and lose weight. The nurse informs the patient that being overweight or obese may result in which conditions? (Select all that apply.)

  a. Diabetes

  b. Hypertension

  c. Hypoglycemia

  d. Hypokalemia

  e. Gallstones

6. A patient who has clinical depression is reluctant to take medication because of a fear of weight gain. What information would the nurse share with the patient?

  a. "The physician will prescribe fluoxetine (Prozac) because it has been shown to promote weight loss in long-term use."

  b. "The physician will prescribe phenelzine (Nardil) because it is associated with weight loss."

  c. "Amitriptyline (Elavil) is the best medication because it leads to decreased appetite and weight loss."

  d. "More patients who have taken bupropion (Wellbutrin) experience weight loss than weight gain."

7. A patient took sibutramine 5 years ago to assist in a 30-pound weight loss. The patient has gained the weight back and is requesting the medication again. What is the nurse's best response to this patient?

  a. "You shouldn't use medication for weight loss because you gained all your weight back again."

  b. "The drug you took 5 years ago is no longer available in the United States. The physician will discuss with you the options that are available at this time."

  c. "Sibutramine is no longer available in the United States. I will give you a Web site where you can get it on the Internet."

  d. "I think it would be a good idea if you just cut calories and exercised more."

8. An 82-year-old patient is approximately 75 pounds overweight. The physician has prescribed orlistat. The nurse is aware that the drug will be used conservatively because what organ function is decreased in older adults? (Select all that apply.)

  a. Renal function

  b. Cardiac function

  c. Pancreatic function

  d. Liver function

  e. Cognitive function

9. A female patient brings her overweight child to the pediatrician's office. She requests medication to help her child lose weight. The physician does not order medication. The nurse will focus the family teaching on what aspect of weight loss?

  a. Decreasing physical activity

  b. Putting the child on a diet

  c. Increasing physical activity

  d. Decreasing the child's BMI

10. A female patient's child exceeds optimal adult weight. The nurse understands that the goal of the treatment plan established with the mother and her child is a weight loss of how many pounds per year until the optimal adult weight is reached?

  a. 10 to 12 pounds

  b. 6 to 8 pounds

  c. 12 to 15 pounds

  d. 25 to 30 pounds

11. A female patient brings her 16-year-old daughter to the physician's office for a weight-loss program. The daughter is 100 pounds overweight, and diets have been unsuccessful in the past. The nurse is aware that the physician will order which medication?

  a. Phentermine

  b. Orlistat

  c. Glucomannan

  d. Guarana

12. A patient comes to the clinic to talk about weight-loss strategies. The patient understands the need to increase exercise and decrease calories. What additional strategy can the nurse share with this patient that will assist in his effort to lose weight?

   a. Do not eat any carbohydrates.

   b. Keep a diary of both food intake and physical activity.

   c. Put a lock on the refrigerator.

   d. Increase water intake to 4 glasses per day.

13. A patient takes orlistat for weight loss. The weight loss is not progressing as quickly as the patient would like, and the patient asks her physician to order phentermine for her. The patient hopes that the combination will decrease her appetite and foster quicker weight loss. The nurse expects the physician to perform what action for this patient?

   a. Order the medication combination

   b. Order a low dose of phentermine to use with the orlistat

   c. Does not order the combination due to possible adverse reactions

   d. Does not order the combination because it does not improve weight loss

14. A male patient is diagnosed with type 2 diabetes. He presents to the physician's office after a weight loss of 25 pounds. The nurse expects the physician to perform what action?

   a. Tell the patient that his diabetes is cured

   b. Decrease the patient's diabetic medications

   c. Increase the patient's diabetic medications

   d. Diagnose the patient with hypoglycemia

15. A male patient is 45 pounds overweight and has heart disease. For a patient with cardio-vascular disease, the nurse identifies the benefits of weight loss as what? (Select all that apply.)

   a. Lower blood pressure

   b. Decreased HDL cholesterol

   c. Increased HDL cholesterol

   d. Lower serum triglycerides

   e. Increased hemoglobin

16. A female patient is 35 pounds overweight with no major health problems. She asks the physician for a referral to a surgeon for bariatric surgery. What would the nurse expect the physician to do for this patient?

   a. Make the referral

   b. Decline to make the referral

   c. Refer the patient to a psychologist

   d. Refer the patient to a pharmacologist for an OTC diet supplement

17. A female patient presents to the physician's office with complaints of weakness, dizziness, and heart palpitations. She takes over-the-counter Super Dieter's Tea. What laboratory tests does the nurse expect the physician to order for this patient?

   a. Serum electrolytes

   b. Hemoglobin and hematocrit

   c. Serum albumin

   d. CO_2

18. A female patient presents to the physician's office with complaints of abdominal pain. During the interview, the nurse discovers that the patient is using guar gum as a weight-loss product. In addition, she limits her fluid intake to reduce retention. The nurse knows that the patient is at risk for what condition?

   a. Pancreatitis

   b. Peptic ulcer disease

   c. Intestinal obstruction

   d. Esophageal varices

19. A patient who is 80 pounds overweight has been diagnosed with metabolic syndrome and has been prescribed medication to assist with the weight loss. The nurse is aware that metabolic syndrome is diagnosed if the patient has three or more of what abnormalities? (Select all that apply.)

   a. Serum triglycerides between 100 and 125 mg/dL

   b. HDL cholesterol below 40 mg/dL

   c. Blood pressure of 150/100 mm Hg or higher

   d. Serum glucose of 110 mg/dL or higher

   e. Central obesity

CHAPTER 35

Drug Therapy for Peptic Ulcer Disease and Gastroesophageal Reflux Disease

Learning Objectives

- Describe the main elements of peptic ulcer disease and gastroesophageal reflux disease (GERD).
- Discuss antacids in terms of the prototype, indications and contraindications for use, routes of administration, and major adverse effects.
- Describe histamine$_2$ receptor antagonists in terms of the prototype, indications and contraindications for use, routes of administration, and major adverse effects.
- Discuss proton pump inhibitors in terms of the prototype, indications and contraindications for use, routes of administration, and major adverse effects.
- Identify the adjuvant medications used to treat peptic ulcer and gastroesophageal reflux disease.
- Understand how to use the nursing process in the care of patients receiving antacids, proton pump inhibitors, and histamine$_2$ receptor antagonists.

SECTION I: ASSESSING YOUR UNDERSTANDING

Activity A FILL IN THE BLANKS

1. _____ is characterized by ulcer formation in the esophagus, stomach, or duodenum, areas of the gastrointestinal (GI) mucosa that are exposed to gastric acid and pepsin.

2. Gastric and _____ ulcers are more common than esophageal ulcers.

3. Peptic ulcers are attributed to an imbalance between cell-destructive and cell-_____ effects.

4. Cell-destructive effects include those of gastric acid (hydrochloric acid), _____, *Helicobacter pylori* infection, and ingestion of nonsteroidal anti-inflammatory drugs (NSAIDs).

5. _____, a strong acid that can digest the stomach wall, is secreted by parietal cells in the mucosa of the stomach antrum, near the pylorus.

Activity B   MATCHING

Match the term in Column A with the definition in Column B.

Column A

____ 1. Antacids

____ 2. H₂RAs

____ 3. PPIs

____ 4. Naturally occurring prostaglandin E

____ 5. Sucralfate

Column B

a. Produced in mucosal cells of the stomach and duodenum, inhibits gastric acid secretion and increases mucus and bicarbonate secretion, mucosal blood flow, and perhaps mucosal repair

b. A preparation of sulfated sucrose and aluminum hydroxide that binds to normal and ulcerated mucosa; used to prevent and treat peptic ulcer disease

c. Inhibits both basal secretion of gastric acid and the secretion stimulated by histamine, acetylcholine, and gastrin

d. Strong inhibitors of gastric acid secretion

e. Alkaline substances that neutralize acids

Activity C   SHORT ANSWERS

Briefly answer the following questions.

1. Explain the mechanism of action of antacids.

2. Explain the effect that histamines have on the gastrointestinal system.

3. What are proton pump inhibitors, and how do they affect the gastrointestinal system?

4. What effect does naturally occurring prostaglandin E have on the gastrointestinal system?

5. What disease process is sucralfate used for, and what is its mechanism of action?

SECTION II: APPLYING YOUR KNOWLEDGE

Activity D   CASE STUDY

Consider the scenario and answer the questions.

Mr. Dinwiddie, a construction worker, self-administers ibuprofen 800 mg four times a day for pain related to arthritis and his work. He presents to the physician's office with stomach pain that has become chronic within the past 2 weeks. The physician orders misoprostol.

1. Why did the physician order misoprostol? What is misoprostol? How will this drug help with the stomach pain?

2. Mr. Dinwiddie asks if misoprostol is safe for his wife. She has chronic back pain and also self-administers NSAIDs prescribed by her physician. Would you refer Mrs. Dinwiddie to her physician for the same treatment?

3. What is the most common adverse reaction related to misoprostol use? What is the most common indication for misoprostol?

SECTION III: PRACTICING FOR NCLEX

Activity E

Answer the following questions.

1. The physician orders sucralfate to assist in the healing of a duodenal ulcer. The nurse is aware that to ensure this medication's effectiveness, it should be administered under what condition?

   a. In an acid pH
   b. In a basic pH
   c. On an empty stomach
   d. On a full stomach

2. The nurse is taking a history of a patient who is complaining of burning pain in the stomach. The nurse knows that which risk factors increase this patient's chance of having a peptic ulcer? (Select all that apply.)

   a. Smoking
   b. Psychological stress
   c. Acetaminophen use
   d. Physiological stress
   e. Sucralfate use

3. A female patient comes to the clinic with complaints of burning pain in the stomach. She states that she thinks she had a virus 48 hours ago and she vomited many times. She hasn't vomited in 24 hours. She asks the physician to give her a prescription for omeprazole because she saw an ad on TV that said it would heal stomach pain. The nurse assists the patient in understanding that PPIs are considered drugs of choice for treatment of what conditions? (Select all that apply.)
   a. Duodenal ulcers
   b. Esophageal varices
   c. Zollinger-Ellison syndrome
   d. Gastric ulcers
   e. Anaphylactic shock

4. A male patient is receiving morphine sulfate for pain after an accident. The physician has also ordered cimetidine IV to assist in preventing a stress ulcer. The nurse will monitor for what effect that is caused by the interaction of these two drugs?
   a. Increased nausea and vomiting
   b. Increased incidence of respiratory depression
   c. Increased symptoms of GERD
   d. Increased complaints of pain

5. A patient is diagnosed with *Helicobacter pylori* infection. The physician will order amoxicillin and what other type of medication?
   a. Proton pump inhibitors
   b. Sucralfate
   c. H₂RAs
   d. Antacids

6. A female patient presents to the physician's office with increasing stomach acidity. She self-administers calcium antacids. She notes that she seems to be having more issues with stomach acid, so she has been taking the calcium antacids more frequently. The nurse suspects that this may have caused what to occur in this patient?
   a. Hypocalcemia
   b. Rebound acidity
   c. Gastric reflux
   d. Hyperactive gastric mucosa

7. A female patient self-administers magnesium antacids. She presents to the office with symptoms of dizziness and weakness. The nurse knows that these symptoms are

secondary to what common adverse effect of magnesium antacids?
   a. Hypercalcemia
   b. Hypocalcemia
   c. Diarrhea
   d. GERD

8. The nurse is caring for a patient with a nasogastric tube. Which PPI would be most appropriate for the physician to order for this patient?
   a. Omeprazole
   b. Lansoprazole
   c. Rabeprazole
   d. Esomeprazole

9. A male patient is overweight and lives a sedentary lifestyle. He presents to the office with complaints of acid regurgitation, especially at night. The nurse is aware that this patient is displaying symptoms of what disorder?
   a. Gastritis
   b. Peptic ulcer disease
   c. Duodenal ulcer disease
   d. Gastroesophageal reflux disease

10. The nurse is preparing to administer misoprostol to a female patient who has osteoarthritis and has developed an ulcer from the use of NSAIDs. What is the nurse's priority assessment with this patient?
    a. The patient's height and weight
    b. The length of time the patient has been taking the NSAID
    c. The date of the start of the patient's last menstrual period
    d. The dosage of the NSAID the patient has been taking

11. The physician has prescribed sucralfate for a patient with a gastric ulcer. The patient asks how long he must take this medication. What is the nurse's best response to this patient?
    a. "You must take this medication for the full 10 days."
    b. "You will need to take this medication for 4 to 8 weeks to ensure healing has occurred."
    c. "You will need to take this medication for the rest of your life."
    d. "You will take it for 5 days, then skip 5 days, then take it for another 5 days and you will be done with it."

12. A female patient is currently taking sucralfate and has been given a prescription for cipro-floxacin for treatment of a urinary tract infection. The nurse will inform the patient that she should take her medication in what way?

   a. "Both medications should be taken together on an empty stomach."

   b. "Take the sucralfate 30 minutes before the ciprofloxacin."

   c. "Take the ciprofloxacin 2 hours before the sucralfate."

   d. "Eat breakfast, then take the sucralfate, and then an hour later take the ciprofloxacin."

13. A female patient is self-administering cimetidine. What is the home care nurse's most important assessment of this patient?

   a. Adverse reactions

   b. Potential drug–drug interactions

   c. Allergic reactions

   d. Toxicity

14. A male patient has liver disease and is diagnosed with esophageal reflux. He asks the physician to prescribe PPIs. The nurse is aware that PPIs given in conjunction with liver disease may result in what issue for this patient?

   a. Decreased absorption of the PPIs

   b. Transient elevations in liver function tests

   c. PPI toxicity

   d. Subtherapeutic levels of PPIs in the bloodstream

15. A female patient's diagnoses include diabetes mellitus, gastric ulcer disease, and chronic renal disease. When the nurse reviews her medications with her, the nurse discover that she self-administers antacids containing magnesium. What statement is true about antacids containing magnesium?

   a. They are an acceptable treatment for gastric ulcer disease.

   b. They are contraindicated for patients with renal disease.

   c. They may cause an exacerbation of her hyperglycemia.

   d. They may cause hypoglycemia for patients with chronic renal disease and diabetes.

16. A 75-year-old patient is diagnosed with type 2 diabetes mellitus, hypertension, osteoporosis, and gastric ulcer disease. She is prescribed PPIs. The nurse is aware that long-term (greater than 1 year) administration of PPIs may lead to what problem for this patient?

   a. Increased risk for gastric cancer

   b. Increased risk for peptic ulcer disease

   c. Increased risk for hip fractures

   d. Increased risk for hypercalcemia

17. An 86-year-old patient has been prescribed ranitidine (Zantac). The nurse knows that an older adult who takes H_2RAs may experience what adverse effect?

   a. Agitation

   b. Lethargy

   c. Hyperplasia

   d. Hypertension

18. A 75-year-old patient is treating his ulcer with antacids. Based on the patient's age, the nurse expects the physician to prescribe a dose of antacid that compares with the average prescribed dose in what way?

   a. Smaller than the average prescribed dose

   b. Larger than the average prescribed dose

   c. The same as the average prescribed dose

   d. No antacids, because they are contraindicated in the elderly

19. The nurse is caring for a male patient in the medical unit. He is fed via a nasogastric tube. The dose of antacid is based on what factors?

   a. Signs and symptoms

   b. The pH of the stomach contents

   c. Patient age

   d. Disease processes

20. A male patient is diagnosed with a duodenal ulcer. The physician chooses to treat the ulcer with PPIs. The patient asks how long he will have to take the medication. The nurse inform him that, although treatment may be extended, most duodenal ulcers heal in about how long?

   a. 6 weeks

   b. 8 weeks

   c. 4 weeks

   d. 21 days

Drug Therapy for Nausea and Vomiting

Learning Objectives

- Identify patients who are at risk for developing nausea and vomiting.
- Discuss the phenothiazines in terms of indications and contraindications for use, routes of administration, and major adverse effects.
- Describe selected antihistamines used to control nausea and vomiting in terms of indications and contraindications for use, routes of administration, and major adverse effects.
- Discuss the 5-hydroxytryptamine$_3$ receptor antagonists in terms of indications and contraindications for use, routes of administration, and major adverse effects.
- Describe the substance P/neurokinin 1 antagonist aprepitant in terms of indications and contraindications for use, routes of administration, and major adverse effects.
- Identify the prototype drug for each drug class.
- Identify nonpharmacologic measures to reduce nausea and vomiting.
- Understand how to use the nursing process in the care of patients receiving drugs for the management of nausea and vomiting.

SECTION I: ASSESSING YOUR UNDERSTANDING

Activity A FILL IN THE BLANKS

1. _____ drugs are used to prevent or treat nausea and vomiting.

2. _____ is an unpleasant sensation of abdominal discomfort accompanied by a desire to vomit.

3. _____ is the expulsion of stomach contents through the mouth.

4. Nausea and vomiting are the most common _____ of drug therapy.

5. Vomiting occurs when the _____, a nucleus of cells in the medulla oblongata, is stimulated.

Activity B MATCHING

Match the term in Column A with the definition in Column B.

Column A

___ 1. Prochlor-perazine (Compazine) phenothiazines

___ 2. Dexamethasone and methyl-prednisolone

Column B

a. Antihistamine thought to relieve nausea and vomiting by blocking the action of acetylcholine in the brain

b. Effective in preventing or treating nausea and vomiting induced by drugs, radiation therapy, surgery, and most other stimuli

_____ **3.** Lorazepam (Ativan)

_____ **4.** Hydroxyzine (Vistaril)

_____ **5.** Ondansetron (Zofran), granisetron (Kytril), dolasetron (Anzemet), and palonosetron (Aloxi)

c. Often prescribed for patients who experience anticipatory nausea and vomiting before administration of anticancer drugs

d. Commonly used in the management of chemotherapy-induced emesis and postoperative nausea and vomiting

e. Antagonize serotonin receptors, preventing their activation by the effects of emetogenic drugs and toxins

Activity C SHORT ANSWERS

Briefly answer the following questions.

1. Identify three drugs most commonly associated with the adverse effects of nausea and vomiting.

2. Identify three causes other than drugs that may produce nausea and vomiting.

3. List five of the receptors located in the vomiting center, CTZ, and GI tract, which are stimulated by emetogenic drugs and toxins.

4. Describe the physiologic processes that occur during vomiting, beginning with the stimulation of the vomiting center and ending with the stomach contents' arriving toward the mouth for ejection.

5. Define the term _anticipatory nausea._

SECTION II: APPLYING YOUR KNOWLEDGE

Activity D CASE STUDY

Consider the scenario and answer the questions.

Mrs. Homan was diagnosed with cancer and subsequently treated with chemotherapeutic agents. She develops moderate nausea and vomiting after chemotherapy; she is losing weight and stamina and has a significant fluid and

electrolyte imbalance. The physician prescribes aprepitant (Emend). You are responsible for the patient's education plan.

1. How does aprepitant decrease nausea and vomiting? How is aprepitant typically used?

2. What can you tell Mrs. Homan about when the effect of the medication begins and how long it lasts?

3. Mrs. Homan wishes to return to work part-time, now that her nausea is managed. What adverse effect may impact her decision?

SECTION III: PRACTICING FOR NCLEX

Activity E

Answer the following questions.

1. A female patient is going on a cruise to Nova Scotia with her husband to celebrate their 15th wedding anniversary. She is concerned because she has experienced severe, debilitating seasickness in the past. What would the nurse expect the physician to order?
   a. Scopolamine
   b. Dexamethasone
   c. Palonosetron
   d. Ondansetron

2. A female patient is receiving chemotherapy to treat her cancer. Several antiemetics have been prescribed, and each has been unsuccessful in treating her nausea and vomiting. The physician chooses to prescribe what cannabinoid drug to manage her symptoms?
   a. Scopolamine
   b. Fosaprepitant
   c. Ondansetron
   d. Dronabinol

3. The nurse is caring for a male patient who has benign prostatic hypertrophy. The nurse would be alert for what complication if this patient is given promethazine for treatment of nausea?
   a. Polyuria
   b. Hematuria
   c. Urinary retention
   d. Dysuria

4. A male patient has developed intractable hiccups after abdominal surgery. The nurse anticipates that the physician will order which medication?

   a. Aprepitant

   b. Ondansetron

   c. Chlorpromazine

   d. Dimenhydrinate

5. The nurse is caring for a patient who is experiencing chemotherapy-induced nausea and vomiting. The physician has prescribed aprepitant as part of a combination therapy. The nurse knows that what other drugs are part of this combination?

   a. Ondansetron and dexamethasone

   b. Ondansetron and promethazine

   c. Dexamethasone and lorazepam

   d. Dexamethasone and dronabinol

6. A female patient prepares to begin her second round of chemotherapy. She tells the physician that she knows that the nausea and vomiting will be worse this time around. The physician orders lorazepam because it has what effect? (Select all that apply.)

   a. Producing relaxation

   b. Relieving anxiety

   c. Inhibiting cerebral cortex input to the vomiting center

   d. Creating a sense of euphoria

   e. Produces amnesia

7. A woman who is 7 weeks pregnant is experiencing morning sickness but does not want to use any medications to treat the nausea. What nonpharmacologic therapy would be helpful to this patient?

   a. Drink a cup of milk every morning before you eat your breakfast.

   b. Wear acupressure wristbands.

   c. Take phosphorated carbohydrate solution.

   d. Eat a sweet roll before getting out of bed in the morning.

8. The nurse is caring for a patient who has just had an episode of vomiting. What is the first intervention that the nurse would complete after the patient has finished vomiting?

   a. Take vital signs.

   b. Help the patient rinse his mouth.

   c. Go prepare an IM injection of an antiemetic.

   d. Weigh the patient.

9. The home care nurse is visiting a patient who is receiving antiemetics. Which actions will the nurse perform to ensure safe and effective treatment for the patient? (Select all that apply.)

   a. Reinforce teaching about dosage.

   b. Encourage the patient to get up and walk after taking the medication.

   c. Take the medication approximately 5 minutes before taking the medication that makes you nauseated.

   d. Encourage patient to sip on clear fluids to prevent dehydration.

   e. Do not drive while taking antinausea medicine.

10. A male patient has been receiving promethazine for nausea that occurred following chemotherapy. Recently it has been discovered that this patient has developed liver dysfunction. The nurse anticipates that the physician will do what to treat this patient's nausea?

    a. Use an alternative medication.

    b. Increase the dose of the medication.

    c. Decrease the dose of the medication.

    d. Maintain the current dose of the medication.

11. The nurse is caring for a patient with a hepatic impairment. The nurse knows that the dose of ondansetron should not exceed what amount?

    a. 8 mg

    b. 6 mg

    c. 10 mg

    d. 12 mg

12. A patient who is receiving chemotherapy is experiencing nausea. The patient has been receiving antiemetics with moderate success but would like to try a nonpharmacologic solution. The nurse knows that which nonpharmacologic technique is most accepted and widely studied in the treatment of nausea?

    a. Use of herbal supplements

    b. Use of acupuncture

    c. Use of acupressure

    d. Use of biofeedback

13. A 75-year-old patient develops nausea and vomiting secondary to administration of a new drug regimen to treat his Parkinson's disease. He is at risk for what adverse effect?

    a. Increased extrapyramidal effects

    b. Fluid and electrolyte imbalance

    c. Prostatitis

    d. Anxiety-induced vomiting

14. A patient has been using dronabinol for the last 6 weeks for management of nausea associated with chemotherapy. What symptoms may be patient experience when the medication is no longer needed? (Select all that apply.)

    a. Insomnia

    b. Lethargy

    c. Irritability

    d. Nightmares

    e. Mania

15. The nurse is caring for a 19-month-old child who has been hospitalized with dehydration secondary to nausea and vomiting. The nurse is aware that promethazine will not be used for this patient because it can cause what in children under the age of 2?

    a. Fatal hypovolemia secondary to hemorrhage

    b. Life-threatening cardiac dysrhythmias

    c. Fatal respiratory depression

    d. Fatal hypertension and subsequent cerebral vascular accident

16. A patient receiving chemotherapy has begun receiving aprepitant. The patient also takes oral contraceptives. What should the nurse tell the patient in regard to birth control?

    a. "Double the dose of the oral contraceptive while you are taking aprepitant."

    b. "Use alternative means of birth control for 1 month after taking aprepitant."

    c. "There is no need to do anything; your oral contraceptive will continue to be effective."

    d. "You should practice abstinence because the aprepitant will cause severe sores in the vagina."

17. The nurse is preparing to pretreat a patient with an antiemetic prior to the beginning of chemotherapy. The nurse knows that pretreatment is used for what reasons? (Select all that apply.)

    a. Increasing patient comfort

    b. Allowing use of lower drug doses

    c. Possibly preventing aspiration

    d. Possibly preventing extrapyramidal symptoms

    e. Decreasing patient anxiety

18. A parent of a child who gets carsick is planning on using dimenhydrate to help the child on a future care trip. When should the nurse tell the parent to administer the medication?

    a. 24 hours before the trip

    b. 12 hours before the trip

    c. 4 hours before the trip

    d. 1 hour before the trip

19. A patient develops labyrinthitis. What would the nurse expect the physician to order?

    a. Scopolamine

    b. Dexamethasone

    c. Aprepitant

    d. Meclizine

20. The nurse is caring for a patient with liver disease who is receiving promethazine for nausea. What adverse effect may occur in this patient?

    a. Drowsiness

    b. Confusion

    c. Cholestatic jaundice

    d. Photosensitivity

Drug Therapy for Constipation and Elimination Problems

Learning Objectives

- Discuss the etiology, physiology, and clinical manifestations for constipation and elimination problems.
- Educate patients about nonpharmacologic measures to prevent or treat constipation.
- Identify the prototype and describe the action, use, contraindications, adverse effects, and nursing implications of the laxatives.
- Identify the prototype and describe the action, use, contraindications, adverse effects, and nursing implications of the cathartics.
- Identify the prototype, indications, dosages, and routes for the miscellaneous agents used to treat constipation and other conditions.
- Understand how to use the nursing process in the care of patients with constipation.

SECTION I: ASSESSING YOUR UNDERSTANDING

Activity A   FILL IN THE BLANKS

1. _____ is infrequent and painful expulsion of hard, dry stools.

2. Chronic constipation causes _____, a mass of hard, dry stool in the rectum.

3. A drug that causes a person to eliminate soft, formed stool is known as a _____.

4. A drug with strong effects, _____ causes the elimination of liquid or semiliquid stool.

5. When the stomach and duodenum are distended with food, the _____ and _____ reflexes cause propulsive movements in the colon, which move feces into the rectum and arouse the urge to defecate.

Activity B   MATCHING

Match the term in Column A with the definition in Column B.

Column A	Column B
____ 1. Psyllium (Metamucil)	a. Increases osmotic pressure in the intestinal lumen and causes water to be retained
____ 2. Mineral oil	b. Acts by irritating the GI mucosa and pulling water into the bowel lumen
____ 3. Docusate sodium	c. Adds bulk and size to the fecal mass that stimulates peristalsis and defecation

_____ **4.** Bisacodyl
(Dulcolax)

_____ **5.** Magnesium
citrate

d. Acts as a detergent to facilitate the admixing of fat and water in the stool

e. Lubricates the fecal mass and slows colonic absorption of water from the fecal mass

Activity C SHORT ANSWERS

Briefly answer the following.

1. Describe the risk factor associated with the development of constipation.

2. How does voluntary control of the urge to defecate contribute to the development of constipation?

3. Describe symptoms usually associated with constipation.

4. Why do older adults complain of constipation more than younger people?

5. What lifestyle changes will promote regular bowel elimination.

SECTION II: APPLYING YOUR KNOWLEDGE

Activity D CASE STUDY

Consider the scenario and answer the questions.

Mrs. Fuller broke her leg last week. She has been taking pain medication to decrease the pain of the fracture and has not had a bowel movement since her injury. The physician has ordered bisacodyl (Dulcolax) to relieve her constipation.

1. Mrs. Fuller asks the nurse how bisacodyl works and how her lack of bowel movement is related to her leg fracture.

2. Mrs. Fuller wants to know what adverse effects she may experience when she takes this medication. What will the nurse tell this patient?

3. Mrs. Fuller prefers drinking milk to drinking water. How will this affect the prescribed drug?

4. What information will the nurse give Mrs. Fuller to help her prevent additional problems with constipation?

SECTION III: PRACTICING FOR NCLEX

Activity E

Answer the following questions.

1. The nurse understands that the drug docusate sodium (Colace) would be most appropriate for what patient?
   a. A 46-year-old patient who has not had a bowel movement in 4 days
   b. A 74-year-old patient who takes bisacodyl daily at home
   c. A 66-year-old patient who is recovering from a heart attack
   d. A 52-year-old patient who is preparing for a colonoscopy

2. The nurse is preparing to administer psyllium (Metamucil) to a patient. The nurse instructs the patient to mix the medication in how much liquid?
   a. 30 mL
   b. 90 mL
   c. 120 mL
   d. 240 mL

3. The nurse is preparing to administer medications to a group of patients. For which patient is bisacodyl contraindicated?
   a. 8-year-old
   b. 17-year-old
   c. 48-year-old
   d. 75-year-old

4. The nurse is aware that critically ill patients are more at risk for constipation for what reasons? (Select all that apply.)
   a. Decreased activity
   b. Decrease in the amount of family interaction
   c. Increased access to a high-fiber diet
   d. Use of opioid medications
   e. Change in bowel routines

5. The nurse is assessing a patient who is complaining of constipation. The use of a medication to treat this problem is contraindicated if the patient complains of what symptom?
   a. Lack of urge to defecate
   b. Abdominal pain and fever
   c. Lack of bowel movement for 5 days
   d. Frequent episodes of flatulence

6. The nurse is conducting a class on nonpharmacologic treatment for occasional constipation. Which treatments will the nurse recommend? (Select all that apply.)
   a. Eat more high-fiber foods
   b. Decrease fluid intake
   c. Use of prebiotics
   d. Use of probiotics
   e. Decrease the amount of daily exercise

7. The nurse is caring for a patient who is diagnosed with hepatic encephalopathy. The nurse knows that which medication will be used to treat the constipation that accompanies this condition?
   a. Bisacodyl
   b. Psyllium
   c. Lactulose
   d. Mineral oil

8. A female patient has dealt with constipation most of her adult life. She has not had relief of symptoms with most medications used in the treatment of this condition. The nurse is aware that this patient will be prescribed which drug?
   a. Sorbitol
   b. Sodium polystyrene sulfonate
   c. Docusate sodium
   d. Lubiprostone

9. The nurse receives a call from a patient who is taking lactulose. The patient complains that he is having two to three soft stools every day and is afraid he is developing diarrhea. What is the nurse's best response to this patient?
   a. "Stop taking the medication immediately."
   b. "That is exactly what the medication is supposed to do."
   c. "You should be having six to ten stools today, double the dose of medication."
   d. "Only take half of your usual dose today and take your regular dose tomorrow."

10. The nurse is giving instructions to a patient who will be having a colonoscopy in the morning. The patient will be taking polyethylene glycol–electrolyte solution for bowel cleaning. What information will help increase the palatability of this medication?
    a. Refrigerate the solution until it is cold.
    b. Add ice cubes to each glass of liquid.
    c. Allow the liquid to warm up before drinking it.
    d. Warm the liquid in the microwave for 25 seconds before using it.

11. The nurse is caring for a patient with chronic idiopathic constipation and knows that it is characterized by what symptoms? (Select all that apply.)
    a. Presence of loose, watery stools
    b. Straining to pass stools
    c. Abnormal GI motility
    d. Severe abdominal pain
    e. Bloating

12. The nurse is caring for a patient with a K+ level of 6.1 mEq/dL. The nurse is prepared to administer what medication to assist in lowering this lab value?
    a. Bisacodyl
    b. Sodium polystyrene sulfonate
    c. Lactulose
    d. Polyethylene glycol solution

13. The nurse is conducting a class on prevention of constipation and informs the participants that constipation is associated with fluid intake that is less than how much per day?
    a. 2000 mL
    b. 3500 mL
    c. 5000 mL
    d. 10,000 mL

14. The nurse is aware that which medications are known to reduce intestinal function and motility and increase the chance of constipation? (Select all that apply.)
    a. Anticholinergics
    b. Antibiotics
    c. Antidepressants
    d. Antivirals
    e. Anticoagulants

15. The nurse is caring for a group of patients and knows that which patient is most at risk for the development of constipation?
    a. The patient with hyperthyroidism
    b. The patient with hypothyroidism
    c. The patient with gastroenteritis
    d. The patient with rheumatoid arthritis

16. The nurse is assisting a patient with chronic constipation to establish a successful bowel routine. The nurse instructs the patient that what is the best time to use the bathroom for establishment of a routine for bowel elimination?

    a. Immediately upon arising from bed in the morning
    b. Immediately after eating breakfast
    c. Immediately after eating lunch
    d. Immediately after eating dinner

17. The nurse is caring for a patient who will need to use a medication to assist in the prevention of constipation for an extended period of time. The nurse is aware that which drug is the most desirable for long-term use?

    a. Bisacodyl
    b. Polyethylene glycol–electrolyte solution
    c. Lactulose
    d. Psyllium

18. The nurse is conducting a pre-colonoscopy class and knows that polyethylene glycol–electrolyte solution will be contraindicated for the patient with which condition?

    a. Chronic constipation
    b. Colitis
    c. Gastroesophageal reflux disease
    d. Oral stomatitis

19. The nurse would caution a patient with which condition against frequent use of milk of magnesia for treatment of constipation?

    a. The patient with constipation caused by the use of opioid analgesics
    b. The patient with decreased renal function
    c. The patient with decreased liver function
    d. The patient with chronic constipation

20. The nurse recognizes that a patient needs additional instruction if the patient makes which comment about treatment for occasional constipation?

    a. "I will make sure to drink an adequate amount of fluid everyday."
    b. "I will choose more foods with fiber."
    c. "I will make sure that I have a bowel movement every day."
    d. "I will obey the urge to have a bowel movement when it occurs."

Drug Therapy for Diarrhea

■ Identify the common causes of diarrhea.
■ Identify patients at risk for development of diarrhea.
■ Describe opioid-related antidiarrheal agents in terms of the prototype, indications and contraindications for use, routes of administration, and major adverse effects.
■ Identify adjuvant drugs used to manage diarrhea.
■ Understand how to use the nursing process in the care of patients receiving drug therapy for diarrhea.

SECTION I: ASSESSING YOUR UNDERSTANDING

Activity A FILL IN THE BLANKS

1. _____ is a symptom of numerous conditions that increase bowel motility, cause secretion or retention of fluids in the intestinal lumen, and cause inflammation or irritation of the gastrointestinal (GI) tract.

2. *Escherichia coli* O157:H7–related hemorrhagic colitis most commonly occurs with the ingestion of undercooked _____.

3. A serious complication of *E. coli* O157:H7 colitis is _____ syndrome (HUS), which is characterized by thrombocytopenia, microangiopathic hemolytic anemia, and renal failure.

4. So-called travelers' diarrhea is usually caused by an _____ strain of *E. coli* (ETEC).

5. Consumption of improperly prepared poultry may result in diarrhea due to infection with _____.

Activity B MATCHING

Match the term in Column A with the definition in Column B.

Column A	Column B
____ 1. Loperamide (Imodium)	a. Structural analog of the antimycobacterial drug, rifampin
____ 2. Octreotide acetate	b. Useful in treating diarrhea due to bile salt accumulation in conditions such as Crohn's disease or surgical excision of the ileum
____ 3. Polycarbophil and psyllium	
____ 4. Cholestyramine or colestipol (bile-binding drugs)	c. Synthetic derivative of meperidine that decreases GI motility by its effect on intestinal muscles
____ 5. Rifaximin (Xifaxan)	d. Synthetic form of somatostatin, a hormone produced in the anterior pituitary gland and in the pancreas
	e. Most often used as bulk-forming laxatives

Activity C SHORT ANSWERS

Briefly answer the following questions.

1. How do people contract *Salmonella*?

2. How do people contract *Shigella*?

3. How does a lack of digestive enzymes or a deficiency of pancreatic enzymes affect digestion?

4. What is the mechanism by which inflammatory bowel disorders cause diarrhea?

5. What are the symptoms of irritable bowel syndrome (IBS)?

SECTION II: APPLYING YOUR KNOWLEDGE

Activity D CASE STUDY

Consider the scenario and answer the questions.

Mrs. North, age 75, was diagnosed 5 years ago with diarrhea-predominant irritable bowel syndrome. She has experienced an overall 40% weight loss since the initial diagnosis. Multiple conventional therapies have been attempted to control her symptoms without success. She states that she has used medications prescribed by three physicians in the past and hopes that she will meet with success this time. After taking a thorough drug history, the physician orders alosetron (Lotronex). You are responsible for the education plan for Mrs. North.

1. Mrs. North asks why this medication has not been available to her in the past. How would you respond? What kind of drug is alosetron?

2. Mrs. North is diagnosed with an obsessive–compulsive disorder and is prescribed fluvoxamine by her psychiatrist. What kind of drug interaction would you expect? What would you expect the physician to do? What are some other contraindications for the use of alosetron?

3. Is Mrs. North's age a factor in the dosing of this drug? What other factors influence the prescription of alosetron?

SECTION III: PRACTICING FOR NCLEX

Activity E

Answer the following questions.

1. A male patient is diagnosed with bacterial gastroenteritis. On what factor will treatment be based?
   a. Symptomatology
   b. Causative agent and susceptibility tests
   c. Number of days with diarrhea
   d. The country in which the organism originates

2. The nurse is aware that diarrhea is a component of what conditions? (Select all that apply.)
   a. Intestinal infections
   b. Hyperthyroidism
   c. Excessive amount of digestive enzymes
   d. Protein-rich foods
   e. Laxative abuse

3. The nurse is caring for a patient with diarrhea who has been prescribed diphenoxylate with atropine and is observing the patient for which adverse effects of this drug?
   a. Bradycardia
   b. Polyuria
   c. Dizziness
   d. Paleness of the face

4. A husband and wife present to the physician's office with traveler's diarrhea. The nurse expects the physician to order what medication?
   a. Cholestyramine
   b. Psyllium
   c. Octreotide acetate
   d. Bismuth subsalicylate

5. A patient is diagnosed with carcinoid syndrome. The nurse would plan to administer what prescribed medication?
   a. Cholestyramine
   b. Octreotide
   c. Bismuth subsalicylate
   d. Psyllium

6. The nurse is aware that diphenoxylate with atropine is contraindicated in a patient with what condition?
   a. Pathogenic *Escherichia coli* intestinal infection
   b. Diarrhea related to stress/anxiety
   c. Diarrhea caused by metformin
   d. Irritable bowel syndrome

7. The nurse is caring for a patient with HIV who has developed diarrhea. The nurse is aware that diarrhea occurs in HIV patients for what most common reasons? (Select all that apply.)
   a. IBS
   b. Antiretroviral drug therapy
   c. Intestinal neoplasms
   d. Intestinal infections
   e. Diverticulitis

8. A female patient is diagnosed with temporary acute diarrhea. Her other diagnoses include diabetes mellitus, dysrhythmia, and hepatic impairment. The physician orders loperamide. Based on her diagnoses, which adverse effect would the nurse observe for in this patient?
   a. Signs of electrolyte imbalance
   b. Signs of hemorrhage
   c. Signs of hypercalcemia
   d. Signs of CNS toxicity

9. A physician orders diphenoxylate to treat a patient who has severe hepatorenal disease. The nurse calls the physician to question this order because of what reason?
   a. It may precipitate hepatic coma.
   b. It may precipitate hyperkalemia.
   c. It may precipitate hypercalcemia.
   d. It may precipitate hyperglycemia.

10. When administering diphenoxylate to children, the nurse should observe for signs of what condition?
    a. Atropine overdose
    b. Opioid overdose
    c. Fluid and electrolyte imbalance
    d. Hypotensive crisis

11. The nurse is caring for a patient who has anorexia nervosa and is being treated for chronic diarrhea. The nurse is aware that the patient's diarrhea is due to what reason?
    a. Binging
    b. Abuse of laxatives
    c. Intestinal infection
    d. Anxiety

12. The physician has ordered an opioid analgesic for the treatment of diarrhea in a patient. The nurse knows that what dose of morphine is considered effective to treat diarrheal episodes?
    a. 2 mg
    b. 4 mg
    c. 6 mg
    d. 1.25 mg

13. The nurse is caring for a patient who has developed severe diarrhea a few days after beginning an antibiotic prescribed for a severe respiratory infection. The nurse is prepared to initiate what initial treatment?
    a. Imodium
    b. Stopping the causative drug
    c. Administering a medication that will slow peristalsis
    d. Administering a low-dose opioid

14. A patient develops antibiotic-induced colitis. The symptoms have worsened within the past 72 hours. The nurse expects the physician to order what medication, which is considered the initial drug of choice?
    a. Loperamide
    b. Bismuth subsalicylate
    c. Metronidazole
    d. Psyllium

15. The nurse is caring for a patient who has just been diagnosed with ulcerative colitis and knows that what drug is the initial drug of choice for this condition?
    a. Loperamide
    b. Psyllium
    c. Metronidazole
    d. Sulfonamide

16. The nurse receives a phone call from a patient who has been out of the country and is now experiencing diarrhea. The nurse knows that the physician will order what medication for relief of the symptoms of this disorder? (Select all that apply.)

    a. Diphenoxylate with atropine

    b. Psyllium

    c. Metronidazole

    d. Loperamide

17. The nurse cautions a patient with what allergy to avoid the use of bismuth salts in the treatment of diarrhea?

    a. Nuts

    b. Eggs

    c. Aspirin

    d. Penicillin

18. The nurse is conducting a first aid class and informs the class that in the case of acute, nonspecific diarrhea in adults where fluid losses are not severe, patients usually need only simple replacement of fluids and electrolytes lost in the stool. The nurse instructs the class to drink how much fluid during the first 24 hours?

    a. 2 to 3 L of clear liquids

    b. 1 to 2 L of clear liquids

    c. 0.5 to 1 L of clear liquids

    d. 3 to 4 L of clear liquids

19. The nurse is aware that antidiarrheal drugs should not be prescribed if diarrhea is caused by which conditions? (Select all that apply.)

    a. Toxic materials

    b. Microorganisms that penetrate intestinal mucosa

    c. Unknown origin

    d. Antibiotic-associated colitis

20. The nurse is caring for a patient with *Giardia lamblia* and anticipates that the physician will order what drug for the treatment of this patient's diarrhea?

    a. Alosetron

    b. Rifaximin

    c. Nitazoxanide

    d. Cholestyramine

Drug Therapy for Diabetes Mellitus

Learning Objectives

- Differentiate between type 1 and type 2 diabetes mellitus.
- Understand the major effects of endogenous insulin on body tissues.
- Identify the clinical manifestations of type 1 and type 2 diabetes mellitus.
- Identify the prototype and describe the action, use, adverse effects, contraindications, and nursing implications for the insulins.
- Discuss characteristics of the various types of insulins and insulin analogs.
- Identify the various prototypes and describe the actions, uses, adverse effects, contraindications, and nursing implications for the oral antidiabetic drugs.
- Identify the different prototypes and describe the actions, uses, adverse effects, contraindications, and nursing implications for the amylin analogs, incretin mimetics, and dipeptidyl peptidase-4 (DPP-4) inhibitors.
- Implement the nursing process in the care of patients receiving medications for the treatment of diabetes mellitus.
  - Explain the benefits of maintaining glycemic control in preventing complications of diabetes.
  - Assist patients or caregivers in learning how to manage diabetes care, including administration of medication agents used to manage diabetes.
  - Assess and monitor patients' adherence to prescribed management strategies.

SECTION I: ASSESSING YOUR UNDERSTANDING

Activity A FILL IN THE BLANKS

1. _____ is a protein hormone secreted by beta cells in the pancreas.
2. _____, a pancreatic hormone secreted with insulin, delays gastric emptying, increases satiety, and suppresses glucagon secretion, thus complementing the effects of insulin on the blood sugar.
3. Insulin is secreted into the portal circulation and transported to the _____, where about half is used or degraded.
4. Liver, muscle, and _____ cells have many insulin receptors and are primary tissues for insulin action.
5. In the kidneys, insulin is filtered by the _____ and reabsorbed by the tubules, which also degrade it.

Activity B MATCHING

Match the term in Column A with the definition in Column B.

Column A	Column B
_____ 1. Regular insulin	a. Oldest and largest group of oral agents
_____ 2. Exubera	b. Inhaled insulin, approved and then removed from the market

___ **3.** Sulfonylureas

___ **4.** Acarbose and miglitol

___ **5.** Metformin

c. Increases the use of glucose by muscle and fat cells, decreases hepatic glucose production, and decreases intestinal absorption of glucose

d. Used to replace endogenous insulin; has the same effects as the pancreatic hormone

e. Inhibits alpha-glucosidase enzymes in the GI tract; delays digestion of complex carbohydrates into simple sugars

Activity C **SHORT ANSWERS**

Briefly answer the following questions.

1. How does the drug metformin help the patient with type 2 diabetes manage his or her disease?

2. How do thiazolidinediones decrease insulin resistance?

3. Identify the characteristics of the drug pramlintide (Symlin) and the mechanism by which it helps the patient to control his or her blood glucose?

4. How does the drug exenatide help the patient to control his or her blood glucose?

5. Identify one supplement that may increase blood glucose levels and describe the supplement's mechanism of action.

SECTION II: APPLYING YOUR KNOWLEDGE

Activity D **CASE STUDY**

Consider the scenario and answer the questions.

Mrs. Ingles, age 45, is diagnosed with type 2 diabetes. She works in an office and leads a sedentary lifestyle. Her vital signs are as follows: BP 140/84, AP 101 regular, and R 20; fasting glucose is 154; height is 5′6″; and weight is 210 pounds. You are responsible for her education plan regarding both her diabetes disease process and the medication ordered by her primary physician.

1. Based on your assessment, what are two indicators that place Mrs. Ingles at high risk for diabetes?

2. What are the signs and symptoms of hyperglycemia?

3. Laboratory tests indicate that Mrs. Ingles is dehydrated. What is the relationship between uncontrolled type 2 diabetes and dehydration?

4. Mrs. Ingles is given a diet and exercise program and revisits her physician 3 months later. Her fasting glucose is 164, and she has not lost weight. She feels that there are not enough hours in the day to adhere to an exercise program and admits that she is not motivated to comply. The physician orders exenatide (Byetta). What can you teach Mrs. Ingles about this medication?

SECTION III: PRACTICING FOR NCLEX

Activity E

Answer the following questions.

1. A male 43-year-old patient weighs 246 pounds and is 5′10″ tall. His occupation is sedentary and he works 50 to 60 hours a week. His fasting glucose test results are 132 and 140 on two separate occasions. What nonmedication methods would the nurse include in the education plan to assist the patient to reduce his blood glucose? (Select all that apply.)

a. Large doses of vitamin C

b. Routine exercise

c. Elimination of simple sugars

d. Lose weight if needed

e. High-carbohydrate diet

2. The nurse is discussing diabetes mellitus with a group of people who are involved in a weight loss program. The nurse relates to the group that the parameters for a diagnosis of diabetes are a fasting plasma glucose test (FPG) greater than or equal to what level on two separate occasions?

a. 130 mg/dL

b. 118 mg/dL

c. 120 mg/dL

d. 126 mg/dL

3. A group of physicians and nurses are establishing parameters for an outpatient clinic geared to diabetes testing and treatment. What is the fastest and most cost-effective test to determine a diagnosis of diabetes?

   a. Fasting plasma glucose test

   b. Preprandial and postprandial blood glucose test

   c. Urine dip test

   d. Capillary random blood glucose

4. A female patient visits the physician's office after routine labs are drawn. The nurse notes that her A1C is 9. How does the nurse interpret this finding?

   a. Patient is in good glycemic control.

   b. Patient's average blood glucose is above normal.

   c. Patient's blood glucose levels are not consistent.

   d. Patient's blood glucose demonstrates long-standing hypoglycemia.

5. A female patient is a newly diagnosed diabetic. She is a stay-at-home mother and responsible for meal planning and management of the home. What will the home care nurse teach this patient? (Select all that apply.)

   a. Instruct the patient to go to the emergency department immediately if she develops a cold or upper respiratory infection.

   b. Assist the patient in making menus that will meet the needs of both the patient and the family.

   c. Watch the patient draw up and administer her insulin.

   d. Reinforce instructions on dealing with hypoglycemia.

   e. Encourage the patient to check her blood glucose every hour.

6. A female patient is admitted into the critical care unit with a diagnosis of myocardial infarct and subsequent bypass grafts. She has had type 1 diabetes for 10 years. The nurse understands that strict control of the patient's hyperglycemia is critical to prevent what outcomes? (Select all that apply.)

   a. Postoperative infections

   b. Increased mortality

   c. Decreased absorption of antibiotics

   d. Hypertensive crisis

   e. Liver damage

7. A 54-year-old patient is diagnosed with chronic renal failure and hyperglycemia. He asks if he can be prescribed sulfonylurea because it works well for his friend. If he were to be given sulfonylurea, this patient's renal impairment may lead to what effect?

   a. Accumulation and hypoglycemia

   b. Accumulation and hyperglycemic reactions

   c. Decreased absorption of the sulfonylurea

   d. Hypersensitivity to sulfonylurea

8. The nurse is caring for a patient who is taking a thiazide diuretic, a corticosteroid, and estrogens. The nurse understands that this patient is at risk for what condition?

   a. Hypoglycemia

   b. Pulmonary hypertension

   c. Congestive heart failure

   d. Hyperglycemia

9. The school nurse identifies more children with type 2 diabetes each year and recognizes that this trend is mainly attributed to what issue?

   a. Working parents

   b. Economics

   c. Obesity and inadequate exercise

   d. Lack of after-school programs due to budget constraints

10. The nurse admitted a 4-year-old child with type 1 diabetes mellitus. The nurse educates the parents that hypoglycemia can occur as an adverse effect of insulin. The nurse helps the parents to understand that in young children, hypoglycemia may manifest as what signs or symptoms? (Select all that apply.)

    a. Irritability

    b. Anorexia

    c. Impaired mental functioning

    d. Hallucinations

    e. Lethargy

11. The nurse is teaching a class to parents of children who have just been diagnosed with type 1 diabetes mellitus. The nurse informs the parents that recognition of hypoglycemia may be delayed in children because signs and symptoms are vague and the children may be unable to communicate them to parents or caregivers. Because of these difficulties, most pediatric diabetologists recommend maintaining blood glucose levels in what range?

    a. Between 90 and 110 mg/dL

    b. Between 100 and 200 mg/dL

    c. Between 120 and 150 mg/dL

    d. Between 110 and 150 mg/dL

12. The nurse is teaching a patient to self-administer insulin. The patient takes a daily dose of 30 units NPH and 20 units of regular insulin. How will the nurse teach this patient to administer this combination of medications?

    a. Draw up the NPH in one syringe and the regular insulin in another syringe and inject in different areas of the body.

    b. Draw up the NPH in one syringe and the regular insulin in another syringe and inject in the same site.

    c. Draw up the regular insulin first and then the NPH insulin in the same syringe.

    d. Draw up the NPH insulin first and then the regular insulin in the same syringe.

13. A 2-month-old male child is diagnosed with diabetes. His parents are having difficulty measuring 2 units of insulin in the U-100 syringe. What would the nurse expect the physician to order?

    a. U-50 (50 units/mL) insulin

    b. U-20 (20 units/mL) insulin

    c. U-30 (30 units/mL) insulin

    d. U-10 (10 units/mL) insulin

14. A 4-year-old female child is diabetic with a blood glucose level of 120 mg/dL. The child's mother brings her to the physician's office with symptoms of the flu and dehydration. What would the nurse expect the physician to order?

    a. Regular sodas, clear juices, and regular gelatin desserts

    b. Diet sodas, clear juices, and regular gelatin desserts

    c. IV Ringer's solution

    d. IV saline 0.9%

15. The nurse is caring for a patient who is taking glyburide as treatment for type 2 diabetes mellitus. The physician has added a corticosteroid to this patient's medication regimen for treatment of a severe allergic reaction. The nurse knows that this drug combination may cause what adverse effect on this patient?

    a. The patient is at risk for hypoglycemia.

    b. The patient is at risk for hyperglycemia.

    c. The patient will experience nausea and vomiting.

    d. The patient will experience rash and fever.

16. The nurse is educating a patient who is beginning therapy with acarbose and tells the patient to take the medication with the first bite of each main meal to help prevent what adverse effect?

    a. Dizziness

    b. Bloating and diarrhea

    c. Nausea and vomiting

    d. Chest pain

17. The nurse is educating a patient who will be adding an injection of pramlintide to his insulin regimen. What information is most important for the nurse to share with this patient to ensure safe medication administration?

    a. Pramlintide should only be injected in the hip.

    b. Inject pramlintide in the same site where insulin is administered.

    c. Do not give pramlintide in the same site where insulin is administered.

    d. Mix pramlintide in the same syringe with insulin.

18. The nurse is educating a newly diagnosed diabetic who must learn how to give himself insulin injections. The nurse tells the patient that insulin is absorbed fastest from which area of injection?

    a. Deltoid

    b. Thigh

    c. Abdomen

    d. Hip

19. The nurse is caring for a patient who receives an injection of irregular insulin before each meal. How many minutes before a meal should regular insulin be injected?

   a. 10 to 15

   b. 30 to 45

   c. 20 to 30

   d. 15 to 20

20. The nurse is caring for a patient with type 2 diabetes who is being treated with a regimen called BIDS. The nurse is aware that this regimen consists of what medications?

   a. Sulfonylurea plus metformin

   b. Sulfonylurea plus a meglitinide

   c. Bedtime insulin plus daytime sulfonylurea

   d. Metformin plus a thiazolidinedione

40 CHAPTER

Drug Therapy for Hyperthyroidism and Hypothyroidism

Learning Objectives

- Understand the physiologic effects of thyroid hormone.
- Describe the etiology, pathophysiology, and clinical manifestations of hyperthyroidism.
- Describe the etiology, pathophysiology, and clinical manifestations of hypothyroidism.
- Identify the prototype and describe the action, use, adverse effects, contraindications, and nursing implications of the drugs administered for the treatment of hyperthyroidism.
- Identify the prototype and describe the action, use, adverse effects, contraindications, and nursing implications of the drugs administered for the treatment of hypothyroidism.
- Implement the nursing process in the care of the patient receiving medications for the treatment of hyperthyroidism or hypothyroidism.

SECTION I: ASSESSING YOUR UNDERSTANDING

Activity A FILL IN THE BLANKS

1. The thyroid gland produces three hormones: _____, triiodothyronine, and calcitonin.

2. Production of T_3 and T_4 depends on the presence of _____ and _____ in the thyroid gland.

3. Thyroid hormones control the rate of _____ and thereby influence the functioning of virtually every cell in the body.

4. _____ occurs when disease or destruction of thyroid gland tissue causes inadequate production of thyroid hormones.

5. _____ occurs when a child is born with a poorly functioning or absent thyroid gland.

Activity B MATCHING

Match the term in Column A with the definition in Column B.

Column A	Column B
____ **1.** Levothyroxine (Synthroid, Levothroid)	**a.** Synthetic preparation of T_4; the drug of choice for long-term treatment of hypothyroidism and serves as the prototype
____ **2.** Sodium iodide ^{131}I (Iodotope)	**b.** Prototype of the thioamide antithyroid drugs
____ **3.** Strong iodine solution (Lugol's solution) and saturated solution of potassium iodide (SSKI)	**c.** Similar to PTU in actions, uses, and adverse reactions; well absorbed with oral administration; rapidly reaches peak plasma levels

162

____ **4.** Propylthioura-
cil (PTU)

d. Radioactive isotope of iodine

____ **5.** Methimazole (Tapazole)

e. Sometimes used in short-term treatment of hyperthyroidism

Activity C **SHORT ANSWERS**

Briefly answer the following questions.

1. Define hyperthyroidism and the various causes of this disease process.

2. Define thyrotoxic crisis, and discuss the various causes of this complication.

3. What are the mechanisms of action for both thyroid and antithyroid medications?

4. What are the indications for use for both thyroid and antithyroid medications?

5. Identify the various contraindications for the use of iodine preparations and thioamide antithyroid drugs.

SECTION II: APPLYING YOUR KNOWLEDGE

Activity D **CASE STUDIES**

Consider the scenarios and answer the questions.

Case Study 1

Ms. Davis, a nursing student, is diagnosed with subclinical hypothyroidism. You are responsible for the education care plan regarding the patient's diagnosis.

1. Ms. Davis asks you to explain the difference between clinical and subclinical hypothyroidism. How would you describe subclinical hypothyroidism?

2. Ms. Davis asks you how long she will need the replacement therapy ordered by the physician. What is the standard duration of this type of therapy? How long does the patient have to be euthyroid before a change in therapy is considered?

Case Study 2

Mrs. Michelson, age 62, is diagnosed with subclinical hyperthyroidism. You are responsible for her education plan.

1. What are the laboratory values of T_3, T_4, and TSH that represent subclinical hyperthyroidism?

2. For Mrs. Michelson's age and sex, what is a risk factor associated with subclinical hyperthyroidism? If this patient has multiple cardiac diagnoses, what new diagnosis is she also at risk for?

SECTION III: PRACTICING FOR NCLEX

Activity E

Answer the following questions.

1. The nurse is caring for a patient who is seeking care for a chronic condition. The nurse is aware that the FDA has issued a black box warning regarding the use of thyroid hormones for the treatment of what condition?

   a. Obesity

   b. Hypotension

   c. Diabetes mellitus type 1

   d. GERD

2. A 25-year-old female patient is diagnosed with hypothyroidism. She is admitted to the hospital for acute gallbladder disease and subsequent surgical intervention. When planning postoperative opioid pain management, the nurse must take into account the fact that the patient is at greater risk for what condition, secondary to the patient's hypothyroidism diagnosis?

   a. Hypotension

   b. Hypertension

   c. Respiratory depression

   d. Atrial fibrillation

3. The nurse is responsible for the education plan for parents of a child born with congenital hypothyroidism. When should drug therapy start for this patient?

   a. Within 72 hours after birth

   b. Within 6 weeks after birth

   c. Within 24 hours after birth

   d. Within 48 hours after birth

4. The nurse is discussing medication therapy with a family whose infant was born with congenital hypothyroidism and informs them that drug therapy will continue for life to prevent what condition?

   a. To prevent cardiac dysrhythmias

   b. To prevent seizure disorder

   c. To prevent chronic hypotension

   d. To prevent mental retardation

5. The nurse educates a patient newly diagnosed with hypothyroidism that replacement therapy usually continues until the patient is euthyroid for how long?

   a. 6 to 12 months

   b. 18 to 24 months

   c. 3 to 6 months

   d. 8 to 12 months

6. The nurse in the newborn nursery is assessing an infant with suspected congenital hypothyroidism. What assessment findings support this diagnosis? (Select all that apply.)

   a. Elevated temperature

   b. Bradycardia

   c. Feeding difficulties

   d. Lethargy

   e. Diarrhea

7. A female patient comes to the physician's office for her annual checkup. Her medications include a regimen to treat her hyperthyroidism. The nurse would be alert for which symptoms or disease processes in this patient?

   a. Hypothyroidism

   b. Hyperthyroidism

   c. Dysrhythmias

   d. Hypertension

8. The nurse is caring for a patient with severe hypothyroidism and knows to contact the physician if which symptoms of myxedema coma occur? (Select all that apply.)

   a. Decreased level of consciousness

   b. Fever

   c. Decreased respirations

   d. High blood glucose level

   e. Decreased blood pressure

9. The home care nurse may be involved in a wide range of activities when caring for the patient with hyperthyroidism or hypothyroidism. What would be included in the patient's plan of care? (Select all that apply.)

   a. Assessing the patient's response to therapy

   b. Teaching about the disease process

   c. Modifying medication dosages based on symptomatology

   d. Preventing and managing adverse drug effects

   e. Provide information for rapid weight loss

10. A patient is admitted to the intensive care unit in thyrotoxic crisis. What would the nurse expect to happen to the patient's medication dosages?

    a. They would decrease in frequency.

    b. They would increase in frequency.

    c. They would be given by the intramuscular route only.

    d. They would be given by the subcutaneous route only.

11. A patient is diagnosed with liver disease. How would this affect the metabolism of the drugs used to treat the patient's hypothyroidism?

    a. It would be unaffected.

    b. It would be rapid.

    c. It would be prolonged.

    d. It would be short-lived.

12. The nurse is assisting a patient who has just begun medication therapy for hypothyroidism. Which nursing assessment is most important in this patient?

    a. Vital signs

    b. Skin

    c. Vision

    d. Pain

13. An 83-year-old patient is diagnosed with hypothyroidism and cardiovascular disease. The patient is given levothyroxine to manage the hypothyroidism. The nurse would be alert for what symptom or disease process after institution of the drug?

    a. Congestive heart failure

    b. Hypertension

    c. Seizures

    d. Anaphylaxis

14. The nurse is preparing to administer methimazole to an 11-year-old patient newly diagnosed with hyperthyroidism. What are the potential risks for the use of methimazole in children? (Select all that apply.)

    a. Cancer caused by radioactive iodine
    b. Chromosome damage
    c. Chronic hypertension
    d. Chronic hypotension
    e. Chronic hypothyroidism

15. A female patient's diagnoses include hyperthyroidism, congestive heart failure, and type 2 diabetes mellitus. What effect will the treatment of hyperthyroidism have on her routine medications?

    a. Metabolism will be slower than normal, and the dose will be increased.
    b. Metabolism will be slower than normal, and the dose will be decreased.
    c. Metabolism will be faster than normal, and the dose will be decreased.
    d. Metabolism will be faster than normal, and the dose will be increased.

16. A patient's physician has ordered a trial discontinuance of the patient's thyroid medication. The nurse is responsible for the patient's medication education plan. The nurse knows that the patient's medication will be discontinued at what point?

    a. With her next prescription
    b. Gradually over weeks or months
    c. Gradually over a week
    d. Gradually over 48 to 72 hours

17. A patient is diagnosed with both hypothyroidism and adrenal insufficiency. If the adrenal insufficiency is not treated first, what may occur with the administration of thyroid hormone?

    a. Hypertensive crisis
    b. Acute congestive heart failure
    c. Acute adrenocortical insufficiency
    d. Life-threatening dysrhythmias

18. The nurse is preparing to administer levothyroxine to a patient. Which assessment finding would cause the nurse to hold the medication?

    a. Respiratory rate of 16
    b. Temperature of 99.3°F
    c. Heart rate of 110 beats per minute
    d. Blood pressure of 107/64

19. The nurse is caring for a patient who is receiving levothyroxine and educates the patient to what adverse effects of this medication? (Select all that apply.)

    a. Lethargy
    b. Fever
    c. Weight gain
    d. Insomnia
    e. Intolerance to heat

20. The nurse is caring for a patient who has a possible thyroid disorder and is aware that what medication will be used in diagnostic testing?

    a. PTU
    b. Levothyroxine
    c. Sodium iodide[131]I
    d. Propranolol

41

Drug Therapy for Pituitary and Hypothalamic Dysfunction

Learning Objectives

- Describe the functions of the anterior and posterior pituitary hormones as well as the hypothalamic hormones.
- Identify the pathophysiology and clinical manifestations of central precocious puberty, acromegaly, growth deficiency in children, and diabetes insipidus.
- Identify the prototype and describe the action, use, adverse effects, contraindications, and nursing implications of the anterior pituitary hormone used to treat growth hormone deficiency in children.
- Identify the prototype and describe the action, use, adverse effects, contraindications, and nursing implications of the posterior pituitary hormone used to treat diabetes insipidus.
- Identify the prototype and describe the action, use, adverse effects, contraindications, and nursing implications of the hypothalamic hormone drugs used to treat precious puberty.
- Identify the prototype and describe the action, use, adverse effects, contraindications, and nursing implications of the hypothalamic hormone drugs used to treat acromegaly.
- Implement the nursing process in the care of the patient receiving specific pituitary and hypothalamic hormones.

SECTION I: ASSESSING YOUR UNDERSTANDING

Activity A FILL IN THE BLANKS

1. The hypothalamus of the brain and the pituitary gland interact to control most metabolic functions of the body and to maintain _____.

2. The hypothalamus and the pituitary gland are anatomically connected by the funnel-shaped _____ stalk.

3. The _____ controls secretions of the pituitary gland.

4. The pituitary gland regulates secretions or functions of other body tissues, called _____.

5. The posterior pituitary is anatomically an extension of the hypothalamus and is composed mainly of _____ fibers.

Activity B MATCHING

Match the term in Column A with the definition in Column B.

Column A	Column B
____ **1.** Thyrotropin-releasing hormone (TRH)	**a.** Also called ACTH; stimulates the adrenal cortex to produce corticosteroids
____ **2.** Gonadotropin-releasing hormone (GnRH)	**b.** Also called somatotropin; stimulates growth of body tissues
____ **3.** Corticotropin	**c.** Causes release of follicle-stimulating hormone (FSH) and luteinizing hormone (LH)
____ **4.** GH	
____ **5.** Thyrotropin	**d.** Also called TSH; regulates secretion of thyroid hormones
	e. Causes release of TSH in response to stress, such as exposure to cold

Activity C SHORT ANSWERS

Briefly answer the following questions.

1. What is the function of FSH in the human body?

2. What is the function of LH in the human body?

3. What is the function of prolactin in the human body?

4. What is the function of the melanocyte-stimulating hormone in the human body?

5. What is the function of oxytocin in the human body?

SECTION II: APPLYING YOUR KNOWLEDGE

Activity D CASE STUDY

Consider the scenario and answer the questions.

Mr. Chasen is diagnosed with end-stage prostate cancer. The physician orders Lupron 1 mg subcutaneously each day. You are responsible for the patient's education regarding his disease process and medication regimen.

1. You explain that leuprolide (Lupron) initially stimulates LH and FSH secretion. After chronic administration of therapeutic doses, however, what does the drug do?

2. Mr. Chasen is concerned when he is told that his medication regimen will decrease his testosterone level and asks whether this change is permanent. How would you respond?

3. Mrs. Chasen, your patient's wife, is hesitant to administer the medication by injection and asks whether her husband can take the medication by mouth. How would you respond? What other information can you give Mrs. Chasen regarding dosing?

4. What information would you give the patient regarding the adverse effects related to Lupron?

SECTION III: PRACTICING FOR NCLEX

Activity E

Answer the following questions.

1. The nurse is caring for a child who has chronic renal insufficiency and is receiving somatropin. The nurse knows that this medication is prescribed at what point?

   a. Prior to renal dialysis

   b. Prior to renal transplantation

   c. After abdominal surgery

   d. After an acute respiratory illness

2. The nurse is caring for a patient who is receiving desmopressin for treatment of neurogenic diabetes insipidus. The nurse will be alert for which symptom that will alert the patient to a serious adverse effect?

   a. Decrease in urine output

   b. Diminished mental status

   c. Increasing urine specific gravity

   d. Decrease in thirst

3. A patient is diagnosed with hyperpituitarism. The nurse knows that this condition is most often treated by what methods? (Select all that apply.)
   a. Medication to reduce pituitary secretion
   b. Antibiotics
   c. Surgery
   d. Radiation
   e. Vascular embolization

4. A female patient is diagnosed with a pituitary hormone deficiency. She complains that her drug dosages are modified frequently. The nurse explains that the dosage of all pituitary hormones must be individualized. The nurse knows that what factor determines the dosage?
   a. The responsiveness of affected tissues, which varies
   b. The age of the patient
   c. The weight of the patient
   d. The responsiveness of affected tissues, which is static

5. A 45-year-old patient is receiving somatropin for treatment of a growth hormone deficiency. The nurse educates the patient that regular laboratory tests will be needed to monitor the patient for which adverse effect?
   a. Leukocytosis
   b. Renal dysfunction
   c. Hyperglycemia
   d. Hyponatremia

6. A 43-year-old female patient has a history of breast cancer, hyperlipidemia, and atrial fibrillation. She has heard that GH will improve her appearance and increase her energy. The nurse understands that, based on the patient's diagnoses, GH would increase her risk for what condition?
   a. Cancer
   b. Gastrointestinal disease
   c. Pancreatitis
   d. Type 2 diabetes

7. The nurse uses caution when administering somatropin to patients with which conditions? (Select all that apply.)
   a. Turner's syndrome
   b. Obesity
   c. Psoriasis

d. Family history of diabetes mellitus
   e. Family history of hepatic dysfunction

8. The nurse is preparing a female patient for oxytocin induction of labor. The patient asks how the IV medication will induce labor. The nurse is aware that this medication is used because of what drug action?
   a. Promotes uterine irritability
   b. Increases oxygenation to the uterus
   c. Causes labor to continue slowly
   d. Promotes uterine contractility

9. The nurse would contact the physician prior to administering desmopressin to a patient with a history of what condition?
   a. Allergy to bananas
   b. Heart attack
   c. Detached retina
   d. Gout

10. A patient is diagnosed with diabetes insipidus. The physician orders desmopressin, which the nurse knows is the synthetic equivalent of what hormone?
    a. PTH
    b. ACTH
    c. ADH
    d. PTCH

11. A male patient is diagnosed with acromegaly. His secondary diagnoses include hypertension, type 2 diabetes, and a status post myocardial infarct in 1992. Based on his diagnoses, the nurse expects the physician to modify the dose of which of his medications?
    a. Hypoglycemic medication
    b. Antihypertensive medication
    c. Antianginal medication
    d. Nitrate medication

12. The nurse is educating the family of a 9-year-old male patient with precocious puberty about which adverse effects of leuprolide acetate? (Select all that apply.)
    a. Flat affect
    b. Vasodilation
    c. Acne
    d. Pain at injection site
    e. Enlargement of genitals

13. The nurse is caring for a patient who is to receive octreotide and understands that octreotide has pharmacologic actions similar to those of somatostatin. The nurse is aware that octreotide is prescribed for which conditions? (Select all that apply.)
    a. Hyperlipidemia
    b. Acromegaly
    c. Hypertension
    d. Diarrhea in AIDS
    e. Postoperative nausea

14. The nurse is caring for a 73-year-old patient who is receiving growth hormone. The nurse understands that this medication is only used in older adults for what condition?
    a. Hypothyroidism
    b. Hyperthyroidism
    c. Removal of pituitary gland
    d. Prostate gland carcinoma

15. The nurse is admitting a patient with a possible diagnosis of diabetes insipidus. The nurse knows that what assessments are necessary before this patient begins drug therapy? (Select all that apply.)
    a. Weight
    b. BMI
    c. Urine specific gravity
    d. Ratio of intake to output
    e. Renal function laboratory tests

16. The nurse is aware that desmopressin is used in the treatment of diabetes insipidus and what other disorder?
    a. Type 2 diabetes mellitus
    b. Type 1 diabetes mellitus
    c. Nocturnal enuresis
    d. Kidney failure

17. The nurse is providing discharge instructions to a patient who will be self-administering octreotide for treatment of acromegaly. The nurse instructs the patient to schedule which follow-up/diagnostic tests while on octreotide? (Select all that apply.)
    a. Blood glucose
    b. Ultrasound of the kidney for kidney stones
    c. Ultrasound of the gallbladder for gallbladder stones
    d. White blood cell count
    e. Octreotide levels

18. A male patient is prescribed GH. He also takes a medication to control his type 2 diabetes. The nurse understands that GH can cause what condition?
    a. Hyperinsulinemia
    b. Hypoinsulinemia
    c. Hypertension
    d. Hyperglycemia

19. The nurse is aware that somatropin is not appropriate for the person who exhibits growth impairment and what other condition?
    a. Skeletal height below the 10th percentile for age
    b. Closure of the epiphyseal plate
    c. Lack of lean body mass
    d. Decreased number of red blood cells

20. The nurse instructs the patient who is taking desmopressin to avoid drinking alcohol because of what reason?
    a. Alcohol increases the diuretic effect.
    b. Alcohol decreases the diuretic effect.
    c. Desmopressin increases the effect of alcohol.
    d. Desmopressin produces intense vomiting when used with alcohol.

42

Drug Therapy to Regulate Calcium and Bone Metabolism

Learning Objectives

- Examine the roles of parathyroid hormone, calcitonin, and vitamin D in regulating calcium metabolism.
- Evaluate the use of calcium and vitamin D supplements, as well as calcitonin, in the treatment of osteoporosis.
- Identify the prototype and describe the action, use, adverse effects, contraindications, and nursing implications of the bisphosphonates used in the treatment of osteoporosis.
- Outline appropriate management strategies of hypercalcemia as a medical emergency.
- Implement the nursing process in the care of the patient receiving drug therapy to regulate calcium and bone metabolism.

SECTION I: ASSESSING YOUR UNDERSTANDING

Activity A FILL IN THE BLANKS

1. Three hormones regulate calcium and bone metabolism: _____, calcitonin, and vitamin D.

2. _____ secretion is stimulated by low serum calcium levels and inhibited by normal or high levels (a negative feedback system).

3. The patient diagnosis related to insufficient production of PTH would be _____.

4. Excessive production of PTH usually related to removal or damage to the parathyroid glands during neck surgery is called _____.

5. Clinical manifestations and treatment of hypoparathyroidism are the same as those of _____.

Activity B MATCHING

Match the term in Column A with the definition in Column B.

Column A	Column B
____ **1.** Vitamin D	**a.** Hormone from the thyroid gland whose secretion is controlled by the concentration of ionized calcium in the blood flowing through the thyroid gland
____ **2.** Calcium and vitamin D	**b.** Used to treat hypocalcemia and to prevent and treat osteoporosis
____ **3.** Calcitonin	**c.** Given for acute, symptomatic hypocalcemia

_____ **4.** An intravenous (IV) calcium salt

_____ **5.** Calcium carbonate or citrate

d. Given for asymptomatic, less severe, or chronic hypocalcemia

e. Fat-soluble vitamin that includes both ergocalciferol and cholecalciferol

Activity C SHORT ANSWERS

Briefly answer the following questions.

1. How is the secretion of PTH regulated?

2. When the serum calcium level falls below the normal range, how does the level normalize?

3. Discuss the causes of hyperparathyroidism.

4. What is the role of calcitonin as it relates to serum calcium?

5. What is the role of vitamin D as it relates to calcium and bone metabolism?

SECTION II: APPLYING YOUR KNOWLEDGE

Activity D CASE STUDY

Consider the scenario and answer the questions.

Mrs. Bates, aged 52, is diagnosed with osteoporosis based on bone density studies. You are responsible for the education plan for both her disease process and her medication regimen.

1. Mrs. Bates confides that her friend told her that osteoporosis is a form of cancer. How would you reply?

2. What causes osteoporosis?

3. Explain the concept of bone remodeling.

4. The physician orders Fosamax for the treatment of Mrs. Bates' osteoporosis. What is the mechanism of action for this drug? What instructions would you give Mrs. Bates about taking the drug with food?

SECTION III: PRACTICING FOR NCLEX

Activity E

Answer the following questions.

1. A patient is being treated with long-term corticosteroids. What effect will these drugs have?
   a. They will decrease testosterone levels.
   b. They will increase testosterone levels.
   c. They will not affect testosterone levels.
   d. They will increase fertility.

2. The nurse is discussing the use of corticosteroids with a group of nursing students and tells that students that both men and women who take corticosteroids are at risk for what side effect?
   a. Infertility
   b. Osteoporosis
   c. Hypertension
   d. Paget's disease

3. The nurse is caring for four patients. Which patient is at the highest risk for osteoporosis?
   a. The patient receiving diuretic therapy
   b. The patient with a diagnosis of renal hypertension
   c. The patient with frequent falls
   d. The female patient aged 76

4. The nurse is caring for a 77-year-old patient and understands that calcium deficiency commonly occurs in the elderly because of what factors? (Select all that apply.)
   a. Impaired absorption of calcium from the intestine
   b. Excessive exposure to ultraviolet rays
   c. Lack of exposure to sunlight
   d. Impaired liver or kidney metabolism of vitamin D
   e. Excessive intake of sodium

5. The nurse is caring for a patient who has hypocalcemia. The patient also has hypomagnesemia. The nurse knows that medications to correct these conditions will be administered in what manner?

   a. The nurse will administer calcium and then magnesium.

   b. The nurse will hold the calcium until the magnesium level is normal.

   c. The nurse will administer both the calcium and the magnesium at the same time.

   d. The nurse will administer IV calcium followed by oral magnesium.

6. The nurse is concerned that a patient has taken too much vitamin D. What symptoms will the patient exhibit who has vitamin D excess? (Select all that apply.)

   a. Muscle pain

   b. Lethargy

   c. Decrease in urine production

   d. Polydipsia

   e. Irritability

7. The nurse is caring for a patient with a vitamin D deficiency and recognizes that this deficiency causes inadequate absorption of what?

   a. Phosphorus

   b. Calcium

   c. Magnesium

   d. Calcium and phosphorus

8. The nurse is admitting a patient who has been diagnosed with hyperparathyroidism and asks the nurse what causes this condition. The nurse tells the patient that hyperparathyroidism can occur because of what reasons? (Select all that apply.)

   a. A tumor of a parathyroid gland

   b. Hypercalcemia

   c. Hyperplasia of a parathyroid gland

   d. Hypocalcemia

   e. Ectopic secretion of PTH

9. A 45-year-old male patient is scheduled for renal dialysis. He develops hypercalcemia. The physician orders a calcium-free solution for his dialysis treatments. What would the physician order to prevent hyperphosphatemia?

   a. Calcium acetate

   b. Calcium and vitamin D

   c. Vitamin D

   d. Magnesium

10. The nurse is caring for a patient with a possible calcium deficiency and reads the patient's history to see if the patient has experienced which common reasons for calcium deficiency? (Select all that apply.)

   a. Long-term dietary deficiencies of calcium and vitamin D

   b. Impaired absorption of calcium from the intestine

   c. Lack of exposure to sunlight

   d. Overexposure to ultraviolet rays

   e. Chronic use of ampicillin

11. A female patient presents to the physician's office for a routine physical examination. The nurse assesses her current over-the-counter drug history and discovers that she takes vitamin D 600 international units daily. The nurse recognizes that the patient is at risk for what condition?

   a. Paget's disease

   b. Hypocalcemia

   c. Hypocalciuria

   d. Hypercalcemia

12. A 45-year-old female patient is diagnosed with osteoporosis. For 10 years, she has been taking phenytoin to control her seizure disorder. What possible effects do anticonvulsant medications have on osteoporosis?

   a. They do not affect calcium metabolism.

   b. They decrease hepatic metabolism of vitamin D, contributing to the development of osteoporosis.

   c. They increase hepatic metabolism of vitamin D, which decreases calcium absorption in the intestine.

   d. They only marginally affect calcium metabolism and reabsorption of calcium in the bone.

13. A 43-year-old male patient takes prednisone 7.5 mg daily to treat his temporal arteritis. His dose varies from 7.5 to 10 mg based on symptoms and laboratory test analysis. His disease process has been managed successfully with this drug regimen for 7 years. To prevent osteoporosis, what would his physician order? (Select all that apply.)
    a. A calcium supplement
    b. Testosterone
    c. A bisphosphonate drug
    d. Regular weight-bearing exercise
    e. A soy supplement

14. The nurse is caring for a patient who would like to increase her phosphorus intake. The nurse instructs the patient to increase the amount of what foods that are high in phosphorus?
    a. Apples
    b. Dairy products
    c. Tomatoes
    d. Potatoes

15. The nurse is caring for a patient who is being monitored for hypercalcemia. The nurse understands that what calcium level is considered a medical emergency?
    a. 8.5 mg/dL
    b. 9.0 mg/dL
    c. 10.5 mg/dL
    d. 12 mg/dL

16. A 54-year-old female patient is diagnosed with atrial fibrillation, which has been effectively controlled by digoxin for 6 years. She has also been self-administering calcium for 6 months. What conditions might the combination of digoxin and calcium preparations cause? (Select all that apply.)
    a. Dysrhythmia
    b. Hypertension
    c. Digoxin toxicity
    d. Subtherapeutic digoxin levels
    e. Pulmonary edema

17. The nurse is caring for a patient who is interested in taking a calcium supplement for bone health. The nurse is aware that calcium is contraindicated if the patient has what condition? (Select all that apply.)
    a. Hypocalcemia
    b. Kidney stones
    c. Cancer with bone metastases
    d. Hyperphosphatemia
    e. Ventricular fibrillation

18. A female patient presents to the emergency department with symptoms and laboratory values indicative of hypercalcemia. What IV solutions would the physician order to treat the hypercalcemia?
    a. Sodium chloride (0.9%)
    b. D5 1/2 normal saline
    c. D5 1/4 normal saline
    d. Lactated Ringer's solution

19. The nurse knows that phosphates should be given only when hypercalcemia is accompanied by hypophosphatemia. Hypophosphatemia is assumed when the serum phosphorus is less than what level?
    a. Less than 5 mg/dL
    b. Less than 10 mg/dL
    c. Less than 4 mg/dL
    d. Less than 3 mg/dL

20. The physician has ordered oral calcium for a patient. The nurse understands that this medication is used to treat or manage which conditions? (Select all that apply.)
    a. Poor digestion
    b. Bone loss
    c. Fractures
    d. Chronic nonemergent hypercalcemia
    e. Heartburn

43 | CHAPTER

Drug Therapy for Addison's Disease and Cushing's Disease

Learning Objectives

- Understand the etiology and pathophysiology of adrenal cortex disorders.
- Identify the major manifestations of Addison's disease and Cushing's disease.
- Explain how corticotropin (ACTH) is used in the diagnosis of adrenocortical insufficiency.
- Explain how cosyntropin (Cortrosyn) is used in the diagnosis of adrenocortical insufficiency.
- Identify the prototypes and describe the action, use, adverse effects, contraindications, and nursing implications for the drugs used in the treatment of Addison's disease.
- Identify the prototypes and describe the action, use, adverse effects, contraindications, and nursing implications for the drugs used in the treatment of Cushing's disease.
- Implement the nursing process in the care of the patient with Addison's disease or Cushing's disease.

SECTION I: ASSESSING YOUR UNDERSTANDING

Activity A FILL IN THE BLANKS

1. _____, also called *glucocorticoids* or *steroids*, are hormones produced by the adrenal cortex, part of the adrenal glands.

2. _____ corticosteroids are used as drugs in a variety of disorders.

3. When plasma corticosteroid levels rise to an adequate level, secretion of corticosteroids _____ or _____.

4. The mechanism by which the hypothalamus and anterior pituitary "learn" that no more corticosteroids are needed is called a _____.

5. _____ are secreted directly into the bloodstream.

Activity B MATCHING

Match the term in Column A with the definition in Column B.

Column A

_____ 1. Hyperaldosteronism

_____ 2. Congenital adrenogenital syndromes and adrenal hyperplasia

Column B

a. Produced by inadequate secretion of corticotrophin, most often caused by prolonged administration of corticosteroids

b. Associated with destruction of the adrenal cortex by disease processes or hemorrhage and with atrophy of the adrenal cortex

____ **3.** Secondary adrenocortical insufficiency

____ **4.** Primary adrenocortical insufficiency (Addison's disease)

____ **5.** Adrenocortical hyperfunction (Cushing's disease)

c. A rare disorder caused by adenoma or hyperplasia of the adrenal cortex cells that produce aldosterone

d. Result from deficiencies in one or more enzymes required for cortisol production

e. May result from excessive corticotrophin or a primary adrenal tumor

Activity C SHORT ANSWERS

Briefly answer the following questions.

1. Discuss the process by which corticosteroid secretion is controlled.

2. How does the stress response affect the sympathetic nervous system?

3. What are glucocorticoids, and how do they affect the body's processes?

4. What are mineralocorticoids, and how do they affect the body's processes?

5. What are adrenal sex hormones, and how do they affect the body's processes?

SECTION II: APPLYING YOUR KNOWLEDGE

Activity D CASE STUDY

Consider the scenario and answer the questions.

You are participating in a study group of nursing students studying the indications for the various uses of corticosteroids.

1. Mr. Janis is diagnosed with systemic lupus erythematosus. Where would you expect to find inflammation in this patient?

2. Name some skin disorders that may be treated with corticosteroids.

3. Corticosteroids are effective in the treatment of neoplastic diseases. What mechanism of action do they have that makes them effective?

4. Mr. Castile received a kidney transplant 6 months ago. He is not comfortable with the changes in his body related to the corticosteroids he must take. He asks why they are necessary. How would you respond?

5. In patients with asthma, what is the effect of corticosteroids? In patients with anaphylactic shock resulting from an allergic reaction, what is the effect of corticosteroids?

SECTION III: PRACTICING FOR NCLEX

Activity E

Answer the following questions.

1. A female patient's physician discontinues her systemic corticosteroid using a sliding scale and orders an inhaler. The patient asks if she can begin flunisolide; her friend uses it and suggested it as a next option. How should the nurse respond?

a. "I will ask the physician to change the original prescription."

b. "Flunisolide is a safe option."

c. "Flunisolide is not the primary medication to treat your disease process."

d. "The physician did not order flunisolide because it may cause death."

2. The nurse is caring for a patient who has been prescribed a course of corticosteroids. The nurse knows that systemic corticosteroids may cause which side effects? (Select all that apply.)

a. Hirsutism

b. Hypertension

c. Glucose intolerance

d. Premature puberty in children

e. Nasal congestion

3. The nurse is aware that dosing strategies to minimize HPA suppression and risks of acute adrenal insufficiency include which corticosteroid administration schedule?

a. Reducing the dose of systematic corticosteroids when the patient on long-term therapy experiences high-stress situations

b. Administering a systemic corticosteroid during high-stress situations in patients on long-term systemic therapy

c. Concurrent use of oral contraceptives and corticosteroids in women to reduce the stress on the adrenal gland

d. Drug holidays for patients with long-term corticosteroid use

4. A patient experiences an acute exacerbation of his asthma secondary to an allergic reaction. The physician orders which type of therapy to minimize HPA suppression and risks of acute adrenal insufficiency?

   a. A short course of systemic therapy

   b. Long-term systemic therapy to prevent future exacerbations of his asthma

   c. Long-term systemic therapy with drug holidays every 6 months

   d. A short course of systemic therapy with a PRN prescription of corticosteroids

5. A patient experiences weight gain secondary to her systemic steroid therapy for temporal arteritis. She calls the physician's office to ask if she can discontinue the medication for 1 week, to fit into her dress for her class reunion. Which response by the nurse is most appropriate?

   a. "A temporary discontinuance will not adversely affect your health."

   b. "I will ask the physician for a change in your prescription."

   c. "Your prescription must be tapered gradually with the physician's order."

   d. "Your prescription must be tapered for 2 days only with the physician's order."

6. A patient develops a mild rash secondary to sensitivity to a new laundry detergent. The physician orders a topical corticosteroid. The patient states that this medication will take too long to work and asks whether he can just take a steroid by mouth. What is the most appropriate response?

   a. "Oral corticosteroids will not reduce the inflammation of contact dermatitis."

   b. "Oral corticosteroids are contraindicated for cases of contact dermatitis."

   c. "Local therapy will resolve the symptoms of the dermatitis quicker than the use of oral corticosteroids."

   d. "Using local rather than systemic corticosteroids reduces adrenal insufficiency."

7. The nurse is caring for a patient with inoperable adrenocortical carcinoma and is aware that the physician will most likely order which medication?

   a. Hydrocortisone cypionate

   b. Fludrocortisone acetate

   c. Ketoconazole

   d. Mitotane

8. A patient is diagnosed with Addison's disease. Which daily medications would the nurse expect to be administered?

   a. Warfarin

   b. Hydrochlorothiazide

   c. Apresoline

   d. Prednisone

9. The nurse is assessing a patient who has developed severe hypoglycemia, and the patient has never had troubles with blood sugar before. What condition does the nurse suspect is causing the hypoglycemia?

   a. Cushing's disease

   b. Cushing's syndrome

   c. Adrenal insufficiency

   d. Hyperadrenalism

10. Which effects are the most frequently desired of exogenous corticosteroids? (Select all that apply.)

    a. Anti-inflammatory

    b. Immunosuppressive

    c. Anticoagulant

    d. Antianxiety

    e. Antibacterial

11. The nurse is working in a home care setting. A patient is prescribed oral corticosteroids by her physician secondary to a diagnosis of Addison's disease. What task is the nurse's responsibility?

    a. Supervising and monitoring the administration of the drug

    b. Administering all doses of the oral medication

    c. Administering all doses of the oral medication for the first month of use

    d. Teaching all family members to administer the medication

12. A patient is diagnosed with pneumocystosis, and his physician orders corticosteroids. What is an accurate statement to include in the nurse's teaching plan for the patient?

a. Corticosteroids may reduce his survival rate but improve his quality of life.

b. Corticosteroids decrease risks of respiratory failure.

c. Corticosteroids decrease cerebral edema associated with pneumocystosis.

d. Corticosteroids decrease the white blood cell count related to pneumocystosis.

13. A patient is diagnosed with septic shock. What would the nurse expect a long course of low-dose corticosteroids to do?

a. Diminish the patient's survival secondary to impaired immunity

b. Improve the patient's survival without causing harm

c. Improve the patient's survival with long-term adrenal insufficiency

d. Diminish the patient's survival secondary to superinfection

14. A patient is diagnosed with adult respiratory distress syndrome. His family asks whether corticosteroids may help him to breathe easier. Which statement about corticosteroids is accurate?

a. They are successfully used for the long-term treatment of ARDS.

b. They are successful for the short-term treatment of ARDS.

c. They are not used when the patient is at risk for *Pneumocystis* pneumonia.

d. They are not a beneficial treatment for ARDS.

15. A patient receives IV methylprednisolone to treat status asthmaticus. Corticosteroid use may increase the risk of what condition for the patient?

a. Pulmonary infection

b. Bronchospasm

c. Pulmonary edema

d. Bronchoconstriction

16. A patient is diagnosed with adrenal insufficiency. She presents to the emergency department with hypotension. What would the nurse expect the physician to prescribe?

a. Vasopressors

b. Corticosteroids

c. ACE inhibitors

d. Beta-blockers

17. The nurse is caring for a patient who has just been admitted to the intensive care unit with a diagnosis of addisonian crisis. The nurse would expect that this patient may exhibit a craving for what element?

a. Salt

b. Pepper

c. Garlic

d. Onion

18. The physician suspects that a patient has Addison's disease. The nurse knows that the physician will perform what test to confirm this diagnosis?

a. MRI of the patient's adrenal glands

b. Biopsy of the adrenal glands

c. ACTH stimulation test

d. Tensilon test

19. The nurse is aware that the use of corticosteroids in older adults may aggravate what conditions? (Select all that apply.)

a. Congestive heart failure

b. Gout

c. Diabetes mellitus

d. Arthritis

e. Macular degeneration

20. The nurse is administering ketoconazole to a patient with Cushing's disease. What assessments are necessary for the nurse to complete on this patient? (Select all that apply.)

a. Blood pressure

b. Blood glucose

c. Sexual dysfunction

d. Bradycardia

e. Respiratory depression

44 CHAPTER

Drug Therapy for Women's Health

Learning Objectives

- Understand the mechanisms of action of endogenous estrogens and progesterone.
- Describe the fundamental workings of the menstrual cycle.
- Identify the prototype drug for the estrogens, progestins, and estrogen–progestin combinations.
- Describe the estrogens in terms of their action, use, contraindications, adverse effects, and nursing implications.
- Describe the progestins in terms of their action, use, contraindications, adverse effects, and nursing implications.
- Describe the estrogen–progestin combinations in terms of their action, use, contraindications, adverse effects, and nursing implications.
- Evaluate the benefits and risks associated with postmenopausal hormone replacement therapy.
- Apply the nursing process to patients taking estrogens, progestins, and estrogen–progestin combinations.

SECTION I: ASSESSING YOUR UNDERSTANDING

Activity A FILL IN THE BLANKS

1. _____ and _____ are the female sex hormones produced primarily by the ovaries and secondarily by the adrenal cortex in nonpregnant women.

2. A significant source of estrogen synthesis in normal premenopausal women is _____.

3. The main function of estrogen is to promote growth in tissue related to _____ and _____ characteristics in women.

4. Three ovarian estrogens, estradiol, estrone, and estriol, are known as _____ estrogens.

5. _____ is the main estrogen because it exerts more estrogenic activity than the other two estrogens combined.

Activity B MATCHING

Match the term in Column A with the definition in Column B.

Column A	Column B
____ 1. Conjugated estrogen (Premarin)	a. This route of administration of exogenous estrogen more closely mimics premenopausal estrogen levels.
____ 2. Transdermal estradiol patches (Climara)	
____ 3. Medroxy-progester-one acetate (Provera)	b. Prototype female hormone replacement medication

_____ **4.** Ethinyl estradiol–nor-ethindrone (Ortho-Novum)

_____ **5.** Estrogen–medroxy-progesterone (Prempro)

c. Prototype hormonal combination of contraceptive medication

d. It is the most commonly used oral estrogen and is used to treat women's health disorders that are caused by low or absent levels of endogenous estrogen

e. It is used to suppress ovarian function in dysmenorrhea, endometriosis, endometrial cancer, and uterine bleeding.

Activity C **SHORT ANSWERS**

Briefly answer the following questions.

1. What is the function of estrogen in the monthly menstrual cycle?

2. What is the function of progesterone in the monthly menstrual cycle?

3. How does progesterone impact lipid metabolism?

4. The use of exogenous estrogen is contraindicated in what conditions?

5. What causes ovulation to occur?

SECTION II: APPLYING YOUR KNOWLEDGE

Activity D **CASE STUDY**

Consider the scenario and answer the questions.

Mrs. Adams, aged 51, comes to the women's health care clinic with complaints of "hot flashes." She states that she has occasional menstrual periods that last approximately 3 days and occur every 4 to 5 months. She asks the nurse for information about the use of hormone replacement therapy.

1. What are the physiologic changes that may be causing this patient's symptoms?

2. What medications are used for hormone replacement therapy?

3. What assessment findings would contraindicate the use of hormone replacement therapy in this patient?

4. What will the nurse share with this patient about the adverse effects of hormone replacement therapy?

5. What will the nurse share in the latest research concerning hormone replacement therapy?

SECTION III: PRACTICING FOR NCLEX

Activity E

Answer the following questions.

1. The nurse is caring for a female patient who is taking medroxyprogesterone and the physician has ordered lab work. The nurse understands that which laboratory test may give inaccurate results in patients who take progestins?

a. Renal function test

b. Liver function test

c. Complete blood count

d. Electrolyte test

2. The nurse is giving discharge instructions to a patient who has begun to take medroxyprogesterone for treatment of irregular vaginal bleeding. The nurse instructs the patient to take this medication at what time to reduce gastrointestinal effects?

a. Before breakfast

b. Between breakfast and lunch

c. Between lunch and dinner

d. At bedtime

3. A patient has been prescribed transdermal estradiol. What important information does the nurse share with this patient?

a. Avoid prolonged sun exposure

b. There is more nausea with this type of administration than the oral route.

c. The estrogen levels with this route of administration mimic menopause.

d. The patient won't feel any effects of this medication for 2 weeks.

4. A 38-year-old female patient has just visited the physician and has received a prescription for birth control pills. The patient calls the nurse and states that she doesn't need birth control pills because she had voluntary sterilization after her third child. The nurse explains that birth control pills may be used for what other reason?
   a. Thrombophlebitis
   b. Menstrual disorders
   c. Breast lumps
   d. Heart rhythm irregularities

5. A female patient has a history of renal impairment and is visiting the family nurse practitioner to discuss the use of estrogen. The nurse knows that this medication will be used only with extreme caution because of what adverse effect associated with estrogen?
   a. Nausea and vomiting
   b. Thromboembolic disorders
   c. Fluid retention
   d. Gallbladder disease

6. The nurse is caring for a woman who takes estrogen and assesses the patient for what central nervous system adverse reactions related to the use of this medication? (Select all that apply.)
   a. Migraine headaches
   b. Anxiety
   c. Dizziness
   d. Paralysis
   e. Depression

7. The nurse is caring for a patient who has cancer and who until recently took estrogen. The nurse knows that estrogen may have increased the risk of development of which types of cancer? (Select all that apply.)
   a. Lung cancer
   b. Melanoma
   c. Breast cancer
   d. Endometrial cancer
   e. Brain cancer

8. The nurse is discussing the use of estrogen with a woman who smokes cigarettes. The nurse informs the patient that patients who take estrogen and continue to smoke are at a greater risk for thromboembolic disorder because of what reasons? (Select all that apply.)
   a. Increased platelet aggregation
   b. Increased chance of thrombocytopenia
   c. Increase in liver production of blood clotting factors
   d. Vasoconstriction of small capillaries
   e. Decreased oxygen content to the lungs

9. The nurse is completing a history on a patient who is new to the women's clinic. What information is most important for the nurse to obtain if the patient is to be prescribed estrogens? (Select all that apply.)
   a. If the patient had any multifetal pregnancies
   b. Any symptoms of cardiovascular disease
   c. Family history of a brain attack
   d. If the patient's grandfather had lung cancer
   e. When was the patient's last menstrual period

10. The nurse is caring for a woman who is receiving estrogen for treatment of amenorrhea. What evidence will the nurse use to indicate that the medication is working properly?
    a. Lack of menstruation
    b. Appearance of secondary sexual characteristics
    c. Occurrence of menstruation
    d. Decrease in hot flashes

11. A female patient asks the nurse about the use of progestins. The nurse shares with the patient that patients who take this medication are at an increased risk for what serious adverse effect?
    a. Cardiovascular complications
    b. Respiratory difficulties
    c. Seizures
    d. Renal failure

12. The nurse is aware that medroxyprogesterone has a black box warning that the use of the medication can lead to what problem?

    a. Pregnancy

    b. Bone breakage

    c. Mental depression

    d. Hypotension

13. The nurse is instructing a woman with type 2 diabetes mellitus who has been prescribed combined estrogen–progestin therapy. The nurse instructs the patient to be alert for what change related to her diabetes?

    a. Decrease in blood glucose

    b. Increase in blood glucose

    c. Development of diabetic ketoacidosis

    d. Rapid weight loss

14. The nurse is discussing contraception with a patient who has been prescribed a triphasic oral contraceptive. The nurse knows that this preparation is used for what reason?

    a. It mimics normal variations of hormone secretions.

    b. It decreases the number of days of the menstrual period.

    c. It decreases the amount of blood lost during the menstrual period.

    d. It is effective for more than one menstrual cycle.

15. A patient calls the women's health clinic and tells the nurse that she went to the dentist for an abscessed tooth. The dentist put her on an antibiotic, and the patient wants to know if it will cause problems with her prescribed oral contraceptives. What is the nurse's best response?

    a. "There is no interaction; you have nothing to worry about."

    b. "Take two pills each day. The physician will call if the additional medication is needed."

    c. "Take a pill every other day to prevent severe adverse effects."

    d. "Use alternate means of birth control until you are finished with the antibiotic."

16. The nurse is discussing the use of Depo-Provera with a 17-year-old female who desires birth control. The nurse recognizes that this medication is used in this patient for what reason?

    a. No vaginal bleeding for 12 months

    b. Birth control for 3 months

    c. No adverse effects usually associated with medroxyprogesterone

    d. Decreases chance of sexually transmitted infections

17. The nurse is discussing the use of vaginal estrogen for a woman with vaginal atrophy. The nurse knows that vaginal estrogen has what advantage over other forms of estrogen?

    a. It takes away all symptoms of menopause.

    b. It treats the vaginal tissue with little systemic effects.

    c. It causes no adverse effects.

    d. It can be used in women of all ages.

18. The physician has prescribed a combination of estrogen and progestin for a patient. The nurse knows that this combination carries an increased risk of which conditions? (Select all that apply.)

    a. Dementia

    b. Multiple myeloma

    c. Rheumatoid arthritis

    d. Blood clots

    e. Myocardial infarction

19. A patient has been prescribed medroxyprogesterone acetate for treatment of dysfunctional uterine bleeding. The nurse instructs the patient to take the medication in what way?

    a. Take orally for 5 days beginning on the 16th day of her cycle

    b. Take orally every day until there is no longer any uterine bleeding

    c. IM every week

    d. SubQ every 3 months

20. The nurse is discussing the effects of menopause with a group of women. The nurse explains that the decreasing estrogen will cause what effect on the skin?

    a. Cause deposition of fat in subcutaneous tissues, especially the breasts

    b. Increases vascularity in the skin

    c. Decrease in subcutaneous fat in the arms and the thighs

    d. Increase in skin warmth

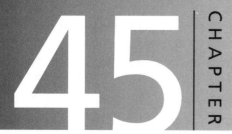

Drug Therapy for Men's Health

Learning Objectives

- Discuss male reproductive problems in terms of etiology, pathophysiology, and clinical manifestations.
- Describe the androgens in terms of prototype, mechanism of action, indications for use, major adverse effects, and nursing implications.
- Identify potential consequences of abusing androgens and anabolic steroids.
- Discuss the phosphodiesterase type 5 inhibitors in terms of prototype, mechanism of action, indications for use, major adverse effects, and nursing implications.
- Describe the 5-alpha reductase inhibitors in terms of prototype, mechanism of action, indications for use, major adverse effects, and nursing implications.
- Describe the alpha-adrenergic blockers in terms of prototype, mechanism of action, indications for use, major adverse effects, and nursing implications.
- Implement the nursing process for men who have reproductive disorders.

SECTION I: ASSESSING YOUR UNDERSTANDING

Activity A FILL IN THE BLANKS

1. _____ is normally the only important androgen.

2. _____, located in the testes, secrete testosterone in response to stimulation by luteinizing hormone from the anterior pituitary gland.

3. The main functions of testosterone are the development of male _____ characteristics, _____, and _____.

4. Testosterone is necessary for normal _____ development.

5. Almost all effects of testosterone result from the increased formation of _____ throughout the body.

Activity B MATCHING

Match the term in Column A with the definition in Column B.

Column A

_____ 1. Anabolic steroids

_____ 2. Testosterone

Column B

a. Synthetic testosterone used in women to prevent or treat endometriosis or fibrocystic breast disease

b. Used in the treatment of androgen deficiency in men and boys

_____ **3.** Danazol

_____ **4.** Sildenafil (Viagra)

_____ **5.** Finasteride (Proscar)

c. Used to enhance a male erection that results from sexual stimuli by increasing blood flow to the penis

d. Used primarily to treat benign prostatic hypertrophy and is used to treat male pattern baldness in lower dosages

e. Synthetic drugs that were developed to modify the masculinizing effects of testosterone while maintaining the tissue-building and growth-stimulating effects

Activity C SHORT ANSWERS

Briefly answer the following questions.

1. What is the difference between primary and secondary hypogonadism?

2. What are the causes of erectile dysfunction?

3. What is the connection between cardiovascular disease and erectile dysfunction?

4. What role does aging have in the development of benign prostatic hypertrophy?

5. Why must great caution be taken by women of childbearing age who handle the drug finasteride?

SECTION II: APPLYING YOUR KNOWLEDGE

Activity D CASE STUDY

Consider the scenario and answer the questions.

Mr. Smith, aged 72, comes to the clinic complaining of problems with urination. He states that he needs to get up at night to urinate and he has a hard time initiating the flow of urine. He also states that he feels like he has to urinate about every 3 hours. He states that these symptoms have been occurring for about 6 months, but

they have only begun to interfere with his lifestyle in the last month. The physician diagnoses the patient with benign prostatic hypertrophy.

1. What are the physiologic changes that may be causing this patient's symptoms?

2. What medications are most effective in treatment of this disorder, and how long will it take for this patient to notice the therapeutic effects?

3. What assessments will the nurse make to ensure that the medication has been effective?

SECTION III: PRACTICING FOR NCLEX

Activity E

Answer the following questions.

1. The nurse is caring for a teenage male who reports using an illegally obtained anabolic steroid to improve his athletic performance. What adverse effects may occur in this patient as a result of taking these substances? (Select all that apply.)

a. Hypotension

b. Jaundice

c. Aggression

d. Testicular hypertrophy

e. Fluid retention

2. A patient has been given a prescription for sildenafil (Viagra) for treatment of erectile dysfunction. The nurse will instruct the patient to take this medication at what time prior to the onset of sexual intercourse?

a. 12 hours

b. 6 hours

c. 30 minutes

d. 5 minutes

3. The nurse instructs the patient taking medication for erectile dysfunction to call the physician if which adverse effect occurs after taking the medication?

a. Lack of erection

b. Flushing of the face

c. Priapism

d. Nasal congestion

4. The patient comes to the clinic with symptoms of BPH and is concerned that the frequency of urination will interfere with a vacation scheduled in 2 ½ weeks. What medication does the nurse anticipate will be prescribed for this patient?

    a. Doxazosin (Cardura)

    b. Alfuzosin (Uroxatral)

    c. Tamsulosin (Flomax)

    d. Finasteride (Proscar)

5. The nurse instructs the patient who is receiving sildenafil to avoid eating which meal immediately prior to taking the medication?

    a. Meatballs and marinara sauce with spaghetti pasta and garden salad

    b. Fried catfish, baked potato with butter, and sour cream and broccoli

    c. Grilled pork chop, corn, and green beans

    d. Baked chicken, rice, and acorn squash

6. The nurse is obtaining a history from a 23-year-old man. The nurse suspects that the patient may be using DHEA if he displays which symptoms?

    a. Hirsutism

    b. Sleepiness

    c. Lethargy

    d. Placidity

7. The nurse is caring for a woman with advanced breast cancer. Which medication that is a derivative of progesterone could be used in this woman's treatment?

    a. Fluoxymesterone

    b. Methyltestosterone

    c. Testolactone

    d. Danazol

8. The nurse is instructing the parents of an 11-year-old male who has testosterone deficiency. Which symptom, if found in this child, would cause the discontinuation of this medication?

    a. Skeletal growth

    b. Enlarged penis

    c. Increased appetite

    d. Improved school skills

9. The nurse is assessing a 22-year-old male. What symptoms would indicate that this patient may be experiencing androgen deficiency? (Select all that apply.)

    a. Very small testicles

    b. Inability to have an erection

    c. Large amount of pubic hair

    d. Low sperm count

    e. Enlarged penis

10. The physician has prescribed testosterone for a 77-year-old patient with a low testosterone level. The nurse will evaluate this patient for what condition that may develop in this patient in response to this medication?

    a. Benign prostatic hypertrophy

    b. Impotence

    c. Fatigue

    d. Breast enlargement

11. The nurse is aware that medications for erectile dysfunction are frequently prescribed because what percentage of men between the ages of 40 and 70 years develop this disorder?

    a. 30%

    b. 50%

    c. 75%

    d. 90%

12. A teenage patient who is using testosterone to treat a hormone deficiency calls the clinic to complain of acne-like skin eruptions on the face. How should the nurse counsel this patient?

    a. Stop taking this drug immediately

    b. Practice frequent and thorough skin cleansing

    c. Make an immediate appointment with a dermatologist

    d. Increase the dose of testosterone

13. The nurse counsels a patient taking sildenafil to avoid which beverage prior to or while using this medication?

    a. Carbonated beverages

    b. Whole Milk

    c. Alcohol

    d. Electrolyte replacement beverage

14. The nurse is instructing a patient with benign prostatic hypertrophy who has been prescribed tamsulosin. The nurse will immediately contact the physician if the patient reports he is also using which medication?

a. Furosemide

b. Warfarin

c. Amoxicillin

d. Propranolol

15. The physician has ordered alprostadil to a patient who has erectile dysfunction. The nurse will instruct the patient to administer this medication in what way?

a. Orally

b. Sublingually

c. Self-injection into the penis

d. Rectal suppository

16. The nurse is aware that a patient receiving which category of medication will not be prescribed vardenafil?

a. Antivirals

b. Antidiuretics

c. Antidysrhythmics

d. Antibiotics

17. A patient is admitted to the hospital with benign prostatic hypertrophy, and the physician prescribed tamsulosin. The nurse knows that other drugs in this class of medications are used to treat which condition?

a. Erectile dysfunction

b. Androgen deficiency

c. Hypertension

d. Heart failure

18. The nurse is instructing a patient who will be taking finasteride for treatment of benign prostatic hypertrophy and gives the patient information about which possible sexual side effects? (Select all that apply.)

a. Reduced libido

b. Impotence

c. Shriveled testicles

d. Decreased volume of ejaculate

e. Priapism

19. The nurse knows that finasteride is used to treat prostatic hypertrophy and in smaller doses is used to treat what condition?

a. Erectile dysfunction

b. Acne

c. Male pattern baldness

d. Neuropathy

20. The nurse is discussing testosterone replacement with a patient and instructs the patient that this medication is not available in what formulation?

a. Intramuscular

b. Oral

c. Transdermal

d. Topical gel

46

Drug Therapy for Myasthenia Gravis and Alzheimer's Disease

Learning Objectives

- Understand the pathophysiology and major manifestations of myasthenia gravis.
- Identify the prototype and describe the action, use, adverse effects, contraindications, and nursing implications for indirect-acting cholinergic drugs used in myasthenia gravis.
- Understand the pathophysiology and major manifestations of Alzheimer's disease.
- Identify the prototype and describe the action, use, adverse effects, contraindications, and nursing implications for reversible indirect-acting cholinergic drugs used in Alzheimer's disease.
- Understand the etiology, pathophysiology, and clinical manifestations of urinary retention.
- Identify the prototype and describe the action, use, adverse effects, contraindications, and nursing implications for direct-acting cholinergic drugs.
- Describe the pharmacologic care of the patient with toxicity of irreversible anticholinesterase agents.
- Be able to implement the nursing process in the care of patients undergoing cholinergic drug therapy for myasthenia gravis, Alzheimer's disease, and urinary retention.

SECTION I: ASSESSING YOUR UNDERSTANDING

Activity A FILL IN THE BLANKS

1. _____ drugs stimulate the parasympathetic nervous system in the same manner as acetylcholine.

2. In normal neuromuscular function, _____ is released from nerve endings and binds to nicotinic receptors on cell membranes of muscle cells to cause muscle contraction.

3. _____ is an autoimmune disorder in which autoantibodies are thought to destroy nicotinic receptors for acetylcholine on skeletal muscle.

4. Alzheimer's disease, the most common type of dementia in adults, is characterized by abnormalities in the cholinergic, serotonergic, noradrenergic, and _____ neurotransmission systems.

5. Acetylcholine stimulates _____ receptors in the gut to promote normal secretory and motor activity.

Activity B MATCHING

Match the term in Column A with the definition in Column B.

Column A

_____ **1.** Bethanechol (Urecholine)

_____ **2.** Neostigmine (Prostigmin)

_____ **3.** Edrophonium (Tensilon)

_____ **4.** Physostigmine salicylate (Antilirium)

_____ **5.** Donepezil (Aricept)

Column B

a. Used to treat mild to moderate Alzheimer's disease

b. Synthetic derivative of choline

c. Short-acting cholinergic drug used to diagnose myasthenia gravis

d. The only anticholinesterase capable of crossing the blood–brain barrier

e. The prototype anticholinesterase agent

Activity C SHORT ANSWERS

Briefly answer the following questions.

1. What is the function of cholinergic drugs on body systems?

2. What is the role of acetylcholine as it relates to normal brain function?

3. What is the role of acetylcholine as it relates to the gastrointestinal system?

4. What is the role of acetylcholine as it relates to the urinary system?

5. What is the mechanism of action for direct-acting cholinergic drugs?

SECTION II: APPLYING YOUR KNOWLEDGE

Activity D CASE STUDY

Consider the scenario and answer the questions.

Mr. Davis, aged 35, presents to the physician's office with complaints of generalized weakness. The physician orders tests to evaluate his condition and diagnoses Mr. Davis with myasthenia gravis. You are responsible for the education plan for both the disease process and the medications prescribed for the condition.

1. Mr. Davis is relieved to understand that the symptoms that he is experiencing are related to a disease process and he can begin treatment. He asks you to explain his diagnosis. How would you respond?

2. How is myasthenia gravis diagnosed? The physician orders neostigmine. How does this fit in?

3. Mr. Davis does not want to self-administer the neostigmine by injection, so the physician prescribes the medication so that it may be administered orally. What can you tell the patient about oral doses of neostigmine? What can you tell him about long-term use of the medication?

SECTION III: PRACTICING FOR NCLEX

Activity E

Answer the following questions.

1. A patient is treated in the critical care unit for overdose of indirect cholinergic drugs. What is the treatment of choice in this situation?

a. An anticholinesterase reactivator

b. Atropine

c. Pralidoxime

d. A cholinesterase reactivator

2. A patient is experiencing paralysis due to overdose of indirect cholinergic drugs. The nurse understands that atropine will reverse muscarinic effects due to overdose of cholinergic drugs, but what will it not reverse?

a. Cholinergic effects of skeletal-muscle weakness or paralysis

b. Nicotinic effects of skeletal-muscle weakness or paralysis

c. Ketoacidosis in the skeletal muscle

d. Lactic acid accumulated in the skeletal muscle

3. The nurse is assessing a patient who has just been diagnosed with myasthenia gravis and the nurse knows to anticipate which symptoms that are characteristic of this disease? (Select all that apply.)

a. Diplopia

b. Stiffness in arms and legs

c. Ptosis

d. Severe nasal congestion

e. Waddling gait

4. The nurse is caring for a patient who is receiving an indirect-acting cholinergic medication and knows it is indicated as a treatment for myasthenia gravis as well as which other condition?
   a. Muscular dystrophy
   b. Musculoskeletal cancer
   c. Alzheimer's disease
   d. Cerebrovascular dementia

5. A female patient had surgery 24 hours ago to repair a hernia. The nurse finds that the patient has not had a bowel movement since the day before the surgery. She is experiencing abdominal distention, and during auscultation the nurse notes an absence of bowel sounds. Further examination and testing reveal a paralytic ileus. The physician orders bethanechol. The nurse is aware that bethanechol is included in which drug classification?
   a. Anticholinergic medication
   b. Direct-acting cholinergic drug
   c. Indirect-acting cholinergic drug
   d. Indirect-acting anticholinergic medication

6. The nurse is caring for a patient with myasthenia gravis and is aware that indirect-acting cholinergic drugs are also used because they stimulate nicotinic receptors in skeletal muscles. The nurse recognizes this will produce what effect?
   a. Increased smooth muscle tone
   b. Decreased musculoskeletal pain
   c. Improved skeletal muscle tone and strength
   d. Decreased muscle spasticity

7. The nurse is caring for a patient who is taking neostigmine and presents to the emergency department with symptoms of respiratory depression. The nurse is aware that this patient has developed which severe complication related to the use of neostigmine?
   a. Addisonian crisis
   b. Myxedema crisis
   c. Cholinergic crisis
   d. Opioid crisis

8. A 75-year-old male patient is diagnosed with myasthenia gravis. How can the home care nurse assist him with medication compliance?
   a. Prepouring his medications 1 week at a time
   b. Ensuring that all medications have safety caps
   c. Persuading his son to call once a week to encourage him to take his medications
   d. Asking the housekeeper to administer the medications

9. A male patient is diagnosed with hepatitis C and myasthenia gravis. His prescriptions include neostigmine. The nurse is concerned because the patient may experience which possible problem?
   a. Increased absorption of the medication
   b. Increased adverse effects
   c. Increased resistance to the medication
   d. Decreased absorption of the medication

10. A 65-year-old male patient takes cholinergic medication. He presents to the emergency department with symptoms associated with GI distress. He is diagnosed with a small-bowel obstruction. What action would the nurse expect the physician to take?
    a. Increase the dose of the cholinergic medication to facilitate peristalsis
    b. Decrease the dose of the cholinergic medication to slow peristalsis
    c. Maintain the same dosage of the cholinergic medication because it will not affect the diagnosis
    d. Discontinue the cholinergic medication to prevent injury to the areas proximal to the obstruction

11. A patient has benign prostatic hypertrophy and has been prescribed neostigmine. The nurse is aware that this patient must be monitored for what adverse effect of this medication?
    a. Pain with urination
    b. Urinary retention
    c. Hematuria
    d. Pyuria

12. A female patient is taking cholinergic medication to control bladder retention. She presents to the emergency department with confusion, shortness of breath, and an apical pulse of 42 beats per minute and irregular. What action would the nurse expect the physician to take?
    a. Increase the cholinergic medication to increase cardiac contractility
    b. Increase the cholinergic medication to increase oxygenation to the heart through vasodilation
    c. Decrease the cholinergic medication to alleviate the symptom of confusion
    d. Discontinue the cholinergic medication secondary to the diagnosis of bradycardia

13. A patient with hyperthyroidism has received a dose of a cholinergic drug. The nurse will monitor this patient for which condition?
    a. Hyperglycemia
    b. Decreases TSH
    c. Increased TSH
    d. Reflex tachycardia

14. The nurse is caring for a patient with asthmatic bronchitis and understands that cholinergic medications are contraindicated because this classification of medication may cause which effect?
    a. Bronchodilation
    b. Decreased secretions
    c. Thickened secretions
    d. Bronchoconstriction

15. The nurse is caring for a patient in the emergency department who has a history of myasthenia gravis. The patient has symptoms that could be interpreted as either myasthenic crisis or cholinergic crisis. The nurse is aware that the physician will order what medication to help determine the type of crisis the patient is experiencing?
    a. Donepezil
    b. Edrophonium
    c. Galantamine hydrobromide
    d. Memantine hydrochloride

16. Direct-acting cholinergic drugs affect the bladder by causing which of the following? (Select all that apply.)
    a. Increased tone and contractility
    b. Relaxation of the sphincter
    c. Increased bladder capacity
    d. Reduction in UTIs
    e. Ability to better empty the bladder

17. The nurse is providing information about how to care for patients during a bioterrorism attack. The nurse knows that which drug will be administered in the case of a sarin attack?
    a. Atropine
    b. Neostigmine
    c. Donepezil
    d. Bethanechol

18. The nurse is preparing a patient for discharge who has moderate to severe Alzheimer's disease. The physician has prescribed memantine hydrochloride (Namenda) and the nurse instructs the family that which preparation for heartburn should not be given to a patient who takes this medication?
    a. Products made with aluminum
    b. Products made with calcium carbonate
    c. Products made with magnesium
    d. Products made with sodium bicarbonate

19. The pharmacology instructor is discussing the drug therapy for Alzheimer's disease with a group of nursing students and states that indirect-acting cholinergic drugs do what to improve symptoms?
    a. Improve cholinergic neurotransmission to the brain
    b. Improve anticholinergic neurotransmission to the brain
    c. Improve medication absorption through the blood–brain barrier
    d. Cause vasodilation of the cerebral arteries

20. The nurse is caring for a patient directly after surgery and anticipates that the anesthesiologist will administer which medication to reverse the effects of tubocurarine used during the surgical procedure?
    a. Edrophonium
    b. Neostigmine
    c. Pyridostigmine
    d. Atropine

47

CHAPTER

Drug Therapy for Parkinson's Disease and Anticholinergics

Learning Objectives

- Describe major characteristics and manifestations of Parkinson's disease.
- Understand the pathophysiology of Parkinson's disease.
- Describe the types of commonly used antiparkinson drugs.
- Identify the prototype and describe the action, use, adverse effects, contraindications, and nursing implications for the dopamine receptor agonists.
- Identify the prototype and describe the action, use, adverse effects, contraindications, and nursing implications for the catechol-*O*-methyltransferase (COMT) inhibitors.
- Identify the prototype and describe the action, use, adverse effects, contraindications, and nursing implications for a COMT inhibitor and decarboxylase inhibitor/dopamine precursor.
- Implement the nursing process in the care of patients undergoing drug therapy for Parkinson's disease.
- Describe the general characteristics of anticholinergic drugs.
- Identify the prototype and describe the action, use, adverse effects, contraindications, and nursing implications for belladonna alkaloids and derivatives.
- Identify the prototype and describe the action, use, adverse effects, contraindications, and nursing implications for centrally acting anticholinergic drugs.

- Identify the prototype and describe the action, use, adverse effects, contraindications, and nursing implications for anticholinergic medications used for gastrointestinal and urinary disorders.
- Implement the nursing process in the administration of anticholinergic agents.

SECTION I: ASSESSING YOUR UNDERSTANDING

Activity A FILL IN THE BLANKS

1. _____ is a chronic, progressive, degenerative disorder of the central nervous system (CNS) characterized by resting tremor, bradykinesia, rigidity, and postural instability.

2. Drugs used in Parkinson's disease help correct the neurotransmitter imbalance by _____ levels of dopamine.

3. Dopaminergic drugs _____ the amount of dopamine in the brain by various mechanisms.

4. When given at high doses, a few anticholinergic drugs are also able to block _____ receptors in autonomic ganglia and skeletal muscles.

190

5. Because cholinergic _____ receptors are widely distributed in the body, anticholinergic drugs produce effects in a variety of locations, including the central nervous system (CNS), heart, smooth muscle, glands, and the eye.

Activity B MATCHING

Match the term in Column A with the definition in Column B.

Column A	Column B
____ 1. Selegiline	a. Combination drug that has the same pharmacokinetics as those of levodopa/carbidopa and entacapone
____ 2. Stalevo	
____ 3. Levodopa	
____ 4. Ipratropium or tiotropium	b. Inhibits metabolism of dopamine by monoamine oxidase
____ 5. Homatropine hydrobromide	c. Most effective drug available for the treatment of Parkinson's disease
	d. A semisynthetic derivative of atropine used as eye drops to produce mydriasis and cycloplegia
	e. May be given by inhalation for bronchodilating effects

Activity C SHORT ANSWERS

Briefly answer the following questions.

1. Explain the roles of dopamine and acetylcholine in Parkinson's disease.

2. Discuss the rationale for the administration of antiparkinson drugs to alleviate the symptoms of Parkinson's disease.

3. Why has the U.S. Food and Drug Administration issued a black box warning regarding selegiline-transdermal?

4. Describe the characteristics of tertiary amines and give examples of two medications in this category.

5. Describe the general characteristics of anticholinergic drugs.

6. How do anticholinergic drugs affect the cardiovascular system?

SECTION II: APPLYING YOUR KNOWLEDGE

Activity D CASE STUDIES

Consider the scenarios and answer the questions.

Case Study 1

Mrs. Genus is diagnosed with idiopathic parkinsonism, and her physician prescribes both levodopa and, as an adjunct therapy, rasagiline. You develop an education plan regarding her drug regimen.

1. Mrs. Genus asks why she must take both drugs, when levodopa works well for her with periodic off times. What answer would you give her?

2. Mrs. Genus asks if she needs to modify her diet. How would you respond?

3. Mrs. Genus' physician tapers her fluoxetine and will discontinue it before beginning the rasagiline. Explain the rationale behind the discontinuance of the medication.

Case Study 2

Mrs. Benz, aged 78, is diagnosed with COPD by her physician. The physician orders tiotropium bromide. You are responsible for her education plan.

1. Mrs. Benz asks you how the medication will help her to breathe easier. How would you respond?

2. Mrs. Benz asks you if it might just be easier to take the capsule by mouth than in the inhalation device. She asks, "Wouldn't it work just as well?" How would you respond? What other patient education concerning this medication is in order?

3. Mrs. Benz then asks if she can take the medication twice on days she goes golfing, so that she will breathe easier. How would you respond to this?

4. Mrs. Benz is later diagnosed with mild to moderate renal insufficiency. What would you expect the physician to do? Would the patient's age be a factor in the physician's decision?

SECTION III: PRACTICING FOR NCLEX

Answer the following questions.

1. The nurse is admitting a patient who has just been diagnosed with Parkinson's disease. The nurse assesses this patient for which symptoms that are considered most characteristic of this disease? (Select all that apply.)

   a. Resting tremor

   b. Activity-generated tremor

   c. Bradykinesia

   d. Rigidity

   e. Postural instability

2. A male patient is diagnosed with Parkinson's disease. The nurse visits him 1 week after hospitalization to assess his progress and medication regimen compliance. He states that there is no significant improvement in his symptoms. What is the best response by the nurse?

   a. "Noticeable improvement may not occur for several weeks after the initial drug dose."

   b. "Noticeable improvement usually occurs 7 to 10 days after the initial drug dose."

   c. "You should have noticed improvement by now; I will notify your physician."

   d. "Are you sure that you are taking the medication as ordered?"

3. A female patient begins tolcapone therapy, and her physician arranges for laboratory testing to be completed on a routine basis. The nurse expects which laboratory study to be ordered by the physician?

   a. CBC

   b. Liver transaminase enzymes

   c. Hemoglobin and hematocrit

   d. BUN and creatinine

4. A male patient is diagnosed with chronic renal failure. He routinely takes amantadine for his Parkinson's disease with success. Why would his physician consider discontinuing the amantadine?

   a. With amantadine, 50% of the drug is excreted via the kidneys.

   b. With amantadine, metabolism occurs in the kidneys.

   c. With amantadine, catabolism occurs in the kidneys.

   d. With amantadine, excretion is primarily via the kidneys.

5. The nurse is caring for an 82-year-old patient who presents with symptoms of Parkinson's disease. The nurse recognizes that the dosage of levodopa/carbidopa may need to be reduced in this patient because of which age-related conditions?

   a. Increase in peripheral AADC, the enzyme that carbidopa inhibits

   b. Decrease in peripheral AADC, the enzyme that carbidopa inhibits

   c. Cardiac incompetency and resultant congestive heart failure

   d. Pulmonary incompetency and resultant chronic obstructive pulmonary disease

6. A female patient is prescribed centrally acting anticholinergics for her Parkinson's disease. Six weeks later, her daughter asks the physician to hospitalize the patient for a psychiatric evaluation. The nurse anticipates that the physician will respond in what way to the daughter's request?

   a. Evaluate the patient for adverse reactions from the centrally acting anticholinergics

   b. Increase the centrally active anticholinergics to decrease the patient's symptoms

   c. Admit the patient to the hospital for a psychological evaluation

   d. Immediately discontinue the centrally acting anticholinergic medication

7. A male patient is prescribed levodopa for his Parkinson's disease. The dosage has been modified on multiple occasions. The patient asks the nurse how the doctor decides what will be the optimal dose. What is the nurse's best response?

   a. "The optimal dose is the highest one that allows the patient to function adequately."

   b. "The optimal dose is the one that allows the patient to function adequately."

   c. "The optimal dose is the lowest one that allows the patient to function adequately."

   d. "The optimal dose is the one that maximizes patient function."

8. A male patient who was diagnosed with Parkinson's disease 8 years ago presents to the physician's office with signs of prominent bradykinesia and rigidity. The physician orders levodopa/carbidopa. As part of the nurse's education plan, what does the nurse tell the patient about the combination of levodopa/carbidopa?

   a. It may be effective with end-stage bradykinesia and rigidity.

   b. It is probably the most effective drug when bradykinesia and rigidity become prominent.

   c. It will provide palliation therapy.

   d. It is the treatment of last resort.

9. A female patient is diagnosed with Parkinson's disease and is having difficulty performing her activities of daily living. Her physician orders pramipexole. Pramipexole may be used alone for which purpose?

   a. To maintain ability to perform activities of daily living

   b. To delay physical impairment related to Parkinson's disease

   c. To delay mental impairment related to Parkinson's disease

   d. To improve motor performance and improve ability to participate in usual activities of daily living

10. A male patient's physician orders levodopa for the treatment of the patient's Parkinson's disease. The patient asks the nurse whether the levodopa will cure his condition. Which of the following is a correct statement about the effects of levodopa?

    a. It does not alter the underlying disease process, but it may improve a patient's quality of life.

    b. It will cure the Parkinson's disease.

    c. It will control the symptoms for 10 to 12 years.

    d. It is the treatment of last resort and may control his symptoms.

11. A male patient is admitted with symptoms of atropine overdose. The nurse is aware that this problem is characterized by which signs and symptoms? (Select all that apply.)

    a. Hyperthermia

    b. Excess salivation

    c. Mydriasis

    d. Urinary retention

    e. Muscle rigidity

12. A 57-year-old female patient has a history of two myocardial infarctions in the past 3 years. She presents to the physician's office with symptoms of an overactive bladder. She requests an anticholinergic medication that she saw advertised on television. What does the nurse expect the physician to do for this patient?

    a. Order the anticholinergic medication

    b. Order blood work to rule out a urinary tract infection and order the medication

    c. Order a urinalysis to rule out a urinary tract infection and order the medication

    d. Explain to the patient that the medication is contraindicated because of her medical history

13. A male patient asks the nurse why he needs the preoperative anticholinergic medication ordered by the anesthesiologist. The nurse explains that anticholinergic drugs are given preoperatively to prevent which anesthesia-associated complication?

    a. Tachycardia

    b. Bradycardia

    c. Hypertension

    d. Dehydration

14. A 75-year-old male patient is experiencing extrapyramidal symptoms secondary to an antipsychotic drug. Which drug would the nurse expect the physician to order to relieve these symptoms?

    a. Beta-blockers

    b. Anticholinergics

    c. ACE inhibitors

    d. Physostigmine salicylate

15. The nurse is caring for an 8-year-old child who is experiencing an exacerbation of asthma. The nurse expects to administer which medication because of its bronchodilation effects in the treatment of asthma and chronic bronchitis?

    a. Ipratropium

    b. Atropine

    c. Hyoscyamine

    d. Scopolamine

16. A male patient is diagnosed with IBS, and the physician orders an antispasmodic. Which drug should the nurse be prepared to administer to this patient?

    a. Atropine

    b. Hyoscyamine

    c. Glycopyrrolate

    d. Ipratropium

17. A male patient is prescribed an anticholinergic drug by his physician. He likes to hike with his grandchildren. The home care nurse instructs the patient that anticholinergic medications have which effect?

    a. Increased sweating and the risk for heat stroke and dehydration

    b. Postural hypotension and increased risk for falls and from exposure to the elements

    c. Bradycardia in older adults, which increases the risk for falls and from exposure to the elements

    d. Prevents sweating and heat loss and increasing the risk of heat stroke

18. An 80-year-old male patient who lives in a long-term care facility is prescribed anticholinergic medications by his physician. Recently, he has complained of blurred vision. The nurse calls the physician regarding these symptoms. The nurse expects to add which intervention to this patient's plan of care?

    a. Falls prevention

    b. Dietary modifications

    c. Use of restraints

    d. Occupational therapy

19. A 45-year-old female patient is diagnosed with overactive bladder, asthmatic bronchitis, and narrow-angle glaucoma. She asks the physician to prescribe the same anticholinergic medication that her friend uses for her overactive bladder. The nurse expects which response by the physician to the patient's request?

    a. Order the medication

    b. Order the medication with scheduled routine blood work

    c. Decline the prescription preference because of the diagnosis of asthmatic bronchitis

    d. Decline the prescription because of the diagnosis of narrow-angle glaucoma

20. A male patient has been a paraplegic for 5 years. He complains of increased incontinence, and the physician orders anticholinergic medication. What is the reason for this decision?

    a. To increase bladder capacity

    b. To strengthen the detrusor muscles

    c. To decrease bladder capacity

    d. To decrease irritation to the wall of the bladder

CHAPTER 48

Drug Therapy With Opioids

Learning Objectives

- Categorize the types of pain.
- Recognize the pathophysiology associated with pain.
- Identify the prototype and describe the action, use, adverse effects, contraindications, and nursing implications for the opioid agonists.
- Identify the prototype and describe the action, use, adverse effects, contraindications, and nursing implications for the opioid agonists/antagonists.
- Discuss administration of preemptive analgesia in the treatment of pain related to surgery.
- Identify the prototype and describe the action, use, adverse effects, contraindications, and nursing implications for the opioid antagonists.
- Understand how to implement the nursing process in the care of the patient receiving opioid medications for pain.

SECTION I: ASSESSING YOUR UNDERSTANDING

Activity A FILL IN THE BLANKS

1. _____, an unpleasant, uncomfortable sensation, usually indicates tissue damage.

2. _____ analgesics are drugs that relieve moderate-to-severe pain.

3. _____ are abundant in arterial walls, joint surfaces, muscle fascia, periosteum, skin, and soft tissues; they are scarce in most internal organs.

4. _____ analgesics are used in the management of both acute and chronic pain; other _____ are used mainly for chronic neuropathic pain or bone pain.

5. Because of the potentially fatal adverse effects and risks of drug abuse and dependence, all of the opioid analgesics have _____.

Activity B MATCHING

Match the term in Column A with the definition in Column B.

Column A	Column B
____ 1. Hydrocodone	a. An opium alkaloid that is mainly used to relieve moderate to severe pain
____ 2. Codeine	b. A schedule III drug that is similar to codeine in its analgesic and antitussive effects
____ 3. Morphine	c. A potent opioid that is widely used for preanesthetic medication, postoperative analgesia, and chronic pain that requires an opioid analgesic

_____ **4.** Fentanyl

_____ **5.** Methadone

    d. A synthetic drug that is similar to morphine but with a longer duration of action

    e. An opium alkaloid and schedule II drug that is used for analgesic and antitussive effects

Activity C SHORT ANSWERS

Briefly answer the following questions.

1. For a person to feel pain, the signal from the nociceptors in peripheral tissues must be transmitted by a certain route. Describe this route and what happens along the way.

2. Causes of tissue damage may be physical or chemical. Explain how physical or chemical damage activates pain receptors.

3. Explain why most opioid oral drug dosages are larger than those injected.

4. Describe the effects that opioids have on the GI tract.

5. Explain why the goal for the postoperative patient is pain relief without sedation.

SECTION II: APPLYING YOUR KNOWLEDGE

Activity D CASE STUDY

Consider the scenario and answer the questions.

Mrs. Leonard is admitted to your unit with severe burns related to a house fire. She is restless, agitated, and complaining of pain: 8 on a scale of 0 to 10. You are responsible for both pain management and the development of an education plan for the patient and her family.

1. The family asks you why you are giving the pain medication through an IV rather than by mouth. Explain your rationale.

2. The family states that the pain is not managed by the current treatment because the patient is agitated. You develop an education plan for the patient's family. Explain the various causes of agitation for this patient.

SECTION III: PRACTICING FOR NCLEX

Activity E

Answer the following questions.

1. A female patient is 12 hours status postappendectomy. Her son asks the nurse to reduce the amount of pain medication that his mother is taking. He states, "When I had my appendix out, I needed half the pain medication that she does." What is the nurse's best response?

    a. "I agree she is taking far too much pain medication."

    b. "You should discuss your mother's pain management with the physician."

    c. "Pain is a subjective experience; we all feel pain differently."

    d. "I will call the physician for an order to decrease the dose and the frequency of your mother's pain medication."

2. A male patient is receiving an opioid analgesic for bone pain related to a fractured femur. On postoperative day 3, he still requests pain medication every 2 to 3 hours. His incision is clean, dry, and intact, and there are no signs or symptoms of an infectious process surrounding the incision. What assessment takes priority in determining how to help this patient?

    a. Drug tolerance

    b. Drug-seeking behavior

    c. Drug addiction

    d. Drug dependence

3. A female patient states that her pain is unbearable. The nurse has an order for one or two tablets of an opioid analgesic for pain relief. What is the best method that the nurse may use to assess the intensity of the pain?

    a. Base the pain level by comparing it with other patients with the same diagnosis

    b. Use a numerical scale of 0 to 10, with 0 being the least amount of pain

    c. Ask the patient to compare her pain with the pain experienced 24 hours ago

    d. Ask the patient to wait for pain medication until she feels that the pain is out of control

4. A male patient presents in the emergency department and states that he is experiencing pain in his shoulder and chest muscles. The physician orders a cardiac diagnostic assessment. The patient asks the nurse why the doctor feels that he has cardiac problems if his shoulder hurts. What is the nurse's best response?

   a. "Cardiac problems are frequently diagnosed. The assessment is a precaution."

   b. "You may have referred pain. Pain of cardiac origin may radiate to the neck, shoulders, chest muscles, and down the arms, often on the left side."

   c. "Your insurance company requires a cardiac diagnostic assessment whenever you present in the emergency department."

   d. "That is how this physician chooses to assess his patients."

5. The nurse administers an oral opioid analgesic to a patient at 6 PM for pain documented as 6 on a scale of 0 to 10. At 6:30 PM, the patient states that the pain level is 3 on a scale of 0 to 10, and that level is acceptable to him. The patient asks the nurse why another assessment was necessary after the administration of the pain medication. What is the nurse's best response to this patient about proper pain management?

   a. "We assess every patient in relation to pain, initially to determine if the medication is the correct dose."

   b. "We assess every patient in relation to pain according to hospital policy."

   c. "We assess every patient in relation to pain and their activity level."

   d. "We assess every patient in relation to pain, initially to determine appropriate interventions and later to determine whether the interventions were effective in preventing or relieving pain."

6. The nurse is preparing to administer 1 mg of morphine to a 4-year-old child who just had surgery. What action should the nurse complete before administering this medication to a child?

   a. Ensure that the child has a respiratory rate greater than 24.

   b. Ask the child to rate the pain on a scale of 1 to 10.

   c. Check the calculation with another licensed nurse.

   d. Make sure that there is a parent directly at the bedside.

7. The nurse is caring for a patient who experienced multiple fractures. The patient has been prescribed morphine 4 mg every 4 hours IM as needed and 2 mg of morphine IV as needed for intense pain. The nurse understands that the 2 mg of morphine is prescribed for the treatment of what type of pain?

   a. Breakthrough pain

   b. Postoperative pain

   c. Preemptive pain

   d. Chronic pain

8. The home care nurse is caring for a patient who has chronic low back pain. The nurse educates the patient that which therapies will be most helpful to this patient? (Select all that apply.)

   a. Morphine by rectal suppository

   b. Physical therapy

   c. NSAIDs

   d. Acetaminophen

   e. Morphine by mouth

9. The nurse is administering opioid analgesics to a patient for postoperative pain. What is the nurse's most important assessment prior to administering the medication?

   a. Apical heart rate

   b. Lying/standing blood pressure

   c. Respiratory rate

   d. Temporal temperature

10. A patient who is receiving morphine complains of nausea after every dose of medication. What is the nurse's best response to this patient?

    a. "I'm sorry. That means you won't be able to have any more pain medication."

    b. "This is a common side effect of the medication. I will try to make sure you have something to eat when you take the morphine."

    c. "I will mark your chart that you are allergic to morphine."

    d. "I will ask the physician if I can give you acetaminophen for the pain instead of the morphine."

11. The nurse receives a phone call from a patient who has become constipated while taking the opioid analgesic prescribed for his pain. The nurse instructs the patient to do what to help relieve this problem? (Select all that apply.)

    a. Eat a diet low in fiber

    b. Drink 2 to 3 quarts of water per day

    c. Take a daily stool softener

    d. Take a laxative twice a day

    e. Try to establish a regular bowel routine

12. The neonatal nursery nurse is caring for a newborn whose mother was addicted to opioids. The nurse will assess the infant for what symptoms that indicate opioid withdrawal? (Select all that apply.)

    a. Decreased muscle tone

    b. Bradycardia

    c. High-pitched screaming

    d. Diarrhea

    e. Decreased body temperature

13. The nurse suspects opioid overdose in a patient after surgery. What interventions must the nurse initiate for this patient? (Select all that apply.)

    a. Administer naloxone

    b. Decrease the patient's IV fluids

    c. Notify the physician

    d. Prepare for endotracheal intubation

    e. Insert a Foley catheter

14. Prior to administering morphine, the nurse checks the patient's medication history. The nurse will contact the physician and hold the morphine if the nurse notes the patient is currently taking which medication?

    a. Antibiotic

    b. Antihypertensive

    c. Monoamine oxidase (MAO) inhibitor

    d. NSAID

15. The nurse is caring for a patient who has been admitted to the emergency department after a fall. An x-ray indicates that the patient has fractured his ankle. Because of a previous stroke, the patient does not speak. What other method will the nurse use to assess this patient's pain? (Select all that apply.)

    a. Patient's gender

    b. Facial expressions

    c. Patient's age

    d. Movement of arms and hands

    e. Guarding of the leg

16. A patient is admitted to the emergency department for an opioid overdose. What would the nurse expect to administer to this patient?

    a. Naloxone

    b. Normeperidine

    c. Corticosteroids

    d. Oxycodone

17. An 80-year-old male patient presents to the emergency department with a fractured ankle and multiple abrasions and contusions. He is admitted to the hospital with an order for oxycodone for pain. Oxycodone may be prescribed for a geriatric patient because the drug has which characteristic?

    a. It has a long half-life and will manage bone pain more effectively.

    b. It is metabolized by the liver.

    c. It is excreted by the kidney.

    d. It has a short half-life and is less likely to accumulate, causing toxicity or overdosage.

18. A 4-year-old child is admitted to the hospital for a fractured tibia. The parents are fearful because their child may not be able to describe his pain in a manner that is necessary for effective pain management. What is an accurate statement to include as part of the nurse's teaching plan for the parents?

    a. "Your child may behave aggressively or complain verbally of discomfort."

    b. "Your child may not experience pain as intensely as an adult."

    c. "Your child may exhibit only nonverbal behavior."

    d. "Your child may become unusually quiet and noncommunicative."

19. A 32-year-old woman in active labor requests opioid analgesics. What is the nurse's best response to this patient?

   a. "Opioids administered during labor and delivery may decrease your pain and speed the progress of your labor."

   b. "Opioids administered during labor and delivery may slow the labor process."

   c. "Opioids administered during labor and delivery may depress fetal and neonatal respiration."

   d. "Opioids administered during labor and delivery may improve fetal and neonatal respiration."

20. The nurse is caring for a patient who is being treated for opioid withdrawal. The nurse notes that the physician has ordered which medication that is also used as an antihypertensive?

   a. Clonidine

   b. Hydrochlorothiazide

   c. Lisinopril

   d. Prazosin

49 CHAPTER

Drug Therapy With Local Anesthetics

Learning Objectives

- Define local anesthesia.
- Describe three types of local anesthesia.
- Identify the prototype and describe the action, use, adverse effects, contraindications, and nursing implications for the amide local anesthetics.
- Identify the prototype and describe the action, use, adverse effects, contraindications, and nursing implications for the ester local anesthetics.
- Implement the nursing process in the care of patients receiving local anesthesia.

SECTION I: ASSESSING YOUR UNDERSTANDING

Activity A   FILL IN THE BLANKS

1. Local anesthetic agents are classified as _____ and _____.

2. _____ anesthesia blocks sensory impulses at the root of the peripheral nerves as they enter the spinal cord.

3. A woman in labor is most likely to request _____ anesthesia for pain control during the labor and delivery process.

4. _____ anesthesia is regional limb anesthesia produced by a local anesthetic and a pneumatic extremity tourniquet.

5. _____ anesthesia involves application of a local anesthetic to skin and mucous membranes.

Activity B   MATCHING

Match the term in Column A with the definition in Column B.

Column A

____ 1. Lidocaine

____ 2. Dibucaine (Nupercainal)

____ 3. Procaine hydrochloride (Novocaine)

____ 4. Benzocaine (Solarcaine)

____ 5. Tetracaine

Column B

a. An ester local anesthetic that is an approved OTC medication for minor skin problems

b. Prototype ester local anesthetic

c. Prototype amide local anesthetic

d. Used prior to rhinolaryngology to provide local anesthesia to the nose and throat

e. Local anesthetic administered topically and considered safe in pregnancy because it is not absorbed systemically

Activity C SHORT ANSWERS

Briefly answer the following questions.

1. What changes are made to go from providing epidural anesthesia to epidural analgesia?

2. Explain the role topical anesthetics play in the care of children.

3. Why is a tourniquet necessary when administering Bier block anesthesia?

4. What is LAST, and what symptoms would the nurse expect to see in a patient with this condition?

5. How is topical cocaine used as a local anesthetic?

SECTION II: APPLYING YOUR KNOWLEDGE

Activity D CASE STUDY

Consider the scenarios and answer the questions.

Jane Ellen, aged 4, has been admitted to the hospital in preparation for surgery to repair renal reflux. The nurse applies EMLA cream to the child's forearm approximately 1 hour prior to the surgery.

1. What is the purpose of applying this cream to the child's forearm?

2. The mother tells the nurse that she wants her daughter to have epidural anesthesia for surgery like she had when she had Jane Ellen. What is the nurse's best response?

3. As the nurse assesses Jane Ellen prior to surgery, what would the nurse observe if this child develops a hypersensitivity reaction to the lidocaine gel?

SECTION III: PRACTICING FOR NCLEX

Activity E

Answer the following questions.

1. The nurse is giving discharge instructions to a patient who will be using a Lido patch for treatment of pain. The nurse instructs the patient to notify the physician if what symptom occurs?

   a. Bradycardia

   b. Anxiety

   c. Numbness at the site of patch

   d. Lethargy

2. The nurse is caring for a patient who is scheduled to receive a local anesthetic. The nurse understands that vital signs should be monitored at what point?

   a. Before the procedure

   b. After the procedure

   c. During the procedure

   d. Before, during, and after the procedure

3. Mr. Walker has just returned from a procedure that required him to gargle with viscous lidocaine. The nurse keeps the patient NPO until what point?

   a. The patient asks for water

   b. The patient is able to swallow

   c. The patient's gag reflex has returned

   d. The patient is able to talk

4. Prior to receiving procaine, the nurse takes the patient's medical history. The nurse will notify the physician immediately when the patient reveals he is being treated for which condition?

   a. Gonorrhea

   b. Presbycusis

   c. Heart failure

   d. GERD

5. The nurse is assessing a patient for the possible development of LAST. The nurse watches for which initial symptoms of this disorder? (Select all that apply.)

   a. Tinnitus

   b. Lethargy

   c. Metallic taste

   d. Severe pain

   e. Circumoral numbness

6. A female patient received a 4% solution of lidocaine by nebulizer in preparation for a bronchoscopy. The nurse assesses this patient for what adverse effect related to this medication's route of administration?

   a. Rash

   b. Bronchospasm

   c. Heart block

   d. Sepsis

7. The nurse is caring for a patient in the emergency department who will need sutures. The physician plans to use lidocaine. The nurse prepares the suture tray and places lidocaine and what other drug on the tray that helps prolong the local anesthetic effects?

   a. Epinephrine

   b. Prednisone

   c. Morphine

   d. Theophylline

8. The nurse is caring for a patient who has been complaining of postherpetic neuralgia. What drug does the nurse anticipate administering to this patient?

   a. IV lidocaine

   b. Topical lidocaine

   c. Epidural lidocaine

   d. Lidocaine for skin infiltration

9. A male patient became hypotensive after receiving procaine. The nurse will check the patient's medication history to see if the patient has been taking which medication?

   a. Vitamin D

   b. Insulin

   c. Diuretics

   d. Sulfonamides

10. A nursing instructor asks the nursing students what problems benzocaine is used to treat. The student who answers correctly identifies which conditions? (Select all that apply.)

    a. Insect bites

    b. Hemorrhoid pain

    c. Severe burns

    d. Mouth ulcers

    e. Deep laceration

11. The nurse is caring for a woman who received epidural anesthesia during the labor and delivery of her baby. The patient is anxious to get up and take a shower. What is the nurse's best action in this situation?

    a. Place the woman in a wheelchair and wheel her to the bathroom.

    b. Ensure the woman has return of normal feelings and movement in the lower extremities.

    c. Inform the woman that she will not be allowed out of bed for the next 24 hours.

    d. Give the woman a bed bath.

12. The nurse is caring for a patient who has developed LAST after receiving lidocaine. What is the most appropriate nursing diagnosis for this patient?

    a. Acute pain related to preoperative illness or surgery

    b. Risk of aspiration related to consumption of food or fluids with facial and mouth numbness

    c. Risk for impaired tissue perfusion related to the onset of local anesthetic systemic toxicity

    d. Deficient knowledge related to anesthesia and surgery

13. A female patient is 24 weeks pregnant. The nurse is aware that which local anesthetic is not absorbed systemically and is considered safe during pregnancy?

    a. Mepivacaine

    b. Lidocaine

    c. Dibucaine

    d. Bupivacaine

14. The nurse is caring for a patient in the emergency department who is scheduled to receive bupivacaine for regional anesthesia. The nurse understands that what drug must be immediately available if the patient develops a cardiac collapse?

    a. IV lidocaine

    b. IV lipid emulsion

    c. IV dibucaine

    d. IV procaine

15. The nurse is instructing a patient in the use of a Lido patch. What statement by the patient indicates understanding of proper medication administration?

    a. "I will take off the old patch and wait 2 hours before putting on a new one."

    b. "I will put on a new patch before taking off the old one."

    c. "I can add patches if my pain increases."

    d. "I will remove the old patch, clean the skin, and then put on a new patch."

16. The nurse is providing discharge instructions to a patient who is recovering from extensive dental work. The patient states he is hungry and wants to eat. What is the nurse's best response?

    a. "You will be allowed to drink in 15 minutes."

    b. "Stop at the local fast food establishment and pick up something on the way home."

    c. "Do not eat or drink anything until the numbness has gone away."

    d. "You may have liquids tonight and progress to oatmeal in the morning."

17. The physician has ordered EMLA cream for a child prior to a venipuncture. How should the nurse apply this cream to ensure adequate lack of feeling to the area?

    a. Apply the cream 1 hour before the procedure, and cover it with an occlusive dressing.

    b. Rub the cream into the skin for 5 full minutes, and put an absorbent dressing over it.

    c. Place ½ inch of cream on the appropriate site and leave open to the air.

    d. Put the cream on an elastic bandage and leave in place for 15 minutes.

18. The nurse is aware that lidocaine may be administered in many ways. What form of administration is considered needle-free and quickly reduces pain at the site of venipunctures?

    a. EMLA cream

    b. Compressed gas

    c. Subcutaneous

    d. Transdermal patch

19. Prior to the administration of a topical local anesthetic, what is the nurse's priority assessment?

    a. Intact skin

    b. Normal body temperature

    c. Adequate subcutaneous fat

    d. Headache

20. The nurse will notify the physician prior to the use of lidocaine if the patient currently takes which medication?

    a. Amoxicillin

    b. Propranolol

    c. Cimetidine

    d. Morphine

50 CHAPTER

Drug Therapy With General Anesthetics

Learning Objectives

- Define general anesthesia.
- Describe the three phases of general anesthesia.
- Describe the fundamental principles of balanced anesthesia.
- Describe how inhalation anesthetics are delivered, and tell how this process is different with intravenous anesthetics.
- Identify the prototype and describe the action, use, adverse effects, contraindications, and nursing implications for the inhalation and intravenous general anesthetic agents.
- Identify the prototype and describe the action, use, adverse effects, contraindications, and nursing implications for the neuromuscular blocking agents.
- Identify the prototype and describe the action, use, adverse effects, contraindications, and nursing implications for the adjuvant medications administered to patients receiving general anesthesia.
- Implement the nursing process in the care of patients receiving general anesthesia.

SECTION I: ASSESSING YOUR UNDERSTANDING

Activity A FILL IN THE BLANKS

1. _____ is defined as a medication-induced reversible unconsciousness with loss of protective reflexes.

2. The concept of using several drugs to achieve a state of physiologic and pharmacologic equilibrium under general anesthesia is called _____.

3. The first phase of general anesthesia is _____, which is rendering the patient unconscious by using inhalation or intravenous anesthetic or both.

4. The administration of a continuous level of general anesthetics until the procedure is complete is called _____.

5. _____ is the concluding phase of general anesthesia where medications are stopped and the patient is permitted to wake up.

Activity B MATCHING

Match the term in Column A with the definition in Column B.

Column A	Column B
____ 1. Isoflurane (Forane)	a. Prototype intravenous anesthetic that is the most widely administered intravenous anesthetic
____ 2. Propofol (Diprivan)	
____ 3. Etomidate (Amidate)	b. Primarily used for paralysis for tracheal intubation for rapid sequence induction

_____ **4.** Vecuronium (Norcuron)

_____ **5.** Succinylcholine (Anectine)

c. Prototype inhalation anesthetic that is an extremely physically stable methyl ethyl ether

d. Short-acting anesthetic that appears to promote cardiovascular stability

e. Prototype nondepolarizing muscle relaxant

Activity C SHORT ANSWERS

Briefly answer the following questions.

1. Describe the four elements of balanced anesthesia.

2. What is the difference between induction of general anesthesia in adults and children?

3. Why is isoflurane not used frequently for inhalation mask inductions?

4. What are the most common adverse effects of inhalation anesthetics?

5. What is monitored anesthesia care, and what is it used for?

SECTION II: APPLYING YOUR KNOWLEDGE

Activity D CASE STUDY

Consider the scenarios and answer the questions.

Ms. Powell, aged 37, is admitted to the outpatient surgery department for an elective surgical procedure that requires general anesthesia. The nurse caring for the patient obtains a CBC and asks the patient to provide a urine specimen.

1. What is the purpose of obtaining a urine specimen? How would this impact the patient's scheduled surgery?

2. What type of medications does the nurse expect to be administered to this patient during the surgical procedure?

3. What preoperative assessment must the nurse obtain before the patient goes to surgery?

SECTION III: PRACTICING FOR NCLEX

Activity E

Answer the following questions.

1. The nurse is caring for a patient with no known medical conditions who will receive general anesthesia through balanced anesthesia. The nurse understands that the patient may receive some or all of what drugs? (Select all that apply.)
   a. Corticosteroids
   b. Benzodiazepines
   c. Antihypertensives
   d. Neuromuscular blocking agents
   e. Opioid analgesics

2. A patient is scheduled for elective surgery with the general anesthetic, isoflurane. The nurse will monitor this patient for what adverse effect if this patient is a smoker?
   a. Sinus congestion
   b. Bronchospasm
   c. Renal failure
   d. Sweating

3. The nurse is caring for a patient who reports that he experienced malignant hyperthermia the last time he had general anesthesia. The nurse knows that the patient's history includes the development of what symptoms associated with this disorder? (Select all that apply.)
   a. Tachycardia
   b. Hypokalemia
   c. Rigid jaw
   d. Alkalosis
   e. Elevated CK level

4. The nurse is assisting in the care of a patient during surgery. The nurse will be prepared to administer which drug if the patient develops malignant hyperthermia?
   a. Acetaminophen
   b. Toradol
   c. Dantrolene sodium
   d. Diazepam

5. The nurse is aware that the anesthesiologist will use what technique for anesthesia during surgery if a patient has a history of severe postoperative nausea and vomiting?

    a. Local anesthetic

    b. Total intravenous anesthesia

    c. Inhalation anesthesia

    d. Hypnosis

6. The nurse is caring for a patient who has been receiving isoproterenol and will receive isoflurane during surgery. The nurse will assess this patient for what adverse effects related to the interaction of the isoproterenol and the anesthesia?

    a. Cardiac dysrhythmias

    b. Bronchospasm

    c. Delayed emergence from anesthesia

    d. Peripheral vasospasm

7. The nurse is caring for a patient in the post-anesthesia care unit (PACU) and is aware that the patient may experience what effects while emerging from inhalation anesthesia? (Select all that apply.)

    a. Sweating

    b. Nausea

    c. Vomiting

    d. Hypotension

    e. Respiratory depression

8. The anesthesiologist plans to use sevoflurane by mask for anesthesia induction of a 4-year-old child. The nurse will assess this child during emergence from anesthesia for what adverse effect associated with the use of sevoflurane in children?

    a. Respiratory depression

    b. Seizure activity

    c. Agitation

    d. Diarrhea

9. The nurse is preparing a patient who will receive intravenous anesthetic during a short surgical procedure. The nurse understands that this patient is most likely to receive which medication?

    a. Diazepam

    b. Nitrous oxide

    c. Isoflurane

    d. Propofol

10. The nurse is caring for a patient who will undergo an emergency repair of an open fracture to the femur that occurred during a motor vehicle accident. Because of the patient's elevated blood alcohol, the nurse expects that the patient may experience what reaction to the use of isoflurane anesthesia?

    a. Decreased effect of isoflurane

    b. Increased effect of isoflurane

    c. Extreme agitation

    d. Profound coma

11. A patient received propofol as anesthesia during a 30-minute diagnostic procedure. The nurse expects that this patient will recover from anesthesia how quickly?

    a. 2 hours

    b. 1 hour

    c. 30 minutes

    d. 10 minutes

12. The nurse understands that propofol differs from isoflurane in what way?

    a. It doesn't produce analgesia.

    b. It doesn't produce amnesia.

    c. It doesn't produce respiratory depression.

    d. It doesn't produce anesthesia.

13. The nurse is caring for a patient in the intensive care unit who is receiving mechanical ventilation and is receiving propofol for sedation. The nurse will assess the patient for what symptoms characteristic of propofol infusion syndrome? (Select all that apply.)

    a. Rhabdomyolysis

    b. Elevated CK level

    c. Respiratory acidosis

    d. Multiorgan failure

    e. Decreased lactic acid level

14. The nurse is admitting a patient in preparation of surgery. The nurse is aware that propofol is contraindicated in a patient who is allergic to what product?

    a. Latex

    b. Pollen

    c. Gluten

    d. Eggs

15. The nurse is caring for a patient immediately prior to the administration of anesthesia. The nurse knows that what equipment must be available when the anesthesiologist administers vecuronium?
    a. Mechanical ventilation
    b. Defibrillator
    c. Intravenous fluids
    d. Cooling blanket

16. The nurse knows that the anesthetist will administer what medication at the end of surgery to ensure that the patient regains skeletal muscle function?
    a. Isoflurane
    b. Vecuronium
    c. Neostigmine
    d. Diazepam

17. The nurse is caring for a group of patients who each received a nonpolarizing neuromuscular block agent and understands that which patient is most at risk for recurarization?
    a. 16-year-old male
    b. 32-year-old female
    c. 53-year-old female
    d. 79-year-old male

18. The nurse in the postanesthesia care unit assesses patients for which symptoms that may signify the development of recurarization? (Select all that apply.)
    a. Sustains head lift off the pillow for 2.5 seconds
    b. Difficulty taking a deep breath
    c. Strong cough
    d. Difficulty swallowing
    e. Blue and green vision deficiencies

19. The nurse is aware that midazolam is administered prior to surgery for what reason?
    a. To produce amnesia
    b. To prevent hyperthermia
    c. To produce analgesia
    d. To prevent respiratory depression

20. A patient received fentanyl during a surgical procedure. The nurse will have what drug available to treat any possible respiratory depression associated with the use of fentanyl?
    a. Vecuronium
    b. Naloxone
    c. Midazolam
    d. Propofol

51

Drug Therapy for Migraines and Other Headaches

Learning Objectives

- Understand the pathophysiology of migraine headaches.
- Identify the major manifestations of tension headaches, cluster headaches, migraine headaches, and menstrual migraine headaches.
- Identify the prototype and describe the action, use, adverse effects, contraindications, and nursing implications for nonsteroidal anti-inflammatory drugs administered as abortive therapy for migraines.
- Describe the action, use, adverse effects, contraindications, and nursing implications for acetaminophen–aspirin–caffeine combinations administered as abortive therapy for headaches.
- Identify the prototypes and describe the action, use, adverse effects, contraindications, and nursing implications for ergot alkaloids administered as abortive therapy.
- Identify the prototypes and describe the action, adverse effects, contraindications, and nursing implications for triptans administered as abortive therapy.
- Identify the prototype and describe the action, use, adverse effects, contraindications, and nursing implications for estrogen administered for menstrual migraines.
- Identify the medications used for the prevention of migraine headaches.

- Describe the action, use, adverse effects, contraindications, and nursing implications for antiemetic drugs used in the treatment of migraine headache.
- Implement the nursing process of care of patients of all ages who suffer from migraine headaches.

SECTION I: ASSESSING YOUR UNDERSTANDING

Activity A   FILL IN THE BLANKS

1. _____ are recurrent, severe, unilateral orbitotemporal headaches that are associated with histamine reactions.

2. Chronic contractions of the scalp muscles that are associated with nervous tension or anxiety are called _____.

3. _____ headaches are unilateral pain in the head that may or may not be accompanied by an aura.

4. An _____ is a subjective sensation that immediately precedes the migraine headache consisting of a breeze, odor, or light.

5. _____ migraine headaches are associated with a drop in circulating estrogen 2 to 3 days prior to the onset of menses.

Activity B MATCHING

Match the term in Column A with the definition in Column B.

Column A

_____ 1. Sumatriptan (Imitrex)

_____ 2. Naproxen sodium (Aleve)

_____ 3. Acetaminophen, aspirin, and caffeine (Excedrin Migraine)

_____ 4. Ergotamine tartrate (Ergomar)

_____ 5. Estradiol

Column B

a. A form of estrogen that is used in the treatment of menstrual migraines

b. Combination of three drugs that act as an analgesic, an inhibitor of the synthesis of prostaglandins, and as a vasoconstrictor

c. Prototype triptans are serotonin 5-HT1B and 5-HT1D that affect the pathophysiologic mechanism of migraine or cluster headaches

d. Produces stimulation of the cranial and peripheral vascular smooth muscles while depressing the effects of the central vasomotor centers

e. Prototype nonsteroidal anti-inflammatory agent prescribed for the treatment of migraine headaches

Activity C SHORT ANSWERS

Briefly answer the following questions.

1. What foods are known to precipitate migraine headaches?

2. Describe how migraines are inherited.

3. What is the difference between a cluster headache and a migraine headache?

4. What are the characteristics of an aura?

5. What is the difference between abortive therapy and preventive therapy in the treatment of migraine headaches?

SECTION II: APPLYING YOUR KNOWLEDGE

Activity D CASE STUDY

Consider the scenarios and answer the questions.

Mr. Atkins comes to the doctor with complaints of bilateral, nonthrobbing head pain that he rates as a 5 on a scale of 1 to 10. He states that it seems to occur at the end of the work day about 3 days a week. The physician diagnoses the patient with tension headaches.

1. What is the physiologic cause of tension headaches?

2. What are the most common medications used in the treatment of tension headaches?

3. What patient teaching would be most appropriate for the nurse to share with the patient to help prevent the headaches from occurring?

SECTION III: PRACTICING FOR NCLEX

Activity E

Answer the following questions.

1. A male patient has a history of migraine headaches. He calls the clinic complaining of symptoms that he states are hard to describe. He states that he is feeling cold and irritable and has had an odd craving for cheeseburgers. The nurse knows that this patient is describing which phase of a migraine headache?

   a. Prodrome

   b. Aura

   c. Headache

   d. Recovery

2. A patient has had symptoms of a migraine headache approximately 2 to 3 days per week for the last 3 months. The nurse is aware that this patient has developed what condition?

   a. Cluster headache

   b. Chronic migraine headache

   c. Tension headache

   d. Brain tumor

3. The nurse is caring for a patient who has received a prescription for naproxen sodium for the treatment of migraine headaches. This patient also takes lithium carbonate for bipolar disorder. The nurse is aware that this patient will be monitored for what condition?
   a. Decreased lithium levels
   b. Decreased naproxen effectiveness
   c. Lithium toxicity
   d. Increased chance of anaphylaxis

4. The nurse in the emergency department is administering a nonsteroidal anti-inflammatory drug to a patient who has a migraine headache. The patient is nauseated, so the nurse obtains an order to administer which NSAID drug IV?
   a. Ibuprofen
   b. Ketorolac tromethamine
   c. Sumatriptan
   d. Acetaminophen

5. A female patient tells the nurse that the first thing she does when she gets a headache is drink a caffeinated beverage. The nurse is aware that caffeine is known to decrease the pain of migraine headaches by what mechanism?
   a. Vasodilation of blood vessels
   b. Vasoconstriction of blood vessels
   c. Inhibits the synthesis of prostaglandins
   d. Satisfies the thirst center in the brain, which aborts the headache

6. The nurse educates the patient who has just been given a prescription for ergotamine to call the physician if the patient develops which symptoms? (Select all that apply.)
   a. Chest pain
   b. Weakness
   c. Palpitations
   d. Jaundice
   e. Hirsutism

7. The nurse is aware that ergotamine is contraindicated in a patient who is taking which medication?
   a. Tetracycline
   b. Ciprofloxacin
   c. Erythromycin
   d. Vancomycin

8. The nurse is giving instructions to a patient who has just been prescribed sumatriptan for the treatment of migraine headaches. The patient will be instructed to take this medication at what time?
   a. Everyday at the same time
   b. At the onset of migraine symptoms
   c. Every 5 minutes until the pain goes away
   d. After other migraine medications have been ineffective

9. The nurse administers almotriptan to a patient because it is not contraindicated with what category of medications?
   a. Benzodiazepines
   b. SSRIs
   c. MAOIs
   d. Phenothiazines

10. A patient has been taking frovatriptan for migraine headaches and has recently begun taking an SSRI for the treatment of depression. The nurse will monitor this patient for what symptoms associated with serotonin syndrome? (Select all that apply.)
    a. Restlessness
    b. Bradycardia
    c. Hypothermia
    d. Hallucinations
    e. Loss of consciousness

11. The nurse is aware that sumatriptan–naproxen sodium has issued black box warnings because it increases the risk of what conditions? (Select all that apply.)
    a. GI bleeding
    b. Blindness
    c. Myocardial infarction
    d. Brain attack
    e. Skin breakdown

12. The nurse is caring for a patient who has symptoms of menstrual migraine headaches. The nurse is aware that estradiol is contraindicated if this patient has a history of what disorder?
    a. Allergy to penicillin
    b. Deep vein thrombosis
    c. Menstrual irregularity
    d. Cluster headaches

13. The physician has prescribed a carboxylic acid derivative medication to a patient in an attempt to prevent migraine headaches. The nurse understands that the patient will most likely receive a prescription for what medication?

a. Naproxen sodium

b. Sumatriptan

c. Valproic acid

d. Ergotamine

14. A female patient calls the clinic and states she has been taking propranolol for the last week to help decrease the incidence of migraine headaches. The patient states that there has been no decrease in the number of headaches yet. What is the nurse's best response?

a. "I'm sorry the medication hasn't worked for you. The physician will try a new medication."

b. "It may take up to 3 months to know whether this medication will be effective in preventing your migraine headaches."

c. "The medication will be more effective if you try to relax a little bit more."

d. "Try to drink more decaffeinated beverages and see if that helps decrease the number of headaches you are having."

15. The nurse is giving instructions to a 28-year-old female patient who has been prescribed candesartan for prevention of her migraine headaches. What information is most important for the nurse to give to this patient?

a. Take this medication every morning at the same time on an empty stomach.

b. Do not chew this medication.

c. Stay out of the sun while you are taking this medication.

d. Use a barrier form of birth control while you are taking this medication.

16. The nurse instructs the patient who will be taking imipramine to prevent migraine and tension headaches to take this medication at which time?

a. Upon arising

b. With lunch

c. Before dinner

d. At bedtime

17. The nurse is planning care for the patient who has been admitted to the emergency department with an acute migraine headache. What is the most appropriate nursing diagnosis for this patient?

a. Fluid volume excess

b. Acute pain

c. Activity intolerance related to muscle pain

d. Fear related to migraine headache

18. The nurse assesses the patient who has frequent migraine headaches. The patient reports that headaches seem to occur more frequently when he eats which foods? (Select all that apply.)

a. Fried chicken

b. Chinese food

c. Diet beverages

d. American cheese

e. Chocolate cake

19. The nurse is educating a patient who will be taking naproxen sodium as treatment for migraine headaches. The nurse instructs the patient to report which symptoms to the physician? (Select all that apply.)

a. Drowsiness

b. Slight nausea

c. Fever

d. Black stools

e. Sore throat

20. The nurse understands that the combination drug of acetaminophen, aspirin, and caffeine is contraindicated in a patient who already takes which medication?

a. Tetracycline

b. Phenytoin

c. Warfarin

d. Digoxin

Drug Therapy for Seizure Disorders and Spasticity

Learning Objectives

- Identify types of seizures as well as the potential causes and pathophysiology of seizures.
- Identify factors that influence the choice of antiepileptic medications in treating seizure disorders.
- Identify the prototypes and describe the actions, uses, adverse effects, contraindications, and nursing implications for antiepileptic drugs in all classes.
- Describe strategies for prevention and treatment of status epilepticus.
- Implement the nursing process in the care of patients undergoing drug therapy for seizure disorders.
- Discuss the common symptoms and disorders for which skeletal muscle relaxants are used.
- Identify the prototypes and describe the actions, uses, adverse effects, contraindications, and nursing implications for the skeletal muscle relaxants.
- Implement the nursing process in the care of patients undergoing drug therapy for muscle spasms and spasticity.

SECTION I: ASSESSING YOUR UNDERSTANDING

Activity A FILL IN THE BLANKS

1. A _____ involves a brief episode of abnormal electrical activity in nerve cells of the brain that may or may not be accompanied by visible changes in appearance or behavior.

2. A _____ is a tonic–clonic type of seizure characterized by spasmodic contractions of involuntary muscles.

3. When seizures occur in a chronic, recurrent pattern, they characterize a disorder known as _____.

4. _____ or cramp is a sudden, involuntary, painful muscle contraction that occurs with musculoskeletal trauma.

5. Spasms may be _____ (alternating contraction and relaxation) or _____ (sustained contraction).

Activity B MATCHING

Match the term in Column A with the definition in Column B.

Column A

____ **1.** Ethosuximide
____ **2.** Diazepam
____ **3.** Phenytoin
____ **4.** Dantrolene
____ **5.** Baclofen

Column B

a. The prototype and one of the oldest and most widely used AEDs

b. The AED of choice for absence seizures; may be used with other AEDs for treatment of mixed types of seizures

c. Used mainly to treat spasticity in MS and spinal cord injuries

d. Acts directly on skeletal muscle to inhibit muscle contraction

e. A benzodiazepine used in seizure disorders

Activity C SHORT ANSWERS

Briefly answer the following questions.

1. Discuss the probable causes for seizure activity in a patient.

2. Describe the characteristics of epilepsy.

3. What is the difference between a tonic–clonic seizure and an absence seizure?

4. What personal and environmental factors may influence the symptoms of multiple sclerosis?

5. Identify two indications for the use of skeletal muscle relaxants.

SECTION II: APPLYING YOUR KNOWLEDGE

Activity D CASE STUDIES

Consider the scenarios and answer the questions.

Case Study 1

Mr. Alphonse is on a business trip to your state. He is brought to the emergency department unconscious with tonic–clonic seizures lasting for several minutes. You find an empty bottle of anticonvulsants in his briefcase. The physician diagnoses Mr. Alphonse with status epilepticus.

1. Identify what other life-threatening signs and symptoms of status epilepticus you must recognize and report to the physician for prompt treatment.

2. What is the probable cause of Mr. Alphonse's seizure activity?

Case Study 2

Mrs. Robb is diagnosed with multiple sclerosis. She is a career woman, active in her community, and a member of the PTA at her children's school. The physician orders muscle relaxants to help her cope with the symptoms that she is experiencing. You are the community health nurse assigned to her case and responsible for the care plan for this patient.

1. Mrs. Robb asks what she might do to improve her mobility and maintain her ability to be self-sufficient. What disciplines would be included in a plan of care involving the patient's safety and functionality?

2. The oral baclofen that the physician orders causes drowsiness and confusion, which interferes with Mrs. Robb's ability to help her children with their homework at night. What information about the absorption of baclofen would assist her to modify her dosage times (with physician approval) to meet her psychosocial goals?

3. Mrs. Robb's symptoms are in remission. She asks you if she can discontinue the baclofen right away. You suggest that she confer with her physician. What explanation would you give her for your suggestion?

SECTION III: PRACTICING FOR NCLEX

Activity E

Answer the following questions.

1. The nurse is caring for an infant who has been diagnosed with secondary seizures. The nurse is aware of which possible causes of seizures that are classified as secondary? (Select all that apply.)
   a. Idiopathic
   b. Metabolic disorders
   c. Birth injury
   d. Inherited from mother
   e. Fever

2. The community health nurse instructs a patient and his family to keep a diary of the occurrence of seizures. How will this diary assist the physician in treating this patient?
   a. Adjust the dosages of the AEDs
   b. Estimate patient compliance with medication
   c. Include the patient in the decision-making process
   d. Keep the patient and the family focused on the symptoms of the disease process

3. The community health nurse also assists the physician in the decision-making process for AED drug titration by performing which function?
   a. Counting the number of pills in the AED drug bottle to ensure compliance
   b. Administering the AED medication to the patient
   c. Ensuring that the patient makes the appointments for serum drug levels
   d. Monitoring the patient for signs and symptoms of seizure activity during the monthly visit

4. The nurse is administering phenytoin to a patient who is also receiving a continuous nasogastric enteral feeding and is aware of what possible effect?
   a. Increasing absorption of the AED
   b. Decreasing the absorption of the AED
   c. Not affecting absorption of the AED
   d. Precipitating signs of overdosage

5. The nurse is giving discharge instructions to patient with a new onset of seizure activity and will be taking phenytoin at home. The nurse instructs the patient to notify the physician for which symptom of phenytoin toxicity?
   a. Seizure activity
   b. Loss of concentration
   c. Memory loss
   d. Nystagmus

6. The nurse in the newborn nursery is caring for a newborn who has exhibited seizure activity and is prepared to administer what drug of choice?
   a. IM phenobarbital
   b. IV phenobarbital
   c. IM phenytoin
   d. PO phenytoin

7. The nurse instructs the parent of a young school-age child with a seizure disorder who takes an AED to be alert for what signs and symptoms?
   a. Poor study habits related to lack of concentration
   b. Hyperactivity and inability to concentrate
   c. Excessive sedation and interference with learning and social development
   d. Anger and agitation in the classroom setting

8. The nurse is caring for an 84-year-old patient who is taking an AED and recognizes that this patient is at increased risk for which condition?
   a. Falls
   b. Seizure activity
   c. Cardiac dysfunction
   d. Renal dysfunction

9. A patient presents in the emergency department with tonic–clonic seizure activity. What is the IV drug of choice for treatment to obtain rapid control of the seizure?
   a. Topiramate
   b. Valproic acid
   c. Zonegran
   d. Benzodiazepine

10. The physician prescribes oxcarbazepine for a patient. What information should be included in the education plan for this patient if she relies on oral contraceptives?

    a. It increases the effectiveness of the oral contraceptive, and the dosage should be reduced.

    b. It is contraindicated with oral contraceptives, and the contraceptive should be discontinued.

    c. It does not affect the absorption of the oral contraceptive.

    d. It decreases effectiveness of oral contraceptives, and a barrier type of contraception is recommended.

11. A female patient's seizure disorder has been successfully controlled by AEDs for years. She and her husband decide that it is time to start a family. She asks the nurse if it is safe for the fetus for her to continue her AEDs as prescribed. What is the nurse's best response?

    a. "They are safe during pregnancy."

    b. "They are considered teratogenic."

    c. "They may interfere with conception."

    d. "They are contraindicated during the third trimester."

12. The nurse understands that certain classifications of drugs may be used to treat more than one condition and knows that what medication may be used for both bipolar and seizure disorders?

    a. Topiramate

    b. Valproic acid

    c. Zonegran

    d. Benzodiazepine

13. A patient has received a prescription for baclofen. The home care nurse would schedule which laboratory tests to monitor this patient?

    a. CBC and electrolytes

    b. Liver function tests

    c. Cardiac function tests

    d. Hemoglobin and hematocrit

14. The nurse's home care teaching for a patient who takes baclofen will include which instructions? (Select all that apply.)

    a. "Limit the amount of alcohol you drink to two beers per day."

    b. "Rise carefully from a seated to a standing position."

    c. "This medication may cause you to have to urinate more frequently."

    d. "You will find that this medication will help you to concentrate better."

    e. "This medicine may give you a headache or make sleeping difficult."

15. A male patient routinely takes baclofen as a skeletal muscle relaxant for a neuromuscular disorder. His last lab results indicate that he is experiencing renal insufficiency. Based on these data, what would the nurse expect the physician to do?

    a. Increase the dose

    b. Titer the dose

    c. Maintain the current dose

    d. Reduce the dose

16. The physician orders short-term skeletal muscle relaxants for an 11-year-old patient. The nurse is responsible for the family education plan and teaches the parents that the medications should be used only under which condition?

    a. When close supervision is available for monitoring drug effects

    b. When the spasms cause uncontrolled pain

    c. When the patient needs to be alert during pain management

    d. During school hours to increase alertness and management of spasms

17. A male patient's physician ordered tizanidine for symptoms related to his spinal cord injury and gave him latitude with dosing. The patient asks the nurse how soon before activities that cause pain should he administer his medication. The nurse states that oral tizanidine begins to act within 30 to 60 minutes and peaks in how long?

    a. 2 to 4 hours

    b. 1 to 3 hours

    c. 1 to 2 hours

    d. 2 to 3 hours

18. A patient presents to the emergency department with severe pain and receives methocarbamol by injection. As part of the nurse's safety care plan, the nurse should instruct the patient that she may experience which common adverse reaction?

   a. Pain at the injection site

   b. Shortness of breath and dizziness

   c. Palpitations and chest pain

   d. Fainting, incoordination, and hypotension

19. A male patient experiences acute musculoskeletal pain. The physician orders carisoprodol, and his pain is adequately managed. He asks if he might take the drug for long-term pain management. Which statement is the correct response?

   a. "Long-term use can cause physical dependence."

   b. "Long-term use is indicated for your disease process."

   c. "Long-term use may facilitate your return to work."

   d. "Long-term use can cause adverse reactions when used with your antiepileptic drug."

20. A male patient works in an auto assembly line. His physician orders a skeletal muscle relaxant for short-term back spasms. Which instruction would be part of the nurse's education plan for this patient?

   a. "Do not take the medication when working with machinery."

   b. "The medication is safe, and you may return to work when your pain is managed."

   c. "You need to take the medication on a full stomach before physical therapy."

   d. "The side effects of skeletal muscle relaxants will not interfere with most activities of daily living, including work."

CHAPTER 53

Drug Therapy to Reduce Anxiety and Produce Hypnosis

Learning Objectives

- Discuss the pathophysiology and clinical manifestations of anxiety.
- Discuss the pathophysiology and clinical manifestations of sleep and insomnia.
- Identify the prototype and describe the action, use, adverse effects, contraindications, and nursing implications for the benzodiazepines.
- Discuss the various nonbenzodiazepines used to reduce anxiety and produce hypnosis in terms of their action, use, contraindications, adverse effects, and nursing implications.
- Implement the nursing process in the care of the patient being treated with benzodiazepines.

SECTION I: ASSESSING YOUR UNDERSTANDING

Activity A FILL IN THE BLANKS

1. _____ drugs (also known as _____ and _____) promote relaxation, and hypnotics produce sleep.

2. The main drugs used to treat insomnia are the _____ and the _____ hypnotics.

3. _____ is a common disorder that may be referred to as nervousness, tension, worry, or other terms that denote an unpleasant feeling.

4. _____ is a normal response to a stressful situation.

5. _____, prolonged difficulty in going to sleep or staying asleep long enough to feel rested, is the most common sleep disorder.

Activity B MATCHING

Match the term in Column A with the definition in Column B.

Column A

____ 1. Ramelteon
____ 2. Eszopiclone
____ 3. Chloral hydrate

Column B

a. The first oral nonbenzodiazepine hypnotic to be approved for long-term use.

b. Used clinically as antianxiety, hypnotic, and anticonvulsant agents.

c. Newest oral nonbenzodiazepine hypnotic indicated for treatment of sleep onset difficulty.

_____ **4.** Benzodiaz-
epines

_____ **5.** Zaleplon

d. Oral nonbenzodi-
azepine hypnotic
approved for the
short-term treat-
ment of insomnia.

e. The oldest sedative–
hypnotic drug, rela-
tively safe, effective,
and inexpensive in
usual therapeutic
doses.

Activity C   **SHORT ANSWERS**

Briefly answer the following questions.

1. Describe the probable physiological cause for
anxiety disorders.

2. Explain the role the serotonin system plays in
anxiety.

3. Discuss the impact of sleep on the biologic
processes of the body.

4. Define insomnia, and discuss the impact
of insomnia on the patient's health and
well-being.

5. Explain the psychological impact that an
excessive amount of norepinephrine may
have on a patient's psychological well-being.

SECTION II: APPLYING YOUR KNOWLEDGE

Activity D   **CASE STUDY**

Consider the scenario and answer the questions.

Mr. Petski, aged 35, suffers from long-term
insomnia, which is affecting both his work and
home life. His profession is high stress, and he
complains that he is unable to stop problem
solving when he goes to bed. He had success
with short-term hypnotics in the past and asks
his physician for a sleep medication. The physician orders eszopiclone. You meet with Mr. Petski
to discuss his medication regimen.

1. What information about Mr. Petski's evening
habits would indicate an impact on the
absorption of the medication as well as its
efficacy?

2. Mrs. Petski calls the office stating that her
husband appears depressed and anxious. You
notify the physician. What is the significance
of Mr. Petski's behavior?

3. What change in Mr. Petski's medications or
diet may cause adverse reactions?

SECTION III: PRACTICING FOR NCLEX

Activity E

Answer the following questions.

1. A female patient, who is a college student, is
diagnosed with insomnia by her physician.
The physician prescribes eszopiclone for
sleep. The patient asks the nurse if she will
develop a tolerance to the medication. What
is the nurse's best response?

a. "If you take the eszopiclone for more than
2 weeks, you may develop a tolerance to
the hypnotic benefits of the medication
and should call your physician."

b. "During drug testing, tolerance to the
hypnotic benefits of eszopiclone was not
observed over a 6-month period."

c. "During drug testing, tolerance to the hypnotic benefits of eszopiclone was observed
after administration of the drug for a
6-month period."

d. "Eszopiclone may be taken indefinitely
without tolerance to the hypnotic benefits
of the medication."

2. A patient asks when eszopiclone should be
taken to promote sleep. What is the nurse's
best response to this patient?

a. "Eszopiclone is rapidly absorbed after oral
administration, reaching peak plasma levels
30 minutes after administration."

b. "Eszopiclone is rapidly absorbed after oral
administration, reaching peak plasma levels
20 minutes after administration."

c. "Eszopiclone is rapidly absorbed after oral
administration, reaching peak plasma levels
1 hour after administration."

d. "Eszopiclone is rapidly absorbed after oral
administration, reaching peak plasma levels
1 to 2 hours after administration."

3. A 76-year-old patient has been diagnosed with generalized anxiety disorder, and the physician has prescribed a benzodiazepine. The nurse understands that the physician will prescribe what medication that is considered the drug of choice for this patient?

   a. Diazepam

   b. Temazepam

   c. Oxazepam

   d. Triazolam

4. A 35-year-old female patient is recently divorced and having difficulty coping. She visits her physician, and he diagnoses her with situational anxiety. She is fearful that the anxiety she feels will become chronic. The nurse gives the patient what information concerning situational anxiety?

   a. A normal response to a stressful situation

   b. An abnormal response to a stressful situation

   c. A method of coping with the divorce

   d. A feeling that will go away on its own

5. A male patient's anxiety is interfering with his ability to perform basic activities of daily living and return to work. The nurse expects that which diagnosis will probably be made by his physician?

   a. Intermittent anxiety disorder

   b. Anxiety disorder

   c. Abnormal anxiety disorder

   d. Chronic anxiety disorder

6. A female patient is prescribed a benzodiazepine for anxiety. She asks the nurse if she can stop the drug when she feels better. What is the nurse's best response?

   a. "Benzodiazepines do not cause physiologic dependence, and withdrawal symptoms will not occur if the drug is stopped abruptly."

   b. "Benzodiazepines may cause physiologic dependence, but withdrawal symptoms will not occur if the drug is stopped abruptly."

   c. "Benzodiazepines may cause physiologic dependence, and withdrawal symptoms will occur if the drug's dosages are tapered."

   d. "Benzodiazepines may cause physiologic dependence, and withdrawal symptoms will occur if the drug is stopped abruptly."

7. A group of nursing students answers correctly if they identify which medication as the prototype benzodiazepine?

   a. Alprazolam (Xanax)

   b. Diazepam (Valium)

   c. Lorazepam (Ativan)

   d. Clonazepam (Klonopin)

8. The physician orders eszopiclone (Lunesta) for a male patient as a treatment for intermittent insomnia. The patient states that he feels the prescription works well as a sleep aid, but he is having difficulty with short-term memory loss. What is this patient experiencing?

   a. An anticipated effect of the drug

   b. An allergic reaction

   c. An adverse reaction

   d. A common side effect

9. A male patient's physician orders ramelteon for his long-term insomnia. The patient is concerned that he will become dependent on the drug and is hesitant to take it. What instructions will the nurse give to this patient?

   a. "Ramelteon may cause physical dependence."

   b. "Ramelteon may cause physical dependence with constant use."

   c. "Ramelteon causes physical dependence only if you have a documented sensitivity to the drug."

   d. "Ramelteon does not cause physical dependence."

10. A male patient asks, "How long before sleep should I take ramelteon?" Which of the following time frames will the nurse give this patient as part of patient teaching?

    a. 15 minutes

    b. 45 minutes

    c. 10 minutes

    d. 20 minutes

11. A male patient is prescribed zaleplon for short-term treatment of his insomnia. He states that it only works once in a while. Upon review of his evening habits, the nurse discovers he is engaging in which behavior that may interfere with the absorption of his prescription?

    a. A late, heavy meal before bedtime

    b. Exercise before bedtime

    c. Fasting before bedtime

    d. Doing paperwork before bedtime

12. A male patient asks the physician about zaleplon to help him sleep. He tells the nurse that he regularly drinks 5 ounces of red wine in the evening. The physician elects not to give this patient the prescription because a combination of zaleplon and alcohol may cause which effect?

    a. Hypertension and respiratory excitement

    b. Respiratory depression and excessive sedation

    c. Cardiac dysrhythmias

    d. A hangover effect

13. A male patient takes over-the-counter drug cimetidine for treatment of acid reflux and asks why the physician will need to adjust his zaleplon dosage. The nurse states that the physician may need to adjust the medication in what way?

    a. Decrease the dose of the zaleplon to 10 mg

    b. Decrease the dose of the zaleplon to 5 mg

    c. Increase the dose of the zaleplon to 15 mg

    d. Increase the dose of the zaleplon to 7 mg

14. A male patient is not only having difficulty falling asleep but wakes up frequently during the night. The physician prescribes zolpidem in the CR form. The patient asks what makes this form of the drug different. What is the nurse's best response to this patient?

    a. "Ambien CR contains a slow-releasing layer of medication, which aids a person in falling asleep, and a second layer, which is released rapidly to promote sleep all night."

    b. "Ambien CR contains a rapid-releasing layer of medication, which aids a person in falling asleep, and a second layer, which is also released rapidly to promote sleep all night."

    c. "Ambien CR contains a slow-releasing layer of medication, which aids a person in falling asleep, and a second layer, which is released even more slowly to promote sleep all night."

    d. "Ambien CR contains a rapid-releasing layer of medication, which aids a person in falling asleep, and a second layer, which is released more slowly to promote sleep all night."

15. A male patient took zolpidem daily for 1 week with good response, then stopped the medication. Two days later, he returns to the physician's office stating that his insomnia is worse than it ever was. The nurse is responsible for the development of a teaching plan for the patient, including adverse reactions. After 1 week of regular use, which adverse reaction may occur with zolpidem?

    a. Chronic insomnia

    b. Short-term insomnia

    c. Rebound insomnia

    d. Long-term insomnia

16. A patient's physician prescribes alprazolam in addition to the patient's antidepressant fluvoxamine. The nurse knows that the patient's benzodiazepine dose will be adjusted in what way?

    a. Reducing the dose by 50%

    b. Increasing the dose by 25%

    c. Tapering the initial doses of the medication

    d. Increasing the dose by 5%

17. A 70-year-old male patient asks why he is receiving a lower dose of zaleplon than his son. As part of the nurse's teaching plan, which explanation will the nurse give this patient?

    a. "Older adults metabolize the drug more quickly, but due to renal dysfunction, the medication must be reduced."

    b. "Older adults metabolize the drug more slowly, and half-lives are longer than in younger adults."

    c. "Older adults metabolize the drug at the same speed as younger adults; I will check the dosage with your physician."

    d. "Older adults do not need as much of the medication for the desired effect as a younger adult does."

18. The medication nurse knows that when benzodiazepines are used with opioid analgesics, the analgesic dose should be adjusted in which way?

    a. It should be increased initially and reduced gradually.

    b. It should be reduced initially and increased gradually.

    c. It should be reduced initially and incrementally thereafter.

    d. It should be increased initially and incrementally thereafter.

19. A female patient's physician prescribes a long-acting antianxiety benzodiazepine. She asks why she should take the medication at night when the morning is more convenient. What teaching would the nurse include in the education plan for this patient?

    a. "If you take the medication in the morning, then you may have difficulty remaining awake at work."

    b. "If you take the medication in the morning, you may have increased anxiety during the day."

    c. "This schedule promotes sleep, and there is usually enough residual sedation to maintain antianxiety effects throughout the next day."

    d. "This schedule is prescribed by the physician and therefore must be followed."

20. The nurse is aware that there is some research that reveals that anxiety may be treated with nutritional and herbal supplements. Which nutritional and or herbal supplement is used in this treatment?

    a. Caffeine

    b. Melatonin

    c. Kava

    d. Whey

Drug Therapy for Depression and Mood Stabilization

Learning Objectives

- Discuss the etiology and pathophysiology of depression and bipolar disorder.
- Describe the major features of various mood disorders.
- Compare and contrast the different categories of antidepressants: tricyclic antidepressants, selective serotonin reuptake inhibitors, mixed serotonin–norepinephrine reuptake inhibitors, monoamine oxidase inhibitors, and other atypical antidepressants.
- Discuss the drugs used to treat depression in terms of prototype, action, indications for use, adverse effects, and nursing implications.
- Discuss the drugs used to treat bipolar disorder in terms of prototype, action, indications for use, adverse effects, and nursing implications.
- Implement the nursing process in the care of patients undergoing drug therapy for mood disorders.

SECTION I: ASSESSING YOUR UNDERSTANDING

Activity A FILL IN THE BLANKS

1. _____ is a major depressive episode occurring after the birth of a child.

2. _____ is associated with impaired ability to function in usual activities and relationships.

3. _____ is characterized by episodes of major depression plus mania and occurs equally in men and women.

4. _____ is characterized by episodes of major depression plus hypomanic episodes and occurs more frequently in women.

5. Sudden termination of most antidepressants results in _____.

Activity B MATCHING

Match the term in Column A with the definition in Column B.

Column A	Column B
____ 1. SSRIs	a. Considered to be third-line medications in the treatment of depression because of a high incidence of food and drug interactions that can potentially lead to hypertensive crisis
____ 2. TCAs	b. Second-line medications in the treatment of depression, producing a high incidence of adverse effects

_____ 3. MAOIs

_____ 4. SNRIs

_____ 5. Antidepressants

c. Similar to SSRIs in terms of therapeutic effects but produce more anticholinergic, CNS sedation, and cardiac conduction abnormalities

d. Must be taken for 2 to 4 weeks before depressive symptoms improve

e. Considered to be first-line medications in the treatment of depression because they have a more favorable side effect profile

Activity C SHORT ANSWERS

Briefly answer the following questions.

1. Discuss the methods used to prevent antidepressant toxicity and the interventions used to treat toxicity.

2. For patients with certain concurrent medical conditions, antidepressants may have adverse effects. Discuss disease-specific adverse reactions related to antidepressants.

3. Why is lithium considered the drug of choice for bipolar disorder?

4. Dosages of antidepressant drugs should be individualized according to clinical response. Discuss the method of dosage adjustment used with SSRIs and venlafaxine.

5. Discuss both the causes and the signs and symptoms of serotonin syndrome.

SECTION II: APPLYING YOUR KNOWLEDGE

Activity D CASE STUDIES

Consider the scenarios and answer the questions.

Case Study 1

Ms. Roth cares for her 70-year-old mother, Millie, in her home. Until recently, Millie was an active member of the household, often helped with the grandchildren's homework, and served as a member of the local senior center. However, since Millie underwent abdominal surgery for a small-bowel obstruction and experienced a routine recovery 1 month ago, she has been refusing to eat and shows little interest in her environment or her grandchildren. The physician prescribes an antidepressant for Millie and orders follow-up care with the community health nurse.

1. One week later, you visit the home. Ms. Roth reports that her mother is the same and states that a larger dose of the antidepressant may be needed. How would you respond?

2. One month later, the physician increases the dose of the antidepressant. What behaviors should the family recognize and report to the physician?

Case Study 2

Mr. Jones' physician ordered fluoxetine 2 months ago for a diagnosis of situational depression. Mr. Jones arrives at the physician's office in an agitated state and complains of chronic insomnia. The physician orders discontinuance of the antidepressant, as recommended by the PDR.

1. What other signs and symptoms might Mr. Jones describe when you take a detailed history before his appointment with the physician?

2. You meet with Mr. Jones 1 week later. He states that he still is experiencing insomnia and agitation. How would you explain this?

SECTION III: PRACTICING FOR NCLEX

Activity E

Answer the following questions.

1. A female patient is prescribed fluoxetine during the third trimester of her pregnancy for depression. After birth, her child exhibits symptoms of neonatal withdrawal syndrome. When would the nurse expect the symptoms to abate?

   a. In a few days

   b. After 6 weeks

   c. In a few hours

   d. With administration of fluoxetine

2. The nurse is caring for a group of patients in a long-term care facility. The nurse is aware that SSRIs are associated with what side effect that is especially undesirable in older adults?

   a. Heart failure

   b. Weight gain

   c. Weight loss

   d. Nocturia

3. The nurse knows that antidepressant therapy is prescribed very carefully for children, adolescents, and young adults aged 18 to 24 because they have an increased risk of what when taking antidepressant medications?

   a. Manic episodes

   b. Suicidal episodes

   c. Somnolence

   d. Postural hypotension

4. The nurse is caring for a patient who has been diagnosed with bipolar disorder type II. The nurse knows that this disorder is characterized by episodes of major depression plus hypomanic episodes and occurs more frequently in what category of patients?

   a. Men

   b. Children

   c. Women

   d. The elderly

5. A 35-year-old male patient is slowly recovering from an abdominal aortic aneurysm repair and cerebral vascular accident 6 weeks ago. His physical condition is unstable at this time. His physician prescribes a low-dose antidepressant for him based on a diagnosis of situational depression. The patient's wife asks if a higher dose might be more beneficial. What would the nurse teach the family regarding this patient's dosage?

   a. Dosage is based on the patient's diagnosis.

   b. Dosage must be titrated based on the patient's weight.

   c. A higher dose may cause postural hypertension.

   d. Dosage must be cautious and slow and the patient's responses carefully monitored.

6. A male patient has a history of hepatic dysfunction secondary to alcoholism. Based on the patient's diagnostic history, what would the nurse expect his physician to order?

   a. A higher dose of the antidepressant

   b. A lower dose of the antidepressant

   c. More frequent doses of the antidepressant

   d. No antidepressants, because they would be contraindicated for this patient.

7. The nurse is interviewing a 75-year-old patient and knows that what antidepressant drug class is the first choice for older adults?

   a. SSRIs

   b. TCAs

   c. MAOIs

   d. Older adults should not receive antidepressant medications.

8. The nurse is assessing a 13-year-old patient who has symptoms of depression and recognizes that what class of antidepressant medication would *not* be a drug of choice for an adolescent?

   a. SSRIs

   b. TCAs

   c. MAOIs

   d. ACE inhibitors

9. The nurse is caring for a 12-year-old child who has been hospitalized with depression, and the physician has elected to treat the child with a TCA. The nurse understands that what laboratory test will be routinely ordered by the physician?

   a. CBC and chemistry panel and plasma drug levels

   b. Hemoglobin and hematocrit and plasma drug levels

   c. Chest x-ray and plasma drug levels

   d. Blood pressure, ECG, and plasma drug levels

10. A male patient asks the physician for anti-depressant therapy for his 14-year-old son. The physician orders a psychiatric consultation before prescribing medication, for what reason?

    a. It is unsafe to administer antidepressants to an adolescent without a psychiatric consultation.

    b. It is probably best to reserve drug therapy for those who do not respond to nonpharmacologic treatments such as cognitive behavioral therapy.

    c. A definitive diagnosis has not been established.

    d. Adolescents require higher doses of antidepressants than adults do.

11. A male African American patient is prescribed a TCA for his depression. He asks the nurse why the dose he receives is lower than that of his Caucasian friend. What response by the nurse is most correct?

    a. "African Americans tend to metabolize TCAs more slowly than Caucasians do."

    b. "African Americans tend to metabolize TCAs more quickly than Caucasians do."

    c. "African Americans experience side effects with higher doses."

    d. "African Americans experience suicidal ideation with higher doses."

12. A female patient's bipolar disorder symptoms have been successfully managed with lithium for many years. She is scheduled for a CABG and is instructed to stop her lithium 1 to 2 days before surgery and resume when full oral intake of food and fluids is allowed. She asks why she must stop the medication. What is the nurse's best response?

    a. "You will not have bipolar symptoms during surgery or immediately afterward because of the anesthetics."

    b. "Lithium will cause hypertension during surgery."

    c. "Lithium may prolong the effects of anesthetics and neuromuscular blocking drugs."

    d. "Lithium may cause cardiac complications during surgery."

13. A female patient discontinues her SSRI abruptly. What signs and symptoms of withdrawal would the nurse expect to see when the patient arrives at the physician's office 1 week later? (Select all that apply.)

    a. Dizziness

    b. Lethargy or anxiety/hyperarousal

    c. Chest pain

    d. Headache

    e. Gastrointestinal upset

14. The nurse is preparing a patient for discharge who is taking phenelzine. The nurse instructs the patient that which foods cause serious complications? (Select all that apply.)

    a. Deer meat

    b. Shrimp

    c. Rice

    d. American cheese

    e. Fava beans

15. The nurse is caring for a patient who has just begun to take lithium for treatment of bipolar disease. The nurse instructs the patient that his lithium level will need to be monitored at what frequency?

    a. Monthly in the morning, 12 hours after the last dose of lithium

    b. Four times weekly in the morning, 12 hours after the last dose of lithium

    c. Weekly in the morning, 12 hours after the last dose of lithium

    d. Two or three times weekly in the morning, 12 hours after the last dose of lithium

16. A patient with type 1 diabetes mellitus has been dealing with feelings of depression for the last month, and the physician has elected to start this patient on fluoxetine. What patient teaching is most important for the nurse to share with this patient?

    a. "You will probably need to increase your usual insulin dosage."

    b. "Increase your monitoring of your blood sugar because there is an increased chance of hypoglycemia."

    c. "Double the carbohydrates you eat daily to prevent hypoglycemia from occurring."

    d. "Decrease your calorie intake by one half by skipping all in-between meals."

17. A male patient wishes to discontinue his antidepressant secondary to sexual dysfunction. What antidepressant medication may be ordered by his physician because it does not interfere with sexual function?

    a. Mirtazapine

    b. Bupropion

    c. Duloxetine

    d. Venlafaxine

18. Because the available drugs have similar efficacy in treating depression, the nurse understands that the choice of an antidepressant depends on what factors? (Select all that apply.)

    a. Cost

    b. Age

    c. Gender

    d. Medical conditions

    e. The specific drug's adverse effects

19. A male patient is taking warfarin and presents to the physician's office with calf pain and a positive Homan's sign. He tells the physician that he has been depressed lately and is taking a herbal remedy. What herbal antidepressant may reduce the effectiveness of his warfarin?

    a. St. John's wort

    b. Feverfew

    c. Watercress

    d. Wallwort

20. The nurse is conducting a preoperative joint replacement session for a patient who is scheduled for a knee replacement in 2 weeks. What instructions will the nurse give this patient regarding the imipramine the patient takes for treatment of depression?

    a. "Take half the dose of imipramine for a week prior to your surgery."

    b. "Stop taking the imipramine 4 days before surgery."

    c. "The physician will order IV imipramine for you while you are in the hospital."

    d. "Stop taking the imipramine until you have surgery."

CHAPTER 55

Drug Therapy for Psychotic Disorders

Learning Objectives

- Discuss common manifestations of psychotic disorders, including schizophrenia.
- Identify the prototype and describe the action, use, adverse effects, contraindications, and nursing implications for the phenothiazines.
- Identify the prototype and describe the action, use, adverse effects, contraindications, and nursing implications for the typical antipsychotics.
- Identify the prototype and describe the action, use, adverse effects, contraindications, and nursing implications for the atypical antipsychotics.
- Compare characteristics of the "atypical" antipsychotics with those of the "typical" antipsychotics.
- Implement the nursing process in the care of the patient being treated with antipsychotics.

SECTION I: ASSESSING YOUR UNDERSTANDING

Activity A FILL IN THE BLANKS

1. Antipsychotic drugs are used mainly for the treatment of _____.

2. _____ are sensory perceptions of people or objects that are not present in the external environment.

3. _____ are false beliefs that persist in the absence of reason or evidence.

4. Deluded people often believe that other people control their thoughts, feelings, and behaviors or seek to harm them; these beliefs are called _____.

5. Antipsychotic drugs, called _____, are derived from several chemical groups.

Activity B MATCHING

Match the term in Column A with the definition in Column B.

Column A	Column B
___ 1. Chlorpromazine	a. Acute dystonia, parkinsonism, and akathisia
___ 2. Neuroleptic malignant syndrome	b. The first drug to effectively treat psychotic disorders
___ 3. Extrapyramidal side effects	c. Blurred vision, constipation, dry mouth, photophobia, tachycardia, and urinary hesitancy
___ 4. Anticholinergic side effects	d. Orthostatic hypotension and CNS depression
___ 5. ___ Anti-adrenergic effects	e. A rare but potentially fatal adverse effect, characterized by rigidity

Activity C SHORT ANSWERS

Briefly answer the following questions.

1. Discuss the signs and symptoms that a patient may experience with the diagnosis of *psychosis* and their impact on the patient's ability to perform activities of daily living and interact within home and work environments.

2. Identify and discuss the factors that may precipitate an acute psychotic episode.

3. Discuss the neurodevelopmental model in relation to the development of schizophrenia.

4. Discuss the role of genetics in the development of schizophrenia.

5. Discuss the impact that the negative symptoms of *schizophrenia* have on a patient's ability to cope within home and work environments.

SECTION II: APPLYING YOUR KNOWLEDGE

Activity D CASE STUDIES

Consider the scenarios and answer the questions.

Case Study 1

Mr. Smith is prescribed clozapine by his physician. You are responsible for his education plan.

1. Mr. Smith asks you whether he will have the same extrapyramidal effects with clozapine that he had with his other antipsychotic medication. How would you reply?

2. Explain the rationale for weekly laboratory tests for this patient.

3. Mr. Smith returns to the office weekly for his blood work. During an interview 1 month later, he states that he feels able to cope within his environment but gets dizzy often. Discuss the elements of your focused assessment, and explain your rationale for this assessment.

Case Study 2

Ms. Case, age 35, is diagnosed with psychosis after an assessment by a psychiatrist in conjunction with her physician. She visits the physician's office with her mother. The physician orders haloperidol. You are responsible for the education plan for this family.

1. Ms. Case's mother states that her daughter is often noncompliant with her medication. After you report this to the physician, how may the medication administration of haloperidol be changed to improve compliance?

2. You discuss signs and symptoms of the extrapyramidal effects of haloperidol. Explain the signs and symptoms in layman's terms.

SECTION III: PRACTICING FOR NCLEX

Activity E

Answer the following questions.

1. The nurse is caring for a patient who has been receiving a prescription for haloperidol for treatment of psychosis. The nurse suspects that the patient is developing neuroleptic malignant syndrome. What assessments would support this? (Select all that apply.)
   a. Severe hypothermia
   b. Confusion
   c. Bradycardia
   d. Dyspnea
   e. Acute renal failure

2. The nurse is caring for a patient who has developed tardive dyskinesia, a late extrapyramidal effect that is generally considered to be irreversible. What is one method used to treat tardive dyskinesia?
   a. Increasing the dosage of the medication
   b. Discontinuing the medication abruptly
   c. Referring the patient to a psychiatrist for evaluation
   d. Reducing the dosage

3. A female patient consults her physician because she can't seem to sit still. She is currently taking antipsychotic medications. Her symptoms may be treated with what class of agent?
   a. Cardiotonics
   b. Antihistamines
   c. Beta-blockers
   d. Antiepileptics

4. A female patient makes an appointment with her physician 2 weeks after beginning her prescription antipsychotic therapy. She states that she is still unable to cope and concentrate at work. What statement would be appropriate to include in the nurse's teaching?

   a. "Antipsychotics may take several weeks to achieve maximum therapeutic effect."

   b. "The medication should be effective by this time; I will consult the physician."

   c. "This medication may need to be changed; I will consult the physician."

   d. "Therapeutic effects of antipsychotics should be evaluated every 2 weeks by your physician."

5. The physician prescribed antipsychotic medication for a female patient 2 months ago. She is noncompliant with her medication regimen and is symptomatic. The nurse is responsible for developing a plan of care to facilitate medication compliance. What would the nurse include in this plan?

   a. A written contract to ensure compliance

   b. Coordination of the efforts of several health and social service agencies or providers

   c. Immediate hospitalization for medication noncompliance lasting 1 week

   d. Administration of daily oral medications by the community health nurse

6. A 13-year-old child is admitted to the mental health unit with symptoms of Tourette's syndrome. The physician orders haloperidol PO. What initial dose would the nurse expect the physician to order?

   a. 7 to 10 mg

   b. 0.3 to 0.5 mg

   c. 20 to 40 mg

   d. 1.5 to 6 mg

7. A male patient is admitted to the emergency department via ambulance. He is attempting to pull out his IV line and is exhibiting symptoms of agitation and thrashing about. The physician orders a benzodiazepine-type sedative. What information is needed prior to administration of the drug?

   a. Whether the patient has a history of agitation

   b. Whether the patient is currently taking antibiotics

   c. Whether the patient is experiencing drug intoxication or withdrawal

   d. Whether the patient is currently taking a diuretic

8. A male patient's physician orders antipsychotic medications for him. He experiences little or no side effects from the medications and is able to function successfully in both his home and work environments. Six weeks later, he is diagnosed with hepatitis B. He begins to experience adverse reactions to his medications. A possible reason for the adverse reactions might be that, in the presence of liver disease, what may happen?

   a. Metabolism may be accelerated and drug elimination half-lives shortened, causing an increased risk of adverse effects.

   b. Metabolism may be slowed and drug elimination half-lives shortened, with resultant accumulation and increased risk of adverse effects.

   c. Metabolism may be slowed and drug elimination half-lives prolonged, with resultant accumulation and increased risk of adverse effects.

   d. Metabolism may be accelerated and drug elimination half-lives prolonged, with resultant accumulation and increased risk of adverse effects.

9. A female patient is diagnosed with renal insufficiency. The nurse develops a teaching plan based on her diagnosis and antipsychotic drug usage. She asks the nurse why it is so important to have renal function tests routinely. The nurse replies that if renal function test results become abnormal, what may be a consequence?

   a. The drug may need to be lowered in dosage or discontinued.

   b. The drug will be discontinued immediately.

   c. The drug will be continued with caution.

   d. The drug dosages will be increased to increase absorption.

10. A male patient presents at the physician's office with yellow sclera. The patient is concerned that he has hepatitis. The patient began a new medication regimen about 1 month ago that includes phenothiazines. The nurse understands that this patient is experiencing what type of event?

    a. An adverse reaction

    b. A hypersensitivity reaction

    c. A rare occurrence

    d. A life-threatening occurrence

11. An African American male patient routinely takes haloperidol to manage his psychosis. Recently, he presented to the physician's office with signs of tardive dyskinesia, and his physician modified the drug regimen over time. The patient will now take the drug olanzapine and discontinue the haloperidol. What will the nurse tell the patient to help decrease his anxiety about the new drug regimen?

    a. "The signs of tardive dyskinesia will diminish over time."

    b. "African Americans always experience tardive dyskinesia with antipsychotics."

    c. "When compared with haloperidol, olanzapine has been associated with fewer extrapyramidal reactions in African Americans."

    d. "The olanzapine does not produce side effects in African American males."

12. A female patient is diagnosed with Alzheimer-type dementia. She resides in a long-term care facility. The patient's daughter asks the physician to prescribe an antipsychotic to control her mother's outbursts of anger and depression. The physician orders a psychiatric consultation for the patient. The patient's daughter asks, "Why doesn't the doctor just order an antipsychotic?" What is the nurse's best response to this family member?

    a. "Patients with dementia routinely become agitated due to their disease process."

    b. "Patients with dementia respond poorly to antipsychotic medications."

    c. "Patients with dementia respond well to antipsychotic medications."

    d. "Use of antipsychotic drugs exposes patients to adverse drug effects and does not resolve underlying problems."

13. A female patient's physician orders a low-dose antipsychotic to manage her acute agitation. Her daughter states that her mother is improved but her cognitive functions are the same, if not worse, than last month. What is the best explanation for this development?

    a. Antipsychotics cause a gradual return of cognitive ability.

    b. Antipsychotics reduce memory loss.

    c. Antipsychotics increase the risk of long-term memory loss.

    d. Antipsychotics do not improve memory loss and may further impair cognitive functioning.

14. A 9-year-old child receives antipsychotics to manage her disease. The child's mother asks why her daughter receives such a high dose of the medication compared with an adult. How will the nurse explain this to the mother?

    a. "Children usually have a slower metabolic rate than adults and may therefore require relatively high doses for their size and weight."

    b. "Children usually have a faster metabolic rate than adults and may therefore require relatively low doses for their size and weight."

    c. "Children usually have a faster metabolic rate than adults and may therefore require relatively high doses for their height and weight."

    d. "Children usually have a faster metabolic rate than adults and may therefore require relatively high doses for their size and weight."

15. A male patient is scheduled for major abdominal surgery in the morning. He is concerned that he is receiving a lower-than-normal dose of his antipsychotic. What is the best response to this patient?

    a. "Antipsychotics potentiate the effects of general anesthetics."

    b. "Antipsychotics diminish the effects of general anesthetics."

    c. "Antipsychotics cause increased tardive dyskinesia when used with anesthetics."

    d. "Antipsychotics cause a hypertensive crisis when combined with anesthetics."

16. The nurse is caring for a patient who has been displaying signs of acute dystonia. The nurse assesses the patient for what characteristics of the disease? (Select all that apply.)

a. Severe spasms of muscles of the face, neck, tongue, or back

b. Oculogyric crisis

c. Opisthotonus

d. Anuria

e. Hypoxia

17. The nurse is caring for a patient with acute dystonia, and the nurse anticipates treating the patient with an intramuscular or intravenous administration of what medication?

a. Cardiotonics

b. Diphenhydramine

c. Cholinergic medications

d. Narcan

18. The nurse is caring for a patient with schizophrenia who has begun to take olanzapine (Zyprexa). The nurse knows that the medication has reached a steady state of concentration in what period of time?

a. 2 days

b. 1 week

c. 1 month

d. 3 months

19. The nurse is caring for a patient who takes clozapine. The nurse would be most concerned if this patient displays what symptom?

a. Temperature of 102°F

b. Blood sugar of 108

c. Weight gain of 1 lb in the last week

d. Blood pressure of 98/64

20. A male patient takes quetiapine for his bipolar disease. His physician orders cimetidine for his GI distress. When used in conjunction with quetiapine, the cimetidine dose will be adjusted in what way?

a. Increased

b. Decreased

c. Remain the same

d. Titrated based on the patient's WBC count

Drug Therapy to Stimulate the Central Nervous System

- Understand the etiology, pathophysiology, and clinical manifestations of attention deficit hyperactivity disorder.
- Understand the etiology, pathophysiology, and clinical manifestations of narcolepsy.
- Describe general characteristics of central nervous system stimulants.
- Identify the prototypes and discuss the action, use, adverse effects, contraindications, and nursing implications for the stimulants used in the treatment of attention deficit hyperactivity disorder and narcolepsy.
- Identify sources and effects of caffeine.
- Implement the nursing process in the care of patients who take central nervous stimulants.

SECTION I: ASSESSING YOUR UNDERSTANDING

Activity A FILL IN THE BLANKS

1. _____ is characterized by persistent hyperactivity, a short attention span, difficulty completing assigned tasks or schoolwork, restlessness, and impulsiveness.

2. _____ is a sleep disorder characterized by daytime "sleep attacks" in which the person goes to sleep at any place or at any time.

3. Two disorders treated with CNS stimulants are _____ and _____.

4. _____ is the most common psychiatric or neurobehavioral disorder in children

5. Studies indicate that children with ADHD are more likely to have _____ _____ , mood disorders, and substance abuse disorders as adolescents and adults.

Activity B MATCHING

Match the terms in Column A with the definition in Column B.

Column A	Column B
____ 1. Amphetamines and methylphenidate	a. Stimulate the cerebral cortex, increasing mental alertness and decreasing drowsiness and fatigue
____ 2. Xanthines	b. Used in the treatment of narcolepsy and ADHD
____ 3. Caffeine	c. Closely related drugs that share characteristics of the amphetamines as a group

_____ **4.** Atomoxetine (Strattera)

_____ **5.** Amphetamine, dextroamphetamine (Dexedrine), and methamphetamine (Desoxyn)

d. Frequently consumed CNS stimulant worldwide, mostly obtained from dietary sources (e.g., coffee, tea, soft drinks) and is the prototype xanthine.

e. Second-line drug for the treatment of ADHD in children and adults, with a low risk of abuse and dependence compared with the other drugs used for ADHD

Activity C SHORT ANSWERS

Briefly answer the following questions.

1. Discuss the psychosocial characteristics of ADHD.

2. Describe the signs and symptoms of narcolepsy.

3. In addition to drug treatments, what might be done to treat narcolepsy?

4. Describe the characteristics of CNS stimulants.

5. How do amphetamines affect brain function?

SECTION II: APPLYING YOUR KNOWLEDGE

Activity D CASE STUDIES

Consider the scenarios and answer the questions.

Case Study 1

Mrs. Stratos, age 35, works in a high-stress job that requires long hours and high levels of concentration. She presents to the physician's office with complaints of palpitations and chronic insomnia. Upon assessment, you note that she is alert and oriented to person, place, and time. Both her blood pressure and pulse are elevated compared with her last office visit. She paces back and forth during the assessment and states that she is unable to sit still. You also note that she has pallor and dark circles under her eyes. She states that she drinks two cups of coffee in the morning and one before she leaves work in order to remain awake while driving home at night.

1. What is the appropriate nursing diagnosis for Mrs. Stratos?

2. What should you explore as part of the patient history?

3. During the history taking, you discover that Mrs. Stratos drinks four energy drinks per day, which results in excessive caffeine intake. What is your plan for this patient?

Case Study 2

Jane, age 7, is placed on medication for ADHD. You are responsible for the education plan for the parents.

1. Jane's mother says to you, "The dose of the medication may be increased by half a tablet in the morning if Jane has difficulty concentrating." How would you respond to the mother?

2. What signs and symptoms should you instruct Jane's mother to report to the physician?

3. In a child taking stimulants, what should you monitor for?

SECTION III: PRACTICING FOR NCLEX

Activity E

Answer the following questions.

1. A college student presents to the emergency department with palpitations and signs and symptoms of CNS stimulation. He states that he has been awake for 72 hours studying and keeps awake using power drinks and caffeine. What statement indicates that his education plan has been effective?

   a. "Caffeine can cause life-threatening health problems with excessive intake."

   b. "Energy drinks do not contain caffeine; if they are not combined with excessive caffeine intake they will not cause adverse side effects."

   c. "Caffeine did not cause my symptoms. I have the flu."

   d. "Caffeine is not an ingredient of energy drinks."

2. The nurse has admitted a patient with a probable diagnosis of narcolepsy. The nurse assesses the patient for what symptoms that are characteristic of this disorder? (Select all that apply.)

   a. Difficult to rouse in the morning

   b. Unpredictable sleep during daytime hours

   c. Transient insomnia

   d. Daytime drowsiness

   e. Cataplexy

3. The nurse is aware that CNS stimulants are prescribed for patients with ADHD because these medications have what effect on behavior and attention?

   a. Restoring

   b. Deteriorating

   c. Improving

   d. Contravening

4. The community health nurse is conducting a class for parents of preschoolers. One of the parents asks if a child with ADHD will always have problems with hyperactivity. What is the nurse's best response?

   a. "ADHD usually starts in childhood and resolves by adolescence."

   b. "ADHD usually starts in childhood and resolves by adulthood."

   c. "ADHD usually starts in childhood and resolves before adolescence."

   d. "ADHD usually starts in childhood and may persist through adulthood."

5. The school nurse is conducting a screening of kindergarten students. The nurse will assess the children for what characteristics of ADHD? (Select all that apply.)

   a. Hyperactivity

   b. Improved retention

   c. Impulsivity

   d. Short attention span

   e. Playing well with others

6. A 75-year-old male patient is given an order for a CNS stimulant secondary to a new diagnosis of narcolepsy. He begins to experience signs and symptoms of excessive CNS stimulation. The nurse knows that the patient is likely to also experience an exacerbation of which preexisting condition?

   a. Diabetes

   b. Cardiac dysrhythmias

   c. Gout

   d. Hyperparathyroidism

7. The nurse is aware that medication dosage for a child with ADHD is stopped occasionally for what reason?

   a. Onset of puberty

   b. Evaluation of treatment regimen

   c. Brain growth

   d. Musculoskeletal growth

8. The nurse understands that methylphenidate is commonly prescribed and usually given daily for the first 3 to 4 weeks for what purpose?

   a. To determine parent and child compliance with the medication regimen

   b. To determine medication blood levels in order to modify the dose

   c. To assess the education plan and modify the plan to meet the patient's needs

   d. To assess beneficial and adverse effects

9. The nurse is aware that drug therapy is prescribed for children with ADHD under which circumstances? (Select all that apply.)

   a. Symptoms are mild to moderate.

   b. Symptoms are moderate to severe.

   c. Symptoms are identified by the parents and teacher.

   d. Symptoms are present for several months.

   e. Symptoms interfere in social, academic, or behavioral functioning.

10. A male patient arrives at the emergency department with signs and symptoms of CNS stimulant toxicity. The nurse anticipates participating in which treatments for this patient? (Select all that apply.)

    a. Monitoring for musculoskeletal changes

    b. Monitoring cardiac function

    c. Increasing sensory stimulation

    d. Minimizing external stimulation

    e. Providing a caffeinated cola drink

11. A patient asks the nurse how quickly a cup of coffee will cause the greatest stimulation to the central nervous system. What is the nurse's best response?

    a. "30 to 45 minutes"

    b. "45 to 60 minutes"

    c. "10 to 15 minutes"

    d. "15 to 20 minutes"

12. The nurse is aware that caffeine may be contraindicated because of what effect?

    a. Decreases analgesia

    b. Decreases anxiety

    c. Reduces dysrhythmias

    d. Increases analgesia

13. A patient tells the nurse that he would like to decrease his caffeine intake and he wants to know what product or beverage has the most caffeine. What is the nurse's best response?

    a. "Brewed coffee"

    b. "Instant coffee"

    c. "Energy drink"

    d. "Brewed tea"

14. A male patient is diagnosed with narcolepsy by his physician. He asks the physician to prescribe modafinil, because it works so well for his friend. The physician will not prescribe the medication because of what aspect of the patient's history?

    a. Gout and a history of tophi

    b. Ischemic changes on his electrocardiograms

    c. Pancreatitis

    d. Cirrhosis of the liver

15. A male patient asks whether a guarana product will keep him awake longer than caffeine. As part of the nurse's education plan, which statement is the most accurate?

    a. "The caffeine content of a guarana product is unknown."

    b. "Guarana is caffeine free."

    c. "The caffeine content of guarana is essentially the same as coffee."

    d. "The amount of caffeine in guarana is higher than in coffee."

16. The nurse understands that the main goal of therapy with CNS stimulants is to relieve symptoms of the disorders for which they are given. What is a secondary goal for their use?

    a. To prevent adverse reactions

    b. To serve as a study aid

    c. To have patients use the drugs appropriately

    d. To prevent side effects

17. The nurse is aware that drinking caffeinated coffee is contraindicated for which individuals? (Select all that apply.)

    a. Long-haul truckers

    b. Patients with depression

    c. Patients diagnosed with cardiac dysrhythmias

    d. Patients diagnosed with gout

    e. Patients with peptic ulcer disease

18. A patient calls the clinic complaining that she is only able to get a 1-month supply of pills for her son who takes a CNS stimulant for ADHD. The nurse understands that these medications are given in limited numbers for what reason?

    a. The cost is prohibitive when prescribed in a large number.

    b. It reduces the likelihood of drug dependence or diversion.

    c. Changes in dosages are common.

    d. HMOs will not reimburse the cost for larger numbers.

19. A parent would like her child to be placed on a medication for symptoms of ADHD. The nurse knows that CNS stimulants are not recommended for ADHD in children younger than what age?

a. 6 years

b. 5 years

c. 4 years

d. 3 years

20. A college student returns home after final examinations during which he drank approximately 6 to 10 cups of coffee a day for the last week. He is concerned about what will happen if he quits drinking coffee. The nurse counsels this patient that he may develop withdrawal symptoms after how many hours without coffee?

a. 4 to 6 hours

b. 8 to 10 hours

c. 12 to 15 hours

d. 18 to 24 hours

CHAPTER 57

Drug Therapy for Substance Abuse Disorders

Learning Objectives

- Describe the etiology, pathophysiology, and clinical manifestations of substance abuse.
- Identify the central nervous system (CNS) depressants of abuse.
- Identify the prototypes and describe the action, use, adverse effects, contraindications, and nursing implications for the treatment of alcohol withdrawal and for the maintenance of sobriety.
- Identify commonly abused CNS stimulants.
- Identify commonly abused psychoactive medications.
- Implement the nursing process for patients who may be abusing CNS depressants, CNS stimulants, or other psychoactive substances.

SECTION I: ASSESSING YOUR UNDERSTANDING

Activity A FILL IN THE BLANKS

1. _____ is a significant health, social, economic, and legal problem. It is often associated with substantial damage to the abuser and society.

2. Most drugs of abuse are those that affect the _____ and alter the state of consciousness.

3. Most drugs of abuse are also associated with _____ if used repeatedly.

4. Many drugs of abuse activate the _____ system in the brain by altering neurotransmission systems.

5. Characteristics of drug _____ include craving a drug, often with unsuccessful attempts to decrease its use, and compulsive drug-seeking behavior.

Activity B MATCHING

Match the term in Column A with the definition in Column B.

Column A	Column B
____ 1. Methadone	a. Provides adequate sedation and has a significant anticonvulsant effect for the patient withdrawing from alcohol
____ 2. Disulfiram (Antabuse)	b. Blocks euphoria produced by heroin, acts longer, and reduces preoccupation with drug use

___ **3.** Chlordiazepox-
ide (Librium)

___ **4.** Naltrexone

___ **5.** Flumazenil

c. Opiate antagonist
that reduces crav-
ing for alcohol and
increases abstinence
rates

d. Given to people
with chronic alco-
holism to maintain
a state of sobriety

e. Specific antidote
that can reverse
benzodiazepine-
induced sedation,
coma, and respira-
tory depression

1. What symptoms might the wife and the
patient describe that would lead the physician
to suspect physical dependence?

2. Mr. Rather's wife also states that when her
husband discusses his friend's death, he takes
more medication. Why would the interdis-
ciplinary team also suspect psychological
dependence?

3. Mr. Rather's wife states that she suspects that
her husband bought the drugs that he is using
on the streets. She states also that he seems to
take more and more as time passes to relieve
the pain. How would you describe tolerance to
Mr. Rather and his wife?

Activity C   **SHORT ANSWERS**

Briefly answer the following questions.

1. Define substance abuse.

2. List commonly abused drugs.

3. What physical or emotional effects are sought
by those who use drugs of abuse?

4. Discuss methods used to obtain drugs of abuse
by the general population.

5. What are the characteristics of drug
dependence?

SECTION II: APPLYING YOUR KNOWLEDGE

Activity D   **CASE STUDY**

Consider the scenario and answer the questions.

Mr. Rather was involved in a motor vehicle
accident 6 months ago in which a friend died.
He received opioid analgesics for his skeletal pain
during his recovery period. He comes to the physician's office today for another prescription for
his pain but refuses any analgesics but opioids.
Based on the care plan for his surgery, he should
not require pain medication, his injuries are
healed, and rehabilitation is complete. His wife
states that he is taking pain medications routinely. The physician suspects drug dependence.

SECTION III: PRACTICING FOR NCLEX

Activity E

Answer the following questions.

1. As an adjunct to a patient's alcohol withdrawal management program, the physician
orders disulfiram. The nurse is responsible for
the patient's education program. When the
patient arrives home after discharge, he pours
himself a beer. What symptoms would he
expect to experience? (Select all that apply.)

a. Flushing, tachycardia, and garlic aftertaste

b. Hypotension, anemia, and confusion

c. Sweating, nausea, and vomiting

d. Paranoia, mania, and depression

e. Blurred vision, headache, and chest pain

2. A male patient returns home after a coronary
artery bypass graft and celebrates his survival
by overindulging in alcohol. He does not
have a history of alcohol abuse. His drug regimen includes warfarin. What adverse reaction
related to the combination of the drugs would
the nurse expect this patient to experience?

a. Decreased anticoagulant effects and
increased risk of clot formation

b. No significant drug reaction related to only
one incident

c. Increased anticoagulant effects and
decreased risk of bleeding

d. Increased anticoagulant effects and risk of
bleeding

3. A female patient has a history of chronic alcohol usage and subsequent liver damage. She develops a deep vein thrombosis and is sent home from the hospital on warfarin. What adverse reactions related to the combination of the drugs would the nurse expect?

   a. Decreased anticoagulant effects and increased risk of clot formation

   b. No significant drug reaction related to only one incident

   c. Increased anticoagulant effects and decreased risk of bleeding

   d. Increased anticoagulant effects and risk of bleeding

4. The nurse is caring for a patient with type 2 diabetes mellitus who takes an oral antidiabetic drug. The nurse cautions the patient against consuming alcohol because of which effect?

   a. It diminishes hypoglycemic effects.

   b. It exacerbates hyperglycemic effects.

   c. It potentiates hypoglycemic effects.

   d. It causes polyuria, polydipsia, and subsequent dehydration.

5. A patient is newly diagnosed with hypertension and has just begun to take an antihypertensive agent. The nurse instructs this patient that drinking alcohol may cause what effect?

   a. It diminishes vasodilation and hypotensive effects.

   b. It potentiates vasodilation and hypotensive effects.

   c. It potentiates vasoconstriction and hypotensive effects.

   d. It causes euphoria, mania, and confusion.

6. A female patient's physician prescribes antianxiety medication. The nurse is responsible for her education plan. The patient asks if she can take the antianxiety medication when she drinks socially with her friends. What is the nurse's best response to this patient?

   a. "If you limit alcohol consumption to two drinks, you should be safe."

   b. "Combining alcohol with antianxiety medication may be lethal and should be avoided."

   c. "The drug and alcohol may be coadministered safely."

   d. "The antianxiety medication will increase your blood alcohol level rapidly; you should use a designated driver."

7. The nurse is caring for a male patient who had abdominal surgery 1 day ago. The patient is reluctant to get up and ambulate because of the pain. The nurse encourages the patient to take the prescribed medication (morphine sulfate) and then ambulate with assistance. The patient refuses because he is afraid of becoming addicted to the medication. What is the nurse's best response to this patient?

   a. "I will only give you half of the dose, so it will decrease your chance of addiction."

   b. "Why are you worried about this? Have you had an addiction problem in the past?"

   c. "Most people who receive pain medications because of a medical reason don't become addicted to the medication."

   d. "I will ask the doctor if I can give you acetaminophen for the pain."

8. When questioned about her alcohol usage, a female patient states that she drinks three martinis a night. What assessment should the nurse make of this statement?

   a. This is the correct amount consumed.

   b. She normally consumes four to six martinis a night.

   c. She is giving information she expects the nurse expects to hear.

   d. She may have understated the amount of alcohol consumed.

9. The nurse works at a hospital-based methadone clinic. When interviewing heroin users, what is the most accurate assessment that the nurse can make concerning the patient's heroin use?

   a. Heroin addicts may overstate the amount used in attempts to obtain higher doses of methadone.

   b. Heroin addicts may understate the amount used due to the adverse effects of the methadone.

   c. Heroin addicts will understate the amount used so that they will experience increased euphoria from an increased dosage of methadone.

   d. Heroin addicts will identify the correct amount of drug abused to maintain the sense of euphoria similar to their current drug.

10. The nurse who is working in the emergency department admits a 14-year-old male who is exhibiting blurred vision, confusion, impaired breathing, muscle twitches, irregular heartbeat, and excessive sweating. His friends who came with him said that he bought a lot of cough syrup and has been drinking it all day. The nurse understands that the patient has overdosed on what over-the-counter medication?

    a. Acetaminophen

    b. Ibuprofen

    c. Dextromethorphan

    d. Guaifenesin

11. Health care professionals are considered to be at high risk for development of substance abuse disorders, at least partly because of what factor?

    a. Easy access

    b. Low cost

    c. Lax regulations related to use

    d. None of the above; health care professionals are considered low risk.

12. The nurse is caring for a patient for whom a psychological therapy has been ordered to assist with recovery from an addictive disorder. The nurse understands that what statement is true about psychological rehabilitation efforts?

    a. They do not make an impact on addiction treatment because it is a physical dependence.

    b. They should be part of any treatment program for a drug-dependent person.

    c. They are rarely covered by health insurance.

    d. They are successful when used in facility-based rehabilitation programs.

13. A female patient presents to the physician's office with her 12-year-old son. She found him in the garage this morning sniffing gasoline to get high. The nurse is assigned the education plan for the family. What would the nurse include as areas of the body where damage might occur?

    a. Heart and lungs

    b. Pancreas and gallbladder

    c. Vascular system

    d. Liver, kidneys, and bone marrow

14. A female patient presents to the emergency department confused and disheveled and states that she was raped. She attended a party earlier in the evening. What substance, often called a date rape drug, might have been added to her drink?

    a. THC

    b. Cocaine

    c. Ketamine

    d. GHB

15. A 19-year-old male patient arrives at the emergency department with his friend. His friend states that they were smoking marijuana and the patient suddenly began having hallucinations, began exhibiting bizarre behavior, and then became unconscious. The nurse finds that the patient is hypertensive and suspects that the marijuana was laced with what substance?

    a. Ketamine

    b. GHB

    c. THC

    d. PCP

16. A 54-year-old male patient recently experienced a myocardial infarction. His medical history indicates that he has been smoking two packs of cigarettes per day since the age of 16. He asks the physician for the nicotine patch. What would the nurse expect the physician to do?

    a. Order the patch

    b. Suggest other methods of nicotine withdrawal

    c. Order a reduced dosage of the patch

    d. State that nicotine cessation at this time may cause further cardiac damage

17. A female patient began using cocaine for the energy rush and uses on a daily basis. She presents to her physician with symptoms of agitation and psychosis and is admitted to the intensive care unit. What medications does the nurse anticipate administering to this patient? (Select all that apply.)

    a. Haloperidol

    b. Diazepam

    c. Propranolol

    d. Caffeine

    e. Nicotine

18. The nurse is caring for a patient who reports having a heroin addiction. The nurse is aware that what is an accurate statement about heroin addicts?

   a. They inject upon waking and cycle throughout the day until sleep.

   b. They inject approximately every 4 to 6 hours to maintain the high.

   c. They inject several times daily, cycling between desired effects and symptoms of withdrawal.

   d. They experience withdrawal symptoms based on the route of administration.

19. The physician orders hospitalization for the patient who withdraws from benzodiazepines. What is the rationale behind this order?

   a. Withdrawal can cause cardiac arrhythmias and subsequent cardiac arrest.

   b. Withdrawal can precipitate renal failure.

   c. Convulsions are more likely to occur during the first 48 hours of withdrawal and delirium after 48 to 72 hours.

   d. Liver failure is a risk for such patients.

20. The nurse working in the emergency department admits a patient who arrived by ambulance and has respirations of 8 to 12 breaths per minute. The EMTs report finding an empty pill container of diazepam next to the patient. The nurse anticipates administering what drug to this patient?

   a. Naloxone

   b. Haloperidol

   c. Chlordiazepoxide

   d. Flumazenil

58 CHAPTER

Drug Therapy for Disorders of the Eye

Learning Objectives

- Describe the basic structures and functions of the eye.
- Understand the pathophysiology of glaucoma as well as ocular infections and inflammation.
- Identify the prototypes and describe the action, use, adverse effects, contraindications, and nursing implications for medications administered for diagnosis and treatment of ocular disorders.
- Identify the prototypes and describe the action, use, adverse effects, contraindications, and nursing implications for medications administered for glaucoma.
- Identify the prototypes and describe the action, use, adverse effects, contraindications, and nursing implications for medications administered for ocular infections and inflammation.
- Understand how to implement the nursing process in the care of the patient with an ocular disorder.

SECTION I: ASSESSING YOUR UNDERSTANDING

Activity A FILL IN THE BLANKS

1. Refractive errors that cause nearsightedness are called _____.

2. Refractive errors that cause farsightedness are called _____.

3. Refractive errors include myopia, hyperopia, _____, and astigmatism.

4. Conditions that cause refractive errors impair vision by interfering with the eye's ability to focus light rays on the _____.

5. Ophthalmic drugs are used only in the _____ of the refractive error conditions; treatment involves prescription of eyeglasses or contact lenses.

Activity B MATCHING

Match the term in Column A with the definition in Column B.

Column A	Column B
____ 1. Conjunctivitis	a. Common eye disorder that may be caused by allergens, bacterial or viral infections, or physical or chemical irritants
____ 2. Blepharitis	
____ 3. Keratitis (inflammation of the cornea)	
	b. Commonly occur and may often be attributed to frequent use of ophthalmic antibiotics and corticosteroids
	c. Chronic infection of glands and lash follicles on the margins of the eyelids, characterized by burning, redness, and itching

_____ **4.** Fungal infections

_____ **5.** Bacterial corneal ulcers

d. Most often caused by pneumococci and staphylococci

e. May be caused by microorganisms, trauma, allergy, ischemia, and drying of the cornea

Activity C SHORT ANSWERS

Briefly answer the following questions.

1. Explain how the eyelids and lacrimal system function to protect the eye.

2. Explain the difference between miosis and mydriasis.

3. Outline the structure of the eyeball.

4. Discuss the process that causes vision to occur.

5. Define refraction.

SECTION II: APPLYING YOUR KNOWLEDGE

Activity D CASE STUDY

Consider the scenario and answer the questions.

Mrs. Lincoln, a 75-year-old African American woman, is diagnosed with primary open-angle glaucoma. She also has hypertension. You are responsible for her education plan.

1. Mrs. Lincoln asks you how glaucoma is diagnosed and how the physician is sure that she has this illness. What is your understanding of a diagnosis of glaucoma? What is the range of intraocular pressure that is characteristic of glaucoma?

2. What are Mrs. Lincoln's risk factors for glaucoma? For which condition is Mrs. Lincoln further at risk because of her glaucoma?

3. As part of your patient teaching, what can you tell Mrs. Lincoln about glaucoma? What type of disease is it? What characterizes the disease?

4. If Mrs. Lincoln were to present to the physician's office with nausea, blurred vision with halo, and, when assessed, increased intraocular pressure and report that she had taken a tricyclic antidepressant, what diagnosis is likely?

SECTION III: PRACTICING FOR NCLEX

Activity E

Answer the following questions.

1. A female patient is diagnosed with cardiac disease. She is also prescribed local eye medications. The nurse cautions Mrs. Young that local eye medications may cause what effect?
 a. Increased visual acuity
 b. Systemic effects
 c. Local effects
 d. Exacerbation of her glaucoma

2. The nurse is giving discharge instructions to a patient who will be using eye medications and counsels the patient to keep the eye medications under what condition?
 a. Refrigerated
 b. Sterile
 c. Clean
 d. In a warm environment

3. A female patient complains that she must administer her eye drops several times because she blinks. How might this influence the therapeutic effects of the drops?
 a. Therapeutic effects depend on administration of the medication on a routine basis.
 b. Therapeutic effects may vary due to blinking.
 c. Therapeutic effects may vary due to the medication schedule.
 d. Therapeutic effects depend on accurate administration.

4. The nurse is caring for a patient with eye disease and is aware that drug therapy of eye disorders is unique because of what factors? (Select all that apply.)
 a. Location of the eye
 b. Structure of the eye
 c. Function of the eye
 d. Proximity of the eye to the brain
 e. Blood–eye barrier

5. What tasks does the role of the home care nurse caring for patients with acute or chronic eye disorders include? (Select all that apply.)

   a. Teaching patients and caregivers reasons for use of drugs

   b. Teaching accurate administration technique of drugs

   c. Assessing therapeutic and adverse drug reactions

   d. Diagnosing eye disorders

   e. Administering all medications

6. A female patient has both heart and eye disease. The nurse will administer the eye medications in what way to prevent exacerbation of her cardiac symptoms?

   a. Schedule eye drugs to coincide with cardiac drugs

   b. Schedule eye drugs 2 hours before cardiac drugs

   c. Occlude the nasolacrimal duct in the inner canthus of the eye

   d. Schedule eye drugs 1 hour before cardiac drugs

7. The nurse is preparing to administer acetazolamide and knows that it may be prescribed to be administered in what ways? (Select all that apply.)

   a. Orally

   b. Subcutaneously

   c. Transdermally

   d. Intravenously

   e. Intranasally

8. The nurse understands that the pediatrician will order which drug when prescribing for children?

   a. Long-acting mydriatics

   b. Cyclopentolate

   c. Gentamicin

   d. Fluoroquinolone

9. When caring for a patient with chronic glaucoma, the nurse sets the goal of drug therapy to slow disease progression by reducing IOP. What are the first-line drugs used to treat glaucoma?

   a. Topical ACE inhibitors

   b. Topical beta-blockers

   c. Antibacterials

   d. Mydriatics

10. A female patient who wears contact lens presents to the physician with a corneal abrasion. The nurse would expect the physician to order which medication for this patient?

    a. Topical ACE inhibitor

    b. Topical beta-blocker

    c. Antipseudomonal antibiotic

    d. Antistaphylococcal antibiotic

11. The nurse is aware that brimonidine is used to produce what physiologic effect in patients with ocular hypertension?

    a. Reduce aqueous humor production

    b. Decrease uveoscleral outflow

    c. Increase IOP

    d. Decrease blood pressure

12. A male patient presents to the physician's office with symptoms of an eye infection. He is diagnosed with a fungal infection. The nurse expects the physician to order which medication for this patient?

    a. Amoxicillin

    b. Natamycin

    c. Penicillin

    d. Nystatin

13. A male patient gets dust in his eyes when he is cleaning his furnace. He flushes his eyes in the sink and 3 days later presents to the physician's office with symptoms of a severe infectious process. The physician orders both a topical and a systemic antibiotic. The nurse knows that what systemic antibiotic is appropriate?

    a. Natamycin

    b. Ampicillin

    c. Erythromycin

    d. Vancomycin

14. The nurse is preparing to administer timolol maleate to a patient who has just been diagnosed with chronic open-angle glaucoma. The nurse will contact the physician before administering the medication if the patient reports a history of which conditions? (Select all that apply.)

    a. Asthma

    b. Tachycardia

    c. Hypovolemic shock

    d. Heart failure

    e. Left ventricular dysfunction

15. A male patient presents to the physician's office with drainage and inflammation in his right eye. What would the nurse expect the physician to do?

    a. Order a topical antibiotic

    b. Refer the patient to an optometrist

    c. Order a systemic antibiotic

    d. Order a culture and sensitivity of the drainage

16. A female patient wears soft contact lenses. She uses eye drops containing benzalkonium. The nurse teaches the patient that the medication should be instilled under what condition?

    a. 15 minutes or longer before inserting soft contacts

    b. While wearing the soft contacts

    c. 15 minutes after application of the soft contacts

    d. 5 minutes before inserting soft contacts

17. The nurse knows that phenylephrine eye drops are contraindicated in patients with what conditions? (Select all that apply.)

    a. Hypotension

    b. Bradycardia

    c. Ventricular tachycardia

    d. Narrow-angle glaucoma

    e. Anaphylactic reaction to penicillin

18. A male patient is prescribed a topical ophthalmic medication. The nurse teaches the patient that the medication should be discarded at what point? (Select all that apply.)

    a. After the expiration date

    b. If it becomes cloudy

    c. If the color changes

    d. If his condition improves

    e. If stinging occurs during administration

19. The physician prescribes medication for a patient's eye disorder. The physician's concern is that the patient requires high concentrations of the drug. The nurse knows that the physician will order the medication in what type of formulation?

    a. Ointment

    b. Drop

    c. Distilled formulation

    d. Suspension

20. The nurse is preparing a patient for an eye examination and administers atropine sulfate (ophthalmic). The nurse instructs the patient that this medication has what effects on the eye? (Select all that apply.)

    a. Produces mydriasis

    b. Produces miosis

    c. Produces pupillary constriction

    d. Produces pupillary dilation

    e. Produces accommodation of near vision

59

Drug Therapy for Disorders of the Ear

Learning Objectives

- Understand the etiology, pathophysiology, and clinical manifestations of both acute otitis externa and necrotizing otitis externa.
- Identify the prototype and describe the action, use, adverse effects, contraindications, and nursing implications for topical medications used to treat otitis externa.
- Identify the prototype and describe the action, use, adverse effects, contraindications, and nursing implications for systemic medications used to treat necrotizing otitis externa.
- Identify the prototype and describe the action, use, adverse effects, contraindications, and nursing implications for systemic medications used to treat otitis media.
- Identify the adjuvant drugs used to treat otitis externa and otitis media.
- Implement the nursing process in the care of the patient with otitis externa or otitis media.

SECTION I: ASSESSING YOUR UNDERSTANDING

Activity A FILL IN THE BLANKS

1. _____ is a disorder of the external ear that produces inflammation, commonly known as swimmer's ear.

2. _____ is an acute infection of the middle ear.

3. Middle ear infections are a result of an alteration in the _____ tube.

4. Symptoms of necrotizing otitis externa are _____, or ear pain, and _____, or purulent drainage.

5. Pharmacological therapy for disorders of the ear is _____ preparations.

Activity B MATCHING

Match the term in Column A with the definition in Column B.

Column A

____ 1. Cortisporin Otic

____ 2. Amoxicillin

____ 3. Coly-Mycin

____ 4. Ofloxacin

____ 5. Ciprofloxacin

Column B

a. A topical otic preparation that is a combination of neomycin, colistin, hydrocortisone, and thonzonium

b. A combination of neomycin–polymyxin and hydrocortisone in a topical preparation used to treat otitis externa

c. Drug of choice for necrotizing otitis externa

d. A topical preparation that is used to treat patients with otitis externa and otitis media and may be used if the patient has a perforated tympanic membrane

e. Drug of choice for the treatment of acute otitis media

Activity C   SHORT ANSWERS

Briefly answer the following questions.

1. Discuss the pathophysiology of otitis externa.

2. Discuss the difference between acute otitis externa and necrotizing otitis externa.

3. What are the symptoms of acute otitis media, and what may cause it to occur?

4. Discuss the use of combination drug therapy in the treatment of otitis externa.

5. Describe how to properly administer ear drops to a patient.

SECTION II: APPLYING YOUR KNOWLEDGE

Activity D   CASE STUDY

Consider the scenario and answer the questions.

Mrs. Parker calls the clinic about her 6-year-old son who woke up this morning complaining of ear pain. The mother states that his ear hurts the most when she touches his ear. She reports that he has been swimming every day for the last week. The physician diagnoses the child with otitis externa.

1. What drug therapy do you expect the physician to order for this child? What teaching will you provide to the mother concerning administration of the medication?

2. Mrs. Parker wants to avoid this infection from recurring in her son. What instructions will you provide to the mother?

3. Mrs. Parker is concerned that this infection will cause her son to lose his hearing. What information will you give the mother to help her understand the difference between otitis externa and otitis media?

SECTION III: PRACTICING FOR NCLEX

Activity E

Answer the following questions.

1. The nurse is caring for a child who has just been diagnosed with otitis media and will be treated with amoxicillin. It is most important for the nurse to instruct the mother to administer this medication on what schedule?
   a. With meals
   b. On an empty stomach
   c. Around the clock
   d. An hour after meals

2. A male patient has been diagnosed with otitis externa. He also has a history of a perforated ear drum. What topical otic preparation does the nurse anticipate the physician ordering for this patient?
   a. Cortisporin Otic
   b. Coly-Mycin S otic
   c. Ofloxacin otic
   d. Cipro HC otic

3. The nurse is caring for a child with otitis externa who also has chickenpox. The nurse knows that which otic medication is contra-indicated for this patient?
   a. Coly-Mycin
   b. Cortisporin
   c. Cipro HC
   d. Ofloxacin

4. The patient with necrotizing otitis externa has been prescribed ciprofloxacin. The nurse instructs the patient to avoid what foods within 2 hours of taking the medication?
   a. Green leafy vegetables
   b. Dairy products
   c. Citrus fruits
   d. Bacon and sausage

5. The nurse is administering ciprofloxacin intravenously to a 60-year-old patient with necrotizing otitis externa who is recently widowed and has type 2 diabetes that is controlled by diet. What factor related to this patient would be of most concern to the nurse?

a. Patient's age

b. Patient's type 2 diabetes

c. Patient's recent loss of wife

d. Patient's diagnosis of necrotizing otitis externa

6. The nurse is admitting a patient with necrotizing otitis externa. The nurse expects the patient to exhibit which symptoms? (Select all that apply.)

a. Shoulder pain

b. Otalgia

c. Pain while chewing

d. Otorrhea

e. Nasal congestion

7. The nurse is giving discharge instructions to a woman who will be taking amoxicillin for treatment of acute otitis media. The nurse teaches the patient that which symptom indicates the development of a superinfection and should be reported to the physician?

a. Nausea

b. Abdominal pain

c. Vaginal itching and discharge

d. Swelling and itching of the throat

8. The nurse is caring for a patient with acute otitis media who is allergic to penicillin. The nurse anticipates that the physician will order which medication?

a. Amoxicillin

b. Cortisporin otic

c. Cefdinir

d. Tetracycline

9. The nurse is evaluating the effectiveness of antibiotic therapy for a patient who has been treated for acute otitis media. What assessments will indicate a resolution of the infection? (Select all that apply.)

a. Presence of otalgia and otorrhea

b. Improved hearing

c. Cherry red and dull tympanic membrane

d. No bulging of the tympanic membrane

e. Normal body temperature

10. The nurse is giving home care instructions to the parent of a 2-year-old child who has been experiencing an increased body temperature and has been diagnosed with otitis media. What instructions will the nurse give the mother concerning antipyretic therapy?

a. Administer aspirin every 4 hours.

b. Alternate acetaminophen and ibuprofen every 4 hours.

c. Administer acetaminophen every 4 hours.

d. Administer ibuprofen every 6 hours.

11. The nurse is performing an assessment of a patient with a suspected ear infection. What would the nurse observe if the patient had otitis media?

a. Pain when the otoscope touches the external ear canal

b. Absence of the cone of light on the ear drum

c. Absence of otalgia

d. Swelling and redness of the external ear canal

12. The nurse is caring for a patient with necrotizing otitis externa. What is the most appropriate nursing diagnosis for this patient?

a. Pain related to inflammation of the middle ear

b. Impaired hearing related to fluid in the middle ear

c. Impaired skin integrity related to auricle lesion

d. Infection related to trauma

13. The nurse is instructing a patient who developed otitis externa. The nurse understands that what is the most important action the patient can take to prevent this infection from recurring?

a. Never allow any water on the head

b. Clean the ear vigorously with a cotton swab every day

c. Take acetaminophen daily

d. Use earplugs when swimming

14. The nurse is conducting a class for new parents and gives what instruction to help prevent the development of otitis media?

   a. "Never let the baby sleep drinking a bottle."

   b. "If the baby takes a bottle to bed, only put water in it."

   c. "Place the baby on his side if he takes a bottle to bed."

   d. "Lie the baby down at least halfway through a feeding to prevent the formula from leaking out of his mouth."

15. The nurse is aware that what is the most common bacterium found in patients with otitis externa?

   a. *Staphylococcus pneumoniae*

   b. *Haemophilus influenzae*

   c. *Streptococcus pyogenes*

   d. *Pseudomonas aeruginosa*

16. The health department nurse is preparing to assist the city in developing policies for reducing otitis externa in the city's public swimming pool. The nurse insists that the city enforce which standard?

   a. Only toilet-trained children are allowed in the swimming pool.

   b. Swimmers must shower before entering the swimming pool.

   c. No suntan lotion will be allowed on persons using the swimming pool.

   d. Swimmers must wear swim shoes while in the swimming pool.

17. A male patient has just begun to use Cortisporin Otic for otitis externa. The nurse knows that the patient will continue this therapy for how long?

   a. 5 days

   b. 10 days

   c. 3 weeks

   d. 6 weeks

18. The nurse is caring for a patient who is taking ciprofloxacin for treatment of necrotizing otitis externa. The nurse instructs the patient to notify the physician immediately if the patient experiences what symptom?

   a. Diarrhea

   b. Dizziness

   c. Tendon pain

   d. Sunburn

19. The nurse will notify the physician immediately if the patient taking amoxicillin for otitis media is also taking what medication?

   a. Tetracycline for acne

   b. Acetaminophen for pain

   c. Aspirin for prevention of blood clots

   d. Ibuprofen for fever

20. A patient with renal impairment has an ear infection. The nurse is aware that dosage reduction is necessary if the patient will be taking which medication?

   a. Amoxicillin

   b. Ofloxacin otic

   c. Ciprofloxacin

   d. Cortisporin Otic

60

Drug Therapy for Disorders of the Skin

Learning Objectives

- Identify the disorders of the skin.
- Identify drug therapy for the treatment of acne vulgaris and drug therapy for other skin disorders.
- Identify the prototype and describe the action, use, adverse effects, contraindications, and nursing implications for the retinoids.
- Implement the nursing process in the care of the patient with disorders of the skin.

SECTION I: ASSESSING YOUR UNDERSTANDING

Activity A FILL IN THE BLANKS

1. Dermatitis is usually characterized by _____, _____, and skin lesions.

2. _____ results from direct contact with irritants or allergens that stimulate inflammation.

3. A disorder that produces wheals and is caused by a histamine release is called _____ (hives).

4. _____ is a skin disorder characterized by erythema, telangiectases, and acne-like lesions of facial skin.

5. Bacterial infections of the skin are most often caused by _____ or _____.

Activity B MATCHING

Match the term in Column A with the definition in Column B.

Column A

_____ 1. Aloe

_____ 2. Azelaic acid (Azelex)

_____ 3. Oralisotretinoin (Accutane)

_____ 4. Coal tar preparations

_____ 5. Hydrocortisone

Column B

a. Has antibacterial activity against *Propionibacterium acnes*

b. Have anti-inflammatory and antipruritic actions and can be used alone or with topical corticosteroids

c. Is often used as a topical remedy for minor burns and wounds (e.g., sunburn, cuts, abrasions) to decrease pain, itching, and inflammation and to promote healing

d. Is the corticosteroid most often included in topical otic preparations

e. May be used for patients with severe acne not responsive to safer drugs

Activity C SHORT ANSWERS

Briefly answer the following questions.

1. What are the most common forms of fungal infections of the skin, and where do they occur?

2. Discuss the four events that take place that are part of the development of acne lesions.

3. Discuss the general treatment for skin disorders.

4. What is the first-line drug treatment for moderate to severe acne, and why is it used?

5. What is the iPLEDGE program, and what drug is it connected to?

SECTION II: APPLYING YOUR KNOWLEDGE

Activity D CASE STUDY

Consider the scenario and answer the questions.

Mrs. Benjamin presents to the physician's office with a red, patchy area on her right forearm that is draining pus. The physician diagnoses the area as atopic dermatitis and prescribes an antibiotic.

1. The patient asks you if the antibiotic will cure the atopic dermatitis. How would you respond?

2. Mrs. Benjamin asks you if she contracted the dermatitis from her brother; she cared for him when he had the chickenpox. What can you tell Mrs. Benjamin about the cause of atopic dermatitis?

3. The physician stages the atopic dermatitis as acute. When you inspect the affected area, what would you expect to find? What other disease process may be evident based on Mrs. Benjamin's diagnosis of atopic dermatitis?

4. You instruct Mrs. Benjamin to avoid possible causes or exacerbating factors. She asks you if she has to give up her job as a financial consultant. What factor related to her profession may cause an exacerbation of her dermatitis?

5. Mrs. Benjamin is concerned and asks you if the red patches on her child's elbows and forearms may be indicative of atopic dermatitis. What should you suggest to her?

SECTION III: PRACTICING FOR NCLEX

Activity E

Answer the following questions.

1. A male patient is prescribed a combination of topical drugs to treat his atopic dermatitis. What statement by the patient indicates that he requires further education regarding his medication regimen?

    a. "The drug therapy will reduce the inflammation caused by my disease."

    b. "The drug therapy may cause dryness of the skin."

    c. "Local drug therapy will not be absorbed systemically."

    d. "The drug therapy may cause adverse effects."

2. The nurse is conducting a class on skin care for adolescents and knows that special precautions are needed for safe use of oral retinoids in what patient population?

    a. Male patients with a history of prostate disease

    b. Children with a diagnosis of type 1 diabetes

    c. Female patients with asthmatic bronchitis

    d. Female patients of childbearing potential

3. The nurse uses special precautions to provide safe use of topical corticosteroids in which group of patients?

    a. Males

    b. Females

    c. Children

    d. Females with comorbidities

4. The physician orders daily topical drugs to treat a patient's dermatitis. What factor is important to teach the patient?

    a. Accurate application to maximize therapeutic effects

    b. PRN usage

    c. Rationale for an open prescription

    d. Alternative medications that are available

5. A 75-year-old male patient develops a red patchy area on his shin. To assist in the diagnosis of the lesion, what must the nurse report to the physician to assist in arriving at a diagnosis for this patient? (Select all that apply.)

   a. Type of lesions

   b. Age of patient

   c. Location of lesions

   d. Sex of the patient

   e. Color of the lesions

6. A female patient comes to the clinic with symptoms of a bacterial skin infection and knows that what are the most common bacterial causes of skin infection? (Select all that apply.)

   a. Staphylococci

   b. Enterococci

   c. *Morganella morganii*

   d. Streptococci

   e. *Pseudomonas*

7. The nurse is caring for a patient who will only use herbal preparations to treat skin conditions. The nurse knows that what topical agent is both safe and effective and considered natural?

   a. Benzoyl peroxide

   b. UVA and UVB radiation

   c. Aloe

   d. Azelaic acid

8. The physician orders a topical corticosteroid for a rash on a patient's elbow. The 75-year-old patient also has hypertension, chronic congestive heart failure, and type 2 diabetes. What concerns the nurse most about this patient and the use of the corticosteroid preparation?

   a. Corticosteroids may be absorbed systemically and exacerbate congestive heart failure symptoms.

   b. Corticosteroids should be used with caution on thin or atrophic skin.

   c. Corticosteroids may diminish signs of infection on the elbow.

   d. Corticosteroids may exacerbate symptoms related to type 2 diabetes.

9. The nurse is giving discharge instructions to parents of an infant with a skin condition and knows that topical agents are used cautiously in infants for what reason?

   a. Diminished absorption of the drug

   b. Infant skin is more permeable

   c. Inconsistent use of the drugs in the health care environment

   d. Infant skin is significantly less permeable

10. The physician has prescribed tacrolimus ointment for a patient with severe atopic dermatitis because the patient's condition has not improved with other medications. The nurse is aware that this medication carries a black box warning that this drug may increase the risk of the development of what condition?

    a. Meningitis

    b. Severe acne

    c. Skin cancer

    d. Full-thickness burn of treated skin

11. The physician orders topical corticosteroids for a 2-year-old patient in the pediatric unit. The nurse would contact the physician if which order for this patient was noted?

    a. The smallest effective dose is ordered.

    b. The open-ended order includes the use of an occlusive dressing.

    c. The order is for the shortest effective time.

    d. The drug is ordered in a topical form.

12. A patient is diagnosed with chronic histamine-induced urticaria. As part of the education plan, when would the nurse teach the patient to administer the antihistamine?

    a. Only when the lesions appear

    b. Before the symptoms appear and PRN thereafter

    c. Before the symptoms appear and round the clock thereafter

    d. When the symptoms appear and round the clock thereafter

13. The nurse is conducting a class to a group of women who are concerned about age-related skin changes. The nurse tells the group that what product is the main component of anti-aging cosmetics?

    a. Salicylic acid

    b. Glycolic acid

    c. Hydrochloric acid

    d. Sulfuric acid

14. The nurse is assessing a 77-year-old patient's skin and understands that what are the most likely skin disorders that occur in this age group? (Select all that apply.)
    a. Skin cancer
    b. Heat rash
    c. Tinea capitis
    d. Actinic keratoses
    e. Dry skin

15. A male patient presents to the physician's office complaining that he has difficulty sleeping because of the intense itching related to his dermatitis. To relieve the itching and promote sleep, the nurse expects the physician to order what medication?
    a. Diphenhydramine
    b. Oral isotretinoin (Accutane)
    c. Corticosteroids
    d. Antibiotic therapy

16. A 17-year-old female patient comes to the clinic with acne, and blood tests reveal that she has a high level of androgens. The nurse expects the physician to order which drug to this patient?
    a. Estrogen
    b. Antiandrogens
    c. Anhydrin
    d. Androgens

17. A female patient is prescribed retinoids for her moderate acne. She returns to the office 1 week later, disappointed because she does not see improvement in her condition. The nurse explains to the patient that improvement may not be seen for up to how many weeks?
    a. 5
    b. 7
    c. 10
    d. 12

18. The nurse is providing instructions to a patient with rosacea about ways to prevent exacerbations of the lesions. The patient understands the instructions when she identifies what actions that cause a worsening of symptoms?
    a. Eating a taco and enchilada dinner
    b. Drinking a carbonated, sweetened beverage
    c. Drinking a glass of beer
    d. Using a suntanning bed
    e. Becoming embarrassed

19. The nurse is discussing acne treatment with a 14-year-old patient and knows that what treatment modality is most effective in treating mild to moderate acne vulgaris?
    a. Clindamycin
    b. Benzoyl peroxide
    c. Topical erythromycin
    d. Topical antibiotic and benzoyl peroxide

20. The nurse is counseling a patient who will be taking isotretinoin for the treatment of acne. The nurse informs the patient that the most common site for adverse effects is which system?
    a. GI
    b. Integumentary
    c. CNS
    d. Endocrine

Answers

CHAPTER 1

SECTION I: ASSESSING YOUR UNDERSTANDING

Activity A FILL IN THE BLANKS

1. Pharmacology
2. Drug therapy
3. medications
4. prototypes
5. Pharmacoeconomics

Activity B MATCHING

1. d   2. e   3. b   4. a   5. c

Activity C SEQUENCING

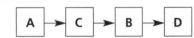

Activity D SHORT ANSWERS

1. Drugs with local effects, such as sunscreen lotions and local anesthetics, act mainly at the site of application.
2. Drugs with systemic effects are taken into the body, circulated through the bloodstream to their sites of action in various body tissues, and eventually eliminated from the body.
3. Synthetic drugs are more standardized in their chemical characteristics, more consistent in their effects, and less likely to produce allergic reactions.
4. The process of biotechnology involves manipulating deoxyribonucleic acid (DNA) and ribonucleic acid (RNA) and recombining genes into hybrid molecules that can be inserted into living organisms (*Escherichia coli* bacteria are often used) and repeatedly reproduced. Each hybrid molecule produces a genetically identical molecule, called a clone.
5. Cloning makes it possible to identify the DNA sequence in a gene and to produce the protein product encoded by the gene, such as insulin. Cloning also allows production of adequate amounts of the drug for therapeutic or research purposes.

SECTION II: APPLYING YOUR KNOWLEDGE

Activity E CASE STUDIES

1. Legally, American consumers have two routes of access to therapeutic drugs. One route is by *prescription* from a licensed health care provider, such as a physician, dentist, or nurse practitioner.
2. Over-the-counter (OTC) is purchase of drugs that does not require a prescription. These routes are regulated by various drug laws.
3. Acquiring and using prescription drugs for non-therapeutic purposes, by persons who are not authorized to have the drugs or for whom they are not prescribed, is illegal.

SECTION III: PRACTICING FOR NCLEX

Activity F

1. **Answer: a.**
   RATIONALE: The FDA approves many new drugs annually. New drugs are categorized according to their review priority and therapeutic potential. A status of "1P" indicates a new drug reviewed on a priority (accelerated) basis and with some therapeutic advantages over drugs already available; a status of "1S" indicates standard review and drugs with few, if any, therapeutic advantages (i.e., the new drug is similar to one or more older drugs currently on the market). Most new drugs are "1S" prescription drugs.
2. **Answer: b, c, and d.**
   RATIONALE: The FDA also approves drugs for OTC availability, including the transfer of drugs from prescription to OTC status, and may require additional clinical trials to determine the safety and effectiveness of OTC use. For prescription drugs taken orally, transfer to OTC status may mean different indications for use and lower doses. FDA approval of a prescription drug to OTC status shifts responsibility from the health care professional to the consumer.
3. **Answer: c.**
   RATIONALE: Having drugs available OTC has potential advantages and disadvantages for consumers. Advantages include greater autonomy, faster and

more convenient access to effective treatment, possibly earlier resumption of usual activities of daily living, fewer visits to a health care provider, and possibly increased efforts by consumers to learn about their symptoms or conditions and recommended treatments. Disadvantages include inaccurate self-diagnoses and potential risks of choosing a wrong or contraindicated drug, delayed treatment by a health care professional, and development of adverse drug reactions and interactions. When a drug is switched from prescription to OTC status, pharmaceutical companies' sales and profits increase and insurance companies' costs decrease. Costs to consumers increase because health insurance policies do not cover OTC drugs.

4. **Answer: a and c.**
RATIONALE: When prevention or cure is not a reasonable goal, relief of symptoms can greatly improve a patient's quality of life and ability to function in activities of daily living. Relief of symptoms does not increase longevity (length of life).

5. **Answer: b.**
RATIONALE: Drugs are classified according to their effects on particular body systems, their therapeutic uses, and their chemical characteristics.

6. **Answer: b.**
RATIONALE: The names of therapeutic classifications usually reflect the conditions for which the drugs are used (e.g., antidepressants, antihypertensives).

7. **Answer: d.**
RATIONALE: Drugs may be prescribed and dispensed by generic name or by trade name.

8. **Answer: c.**
RATIONALE: A new drug is protected by patent for several years, during which time only the pharmaceutical manufacturer that developed it can market it. This is seen as a return on the company's investment in developing a drug, which may require years of work and millions of dollars, and as an incentive for developing other drugs. Other pharmaceutical companies cannot manufacture and market the drug until the patent expires.

9. **Answer: b.**
RATIONALE: Current drug laws and standards have evolved over many years. Their main goal is to protect the public by ensuring that drugs marketed for therapeutic purposes are safe and effective.

10. **Answer: a, c, and d.**
RATIONALE: Synthetic drugs are more standardized in their chemical characteristics, more consistent in their effects, and less likely to produce allergic reaction. Biotechnology produces cloned drugs. These are not considered synthetic. These drugs have increased uses for treatment.

11. **Answer: c.**
RATIONALE: The Comprehensive Drug Abuse Prevention and Control Act was passed in 1970. Title II of this law, called the Controlled Substances Act, regulates the manufacture and distribution of narcotics, stimulants, depressants, hallucinogens, and anabolic steroids. These drugs are categorized according to therapeutic usefulness and potential for abuse and are labeled as controlled substances (e.g., morphine is a C-II or Schedule II drug).

12. **Answer: a, c, and d.**
RATIONALE: Nurses are responsible for storing controlled substances in locked containers, administering them only to people for whom they are prescribed, recording each dose given on agency narcotic sheets and on the patient's medication administration record, maintaining an accurate inventory, and reporting discrepancies to the proper authorities. The nurse is responsible for administering a controlled substance only to the patient for whom it has been prescribed.

13. **Answer: a, b, and d.**
RATIONALE: The Drug Enforcement Administration (DEA) enforces the Controlled Substances Act. People and companies that are legally empowered to handle controlled substances must be registered with the DEA, keep accurate records of all transactions, and provide for secure storage. Prescribers are assigned a number by the DEA and must include the number on all prescriptions they write for a controlled substance. Prescriptions for Schedule II drugs cannot be refilled; a new prescription is required. People and companies that are legally empowered to handle narcotics do not have to educate health care professionals about their adverse effects.

14. **Answer: b.**
RATIONALE: Historically, drug research was done mainly with young, white males as subjects. In 1993, Congress passed the National Institutes of Health (NIH) Revitalization Act, which formalized a policy of the NIH that women and minorities must be included in human subject research studies funded by the NIH and in clinical drug trials.

15. **Answer: a.**
RATIONALE: Since 1962, newly developed drugs have been extensively tested before being marketed for general use. Initially, drugs are tested in animals, and the FDA reviews the test results. Next, clinical trials in humans are done, usually with a randomized, controlled experimental design that involves selection of subjects according to established criteria, random assignment of subjects to experimental groups, and administration of the test drug to one group and a control substance to another group.

16. **Answer: b.**
RATIONALE: FDA approval of a drug for OTC availability involves evaluation of evidence that the consumer can use the drug safely, using information on the product label, and shifts primary responsibility for safe and effective drug therapy from health care professionals to consumers. With prescription drugs, a health care professional

diagnoses the condition, often with the help of laboratory and other diagnostic tests, and determines a need for the drug.

17. **Answer: b.**
    RATIONALE: There are many sources of drug data, including pharmacology and other textbooks, drug reference books, journal articles, and Internet sites. For the beginning student of pharmacology, a textbook is the best source of information, because it describes groups of drugs in relation to therapeutic uses.

18. **Answer: b.**
    RATIONALE: During Phase IV of a drug trial, it is the manufacturer's responsibility to continue to monitor the drug's effects while the drug has been placed in general use. During Phase I, healthy volunteers are found to test the drug. In Phase II, patients with a disease are divided into two groups, and one receives the new drug and the other receives a placebo. During Phase III, it is determined if the drug's benefits outweigh the adverse effects.

19. **Answer: c.**
    RATIONALE: The Durham-Humphrey Amendment designates drugs that must be prescribed by a licensed physician or nurse practitioner and dispensed by a pharmacist.

20. **Answer: c.**
    RATIONALE: Disadvantages of using an OTC include inaccurate self-diagnoses and potential risks of choosing a wrong or contraindicated drug, delayed treatment by a health care professional, and development of adverse drug reactions and interactions. Advances include greater autonomy, faster and more convenient access to effective treatment, possibly earlier resumption of usual activities of daily living, fewer visits to a health care provider, and possibly increased efforts by consumers to learn about their symptoms/conditions and recommended treatments.

CHAPTER 2

SECTION I: ASSESSING YOUR UNDERSTANDING

Activity A FILL IN THE BLANKS

1. Drugs
2. cell membrane
3. Pharmacokinetics
4. Absorption
5. faster
6. Additive effects
7. Synergism
8. Interference
9. Displacement
10. antidote

Activity B MATCHING

1. e   2. b   3. a   4. d   5. c

Activity C SEQUENCING

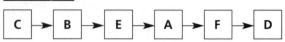

Activity D SHORT ANSWERS

1. To act on body cells, drugs given for systemic effects must reach adequate concentrations in the blood and other tissue fluids surrounding the cells. Therefore, they must enter the body and be circulated to their sites of action (target cells). After they act on cells, they must be eliminated from the body.

2. Although cells differ from one tissue to another, their common characteristics include the ability to perform the following functions:
   - Exchange materials with their immediate environment.
   - Obtain energy from nutrients.
   - Synthesize hormones, neurotransmitters, enzymes, structural proteins, and other complex molecules.
   - Duplicate themselves (reproduce).
   - Communicate with one another via various biologic chemicals, such as neurotransmitters and hormones.

3. Numerous factors affect the rate and extent of drug absorption, including dosage form, route of administration and blood flow to the site of administration, gastrointestinal function, the presence of food or other drugs, and other variables.

4. Rapid movement through the stomach and small intestine may increase drug absorption by promoting contact with absorptive mucous membrane; it also may decrease absorption, because some drugs may move through the small intestine too rapidly to be absorbed. For many drugs, the presence of food in the stomach slows the rate of absorption and may decrease the amount of drug absorbed.

5. Drug distribution into the CNS is limited because the blood–brain barrier, which is composed of capillaries with tight walls, limits movement of drug molecules into brain tissue. This barrier usually acts as a selectively permeable membrane to protect the CNS.

SECTION II: APPLYING YOUR KNOWLEDGE

Activity E CASE STUDIES

1. A *serum drug level* is a laboratory measurement of the amount of a drug in the blood at a particular time; it reflects dosage, absorption, bioavailability, half-life, and the rates of metabolism and excretion. A minimum effective concentration (MEC) must be present before a drug exerts its pharmacologic action on body cells; this is largely determined by the drug dose and how well it is absorbed into the bloodstream.

2. A toxic concentration is an excessive level at which toxicity occurs. Toxic concentrations may stem from a single large dose, repeated small doses, or slow metabolism that allows the drug to accumulate in the body.

3. Between low and high concentrations is the therapeutic range, which is the goal of drug therapy—that is, enough drug to be beneficial, but not enough to be toxic.

SECTION III: PRACTICING FOR NCLEX

Activity F

1. **Answer: d**
   RATIONALE: Bioavailability is the portion of a dose that reaches the systemic circulation and is available to act on body cells.

2. **Answer: c**
   RATIONALE: An intravenous drug is virtually 100% bioavailable. An oral drug is almost always less than 100% bioavailable, because some of it is not absorbed from the gastrointestinal tract and some goes to the liver and is partially metabolized before reaching the systemic circulation.

3. **Answer: c**
   RATIONALE: With chronic administration, some drugs stimulate liver cells to produce larger amounts of drug-metabolizing enzymes (called *enzyme induction*). Enzyme induction accelerates drug metabolism, because larger amounts of the enzymes (and more binding sites) allow larger amounts of a drug to be metabolized during a given time. As a result, larger doses of the rapidly metabolized drug may be required to produce or maintain therapeutic effects. Rapid metabolism may also increase the production of toxic metabolites with some drugs (e.g., acetaminophen). Drugs that induce enzyme production also may increase the rate of metabolism for endogenous steroidal hormones (e.g., cortisol, estrogens, testosterone, vitamin D). However, *enzyme induction does not occur for 1 to 3 weeks after an inducing agent is started*, because new enzyme proteins must be synthesized.

4. **Answer: a and d**
   RATIONALE: Metabolism also may be decreased or delayed in a process called *enzyme inhibition*, which most often occurs with concurrent administration of two or more drugs that compete for the same metabolizing enzymes. In this case, smaller doses of the slowly metabolized drug may be needed to avoid adverse effects and toxicity from drug accumulation. *Enzyme inhibition occurs within hours or days of starting an inhibiting agent.* Cimetidine, a gastric acid suppressor, inhibits several CYP enzymes (e.g., CYP1A, CYP2C, CYP2D, CYP3A) and can greatly decrease drug metabolism.

5. **Answer: a**
   RATIONALE: When drugs are given orally, they are absorbed from the gastrointestinal tract and carried to the liver through the portal circulation.

Some drugs are extensively metabolized in the liver, with only part of a drug dose reaching the systemic circulation for distribution to sites of action. This is called the *first-pass effect* or presystemic metabolism.

6. **Answer: a**
   RATIONALE: Some drugs or metabolites are excreted in bile and then eliminated in feces; others are excreted in bile, reabsorbed from the small intestine, and then returned to the liver in a process called *enterohepatic recirculation*.

7. **Answer: c**
   RATIONALE: For most drugs, serum levels indicate the onset, peak, and duration of drug action. After a single dose of a drug is given, onset of action occurs when the drug level reaches the MEC.

8. **Answer: a, c, e, and f**
   RATIONALE: In clinical practice, measurement of serum drug levels is useful in several circumstances:
   - When drugs with a narrow margin of safety are given, because their therapeutic doses are close to their toxic doses (e.g., digoxin, aminoglycoside antibiotics, lithium)
   - To document the serum drug levels associated with particular drug dosages, therapeutic effects, or possible adverse effects
   - To monitor unexpected responses to a drug dose, such as decreased therapeutic effects or increased adverse effects
   - When a drug overdose is suspected

9. **Answer: d**
   RATIONALE: Systemic absorption from the skin is minimal but may be increased when the skin is inflamed or damaged. Severe sunburn would be an example of inflamed skin. Multiple nevi (moles) and a port wine stain of the face are not examples of skin disorders that would increase absorption of topical medication. Rosacea is an example of an inflammatory skin condition of the face, but it rarely causes systemic absorption because most of the medications prescribed to treat it are topical.

10. **Answer: c**
    RATIONALE: When a drug is given at a stable dose, 4 to 5 half-lives are required to achieve steady-state concentrations and develop equilibrium between tissue and serum concentrations. Because maximal therapeutic effects do not occur until equilibrium is established, some drugs are not fully effective for days or weeks. To maintain steady-state conditions, the amount of drug given must equal the amount eliminated from the body. When a drug dose is changed, an additional 4 to 5 half-lives are required to reestablish equilibrium; when a drug is discontinued, it is eliminated gradually over several half-lives.

11. **Answer: a**
    RATIONALE: Pharmacodynamics involves drug actions on target cells and the resulting alterations in cellular biochemical reactions and functions (i.e., "what the drug does to the body").

12. Answer: a, c, and d

RATIONALE: Relatively few drugs act by mechanisms other than combination with receptor sites on cells. Drugs that do not act on receptor sites include the following:

- Antacids, which act chemically to neutralize the hydrochloric acid produced by gastric parietal cells and thereby raise the pH of gastric fluid.
- Osmotic diuretics (e.g., mannitol), which increase the osmolarity of plasma and pull water out of tissues into the bloodstream.
- Drugs that are structurally similar to nutrients required by body cells (e.g., purines, pyrimidines) and that can be incorporated into cellular constituents, such as nucleic acids. This interferes with normal cell functioning. Several anticancer drugs act by this mechanism.
- Metal chelating agents, which combine with toxic metals to form a complex that can be more readily excreted.

13. Answer: a

RATIONALE: Dosage refers to the frequency, size, and number of doses; it is a major determinant of drug actions and responses, both therapeutic and adverse. If the amount is too small or is administered infrequently, no pharmacologic action occurs, because the drug does not reach an adequate concentration at target cells. If the amount is too large or is administered too often, toxicity (poisoning) may occur. Overdosage may occur with a single large dose or with chronic ingestion of smaller doses.

14. Answer: b

RATIONALE: Most drug–diet interactions are undesirable because food often slows absorption of oral drugs by slowing gastric emptying time and altering gastrointestinal secretions and motility. Giving medications 1 hour before or 2 hours after a meal can minimize interactions that decrease drug absorption.

15. Answer: b

RATIONALE: An interaction occurs between tyramine-containing foods and monoamine oxidase (MAO) inhibitor drugs. Tyramine causes the release of norepinephrine, a strong vasoconstrictive agent, from the adrenal medulla and sympathetic neurons. Normally, norepinephrine is quickly inactivated by MAO. However, because MAO inhibitor drugs prevent inactivation of norepinephrine, ingestion of tyramine-containing foods with an MAO inhibitor may produce severe hypertension or intracranial hemorrhage. MAO inhibitors include the antidepressants isocarboxazid and phenelzine and the antiparkinson drugs rasagiline and selegiline. Tyramine-rich foods to be avoided by patients taking MAO inhibitors include aged cheeses, sauerkraut, soy sauce, tap or draft beers, and red wines.

16. Answer: c

RATIONALE: An interaction may occur between warfarin (Coumadin), an oral anticoagulant, and foods containing vitamin K. Because vitamin K antagonizes the action of warfarin, large amounts of spinach and other green leafy vegetables may offset the anticoagulant effects and predispose the person to thromboembolic disorders.

17. Answer: a

RATIONALE: Grapefruit contains a substance that strongly inhibits the metabolism of drugs normally metabolized by the cytochrome P450 CYP3A4 enzyme. This effect greatly increases the blood levels of some drugs (e.g., the widely used "statin" group of cholesterol-lowering drugs), and the effect lasts for several days. Patients who take medications metabolized by the CYP3A4 enzyme should be advised against eating grapefruit or drinking grapefruit juice.

18. Answer: d

RATIONALE: In older adults (65 years and older), physiologic changes may alter all pharmacokinetic processes. Changes in the gastrointestinal tract include decreased gastric acidity, decreased blood flow, and decreased motility. Despite these changes, however, there is little difference in drug absorption. Changes in the cardiovascular system include decreased cardiac output and therefore slower distribution of drug molecules to their sites of action, metabolism, and excretion. In the liver, blood flow and metabolizing enzymes are decreased. Therefore, many drugs are metabolized more slowly, have a longer action, and are more likely to accumulate with chronic administration. In the kidneys, there is decreased blood flow, decreased glomerular filtration rate, and decreased tubular secretion of drugs; all of these changes tend to slow excretion and promote accumulation of drugs in the body. Impaired kidney and liver function greatly increases the risks of adverse drug effects. In addition, older adults are more likely to have acute and chronic illnesses that require the use of multiple drugs or long-term drug therapy. Therefore, possibilities for interactions among drugs and between drugs and diseased organs are greatly multiplied.

19. Answer: b

RATIONALE: Most drug information has been derived from clinical drug trials using white men. Interethnic variations became evident when drugs and dosages developed for Caucasians produced unexpected responses, including toxicity, when given to people from other ethnic groups. One common variation is that African Americans respond differently to some cardiovascular drugs. For example, for African Americans with hypertension, angiotensin-converting enzyme (ACE) inhibitors and beta-adrenergic blocking drugs are less effective, and diuretics and calcium channel blockers are more effective. Also, African Americans with heart failure seem to respond better to a combination of hydralazine and isosorbide than do Caucasian patients with heart failure.

20. **Answer: b**
    RATIONALE: Drug *tolerance* occurs when the body becomes accustomed to a particular drug over time, so that larger doses must be given to produce the same effects. Tolerance may be acquired to the pharmacologic action of many drugs, especially opioid analgesics, alcohol, and other CNS depressants. Tolerance to pharmacologically related drugs is called *cross-tolerance*. For example, a person who regularly drinks large amounts of alcohol becomes able to ingest even larger amounts before becoming intoxicated—this is tolerance to alcohol. If the person is then given sedative-type drugs or a general anesthetic, larger-than-usual doses are required to produce a pharmacologic effect—this is cross-tolerance.

CHAPTER 3

SECTION I: ASSESSING YOUR UNDERSTANDING

Activity A   FILL IN THE BLANKS

1. unit-dose
2. Controlled drugs
3. Medication reconciliation
4. cognitive and psychomotor
5. Assessment

Activity B   MATCHING

1. c   2. b   3. a   4. e   5. d

Activity C   SEQUENCING

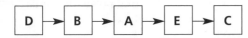

Activity D   SHORT ANSWERS

1. Medication errors commonly reported include giving an incorrect dose, not giving an ordered drug, and giving an unordered drug.
2. Medication orders should include the full name of the patient; the name of the drug (preferably the generic name); the dose, route, and frequency of administration; and the date, time, and signature of the prescriber.
3. Assessment involves collecting data about patient characteristics known to affect drug therapy. This includes observing and interviewing the patient, interviewing family members or others involved in patient care, completing a physical assessment, reviewing medical records for pertinent laboratory and diagnostic test reports, and other methods. Initially (before drug therapy is started or on first contact), assess age, weight, vital signs, health status, pathologic conditions, and ability to function

in usual activities of daily living.
4. Planning/goals involves the expected outcomes of prescribed drug therapy. As a general rule, goals should be stated in terms of patient behavior, not nurse behavior (e.g., "The patient will....").
5. This step involves evaluating the patient's status in relation to stated goals and expected outcomes. Some outcomes can be evaluated within a few minutes of drug administration (e.g., relief of acute pain after administration of an analgesic), but most require longer periods of time. Over time, the patient is likely to experience brief contacts with many health care providers, which increases the difficulty of evaluating outcomes of drug therapy.

SECTION II: APPLYING YOUR KNOWLEDGE

Activity E   CASE STUDIES

Case Study 1

1. Occasionally, verbal or telephone orders are acceptable. When taken, they should be written on the patient's order sheet, signed by the person taking the order, and later countersigned by the prescriber.
2. Prescriptions for Schedule II controlled drugs cannot be refilled.
3. For discharge education, the following information should be part of the nurse's education plan: instructions for taking the drug (e.g., dose, frequency) and whether the prescription can be refilled.

Case Study 2

1. **Answer: b**
   RATIONALE: Assessment includes observing and interviewing the patient, interviewing family members or others involved in patient care, completing a physical assessment, reviewing medical records for pertinent laboratory and diagnostic test reports, and other methods. Initially (before drug therapy is started or on first contact), assess age, weight, vital signs, health status, pathologic conditions, and ability to function in usual activities of daily living.
2. **Answer: a**
   RATIONALE: Subjective assessment includes the patient's response to the interview. Subjective data are facts about the patient that cannot be directly observed by the nurse.
3. **Answer: b**
   RATIONALE: Objective data are facts that can be directly observed by the nurse.

SECTION III: PRACTICING FOR NCLEX

Activity F

1. **Answer: c**
   RATIONALE: The sixth "right" is documentation.
2. **Answer: c**
   RATIONALE: Minimize the use of abbreviations for drug names, doses, routes of administration, and times of administration. This promotes safer administration and reduces errors. When

abbreviations are used by prescribers or others, interpret them accurately or question the writer about the intended meaning.

3. **Answer: c**
   RATIONALE: Measure doses accurately. Ask a colleague to double-check measurements of insulin and heparin, unusual doses (i.e., large or small), and any drugs to be given intravenously.

4. **Answer: b**
   RATIONALE: The nurse may be held liable for not giving a drug or for giving a wrong drug or a wrong dose. In addition, the nurse is expected to have sufficient drug knowledge to recognize and question erroneous orders. If, after questioning the prescriber and seeking information from other authoritative sources, the nurse considers that giving a drug is unsafe, the nurse must refuse to give the drug. The fact that a physician wrote an erroneous order does not excuse the nurse from legal liability if he or she carries out that order.

5. **Answer: a, c, and e**
   RATIONALE: Specific drugs often associated with errors and adverse drug events (ADEs) include insulin, heparin, and warfarin. The risk of ADEs increases with the number of drugs a patient uses.

6. **Answer: c**
   RATIONALE: The bar code on the drug label contains the identification number, strength, and dosage form of the drug, and the bar code on the patient's identification band contains the MAR, which can be displayed when a nurse uses a handheld scanning device. When administering medications, the nurse scans the bar code on the drug label, on the patient's identification band, and on the nurse's personal identification badge. A wireless computer network processes the scanned information; gives an error message on the scanner or sounds an alarm if the nurse is about to give the wrong drug or the right drug at the wrong time; and automatically records the time, drug, and dose given on the MAR.

7. **Answer: a**
   RATIONALE: Enteric-coated tablets and capsules are coated with a substance that is insoluble in stomach acid. This delays dissolution until the medication reaches the intestine, usually to avoid gastric irritation or to keep the drug from being destroyed by gastric acid.

8. **Answer: c**
   RATIONALE: Several controlled-release dosage forms and drug delivery systems are available, and more continue to be developed. These formulations maintain more consistent serum drug levels and allow less frequent administration, which is more convenient for patients. Controlled-release oral tablets and capsules are called by a variety of names (e.g., timed release, sustained release, extended release), and their names usually include CR, SR, XL, or other indications that they are long-acting formulations.

9. **Answer: b**
   RATIONALE: Because controlled-release tablets and capsules contain high amounts of drug intended to be absorbed slowly and act over a prolonged period of time, they should never be broken, opened, crushed, or chewed. Such an action allows the full dose to be absorbed immediately and constitutes an overdose, with potential organ damage or death.

10. The correct answer is two tablets. In this case, the answer can be readily calculated mentally. This is a simple example that also can be used to illustrate mathematical calculations. This problem can be solved by several acceptable methods; the following formula is presented because of its relative simplicity for students lacking a more familiar method:

$$\frac{D}{H} = \frac{X}{V}$$

11. The correct answer is 0.8 mL.

$$\frac{8\,mg}{10\,mg} = \frac{X}{1\,mL}$$

12. The correct answer is one tablet.
    1 g = 1,000 mg; 0.5 g = 500 mg

13. **Answer: c**
    RATIONALE: The American Society of Anesthesiologists recommends that all herbal products be discontinued 2 to 3 weeks before any surgical procedure. Some products (e.g., echinacea, feverfew, garlic, gingko biloba, ginseng, valerian, St. John's wort) can interfere with or increase the effects of some drugs, affect blood pressure or heart rhythm, or increase risks of bleeding; some have unknown effects when combined with anesthetics, other perioperative medications, and surgical procedures.

14. **Answer: a**
    RATIONALE: Most herbal and dietary supplements should be avoided during pregnancy or lactation and in young children.

15. **Answer: d**
    RATIONALE: If taking a liquid medication (or giving one to a child), measure with a calibrated medication cup or measuring spoon. A dose cannot be measured accurately with household teaspoons or tablespoons because they are different sizes and deliver varying amounts of medication. If the liquid medication is packaged with a measuring cup that shows teaspoons or tablespoons, that should be used to measure doses, for adults or children.

16. **Answer: b**
    RATIONALE: If a dose is missed, most authorities recommend taking the dose if remembered soon after the scheduled time, or omitting the dose if it is not remembered.

17. **Answer: c**
    RATIONALE: The nurse must have a physician's order to change the method of administration of a medication. It would not be appropriate to ask the patient to wait for administration of a pain medication.

18. Answer: d
RATIONALE: Extended-release medications should never be opened and the powder contained in that medication mixed with water for administration via gastrostomy tube because it will cause the patient to absorb the total dosage of medication too quickly. Also it should never be crushed for administration for the same reason. The medication may or may not clog the tube. The most appropriate action is to call the physician and ask for a different formulation of the medication.

19. Answer: c
RATIONALE: Subcutaneous heparin injections should never be aspirated. The use of a 25-gauge needle inserted at a 45-degree angle and pressure applied to the injection site for a few seconds after injection are all appropriate actions by the nurse.

20. Answer: b
RATIONALE: The nurse should notify the physician that a suitable vein can't be located. Patients who have had mastectomies should not have IV inserted on the side of the mastectomy. It would not be appropriate to use the feet unless ordered by a physician. The nurse can't change the route of administration without an order from the physician.

CHAPTER 4

SECTION I: ASSESSING YOUR UNDERSTANDING

Activity A FILL IN THE BLANKS
1. pharmacodynamic, pharmacokinetic
2. younger
3. total body water
4. caring
5. puberty

Activity B MATCHING
1. c   2. a   3. d   4. e   5. b

Activity C SHORT ANSWERS
1. Drug dosages in children may be calculated by weight only or by determining the child's body surface area (BSA). The prescriber uses the child's weight and calculates the dose based on a known adult dose by using an equation.
2. Drug effectiveness in the pediatric population is influenced by total body water, fat stores, and protein amounts. Thalidomide is a drug that works differently depending upon the patient's age. It was a very effective antiemetic for pregnant women experiencing morning sickness, but it caused tragic limb abnormalities and even death in the fetus.
3. Drug absorption in the pediatric population is affected by the age of the child, gastric emptying, intestinal motility, routes of administration, and skin permeability.

4. Toddlers are mobile and curious. They have a short attention span, but they also want to be independent. The nurse should involve the toddler in medication administration by having the toddler hold items or choose the bandage or cup to be used. Explanations should be very short and simple. The nurse may flavor oral medications with syrups. Toddlers with a developed muscle mass may have IM injections in the ventrogluteal instead of the vastus lateralis.
5. The nurse should assess adolescents for risky behavior related to the use of laxatives in eating disorders; drug experimentation; and the use of illicit, prescription, or over-the-counter medications.

SECTION II: APPLYING YOUR KNOWLEDGE
Activity D CASE STUDY
1. Dehydration occurs more quickly in children than in adults because children (especially neonates and infants) have a higher percentage of body water than do adults. Adults are 60% total body water and neonates are 80% water.
2. IM injections in neonates are less effective because of low blood flow to skeletal muscles and weak muscle contractions that contribute to erratic absorption of an IM injection.
3. The nurse should recommend that the mother provide comfort care for her daughter after the IV is started. The mother should hold and cuddle the baby and offer her a pacifier.

SECTION III: PRACTICING FOR NCLEX
Activity E
1. **Answer: c**
RATIONALE: Newborn infants process drugs inefficiently. By age 12, children have grown and matured sufficiently to develop pharmacokinetic responses that resemble those of adults.
2. **Answer: d**
RATIONALE: Infants have highly permeable skin tissue, which increases the rate of absorption of topical drugs. Infants have low (not high) blood flow to skeletal muscles, have weak (not strong) muscle contraction, and have a larger (not smaller) percentage of total body water as compared to adults.
3. **Answer: a**
RATIONALE: In infants, immature liver function leads to very low plasma protein levels, which limits the amount of protein binding by drugs such as phenytoin, which is highly protein bound. This may cause toxicity to occur. Immaturity in the other organs would not lead to drug toxicity.
4. **Answer: c**
RATIONALE: Oral medications are best administered with a dropper or oral syringe into the inner aspect of the cheek, giving children time to swallow the medication as it is instilled. The infant may choke if the medication is placed

on the back of the tongue, and there is less of a chance for the infant to swallow the medication effectively if placed between the cheek and gums or under the tongue.

5. **Answer: b**
RATIONALE: Infants lack well-developed muscles. The nurse should use the smallest possible needle and inject the medication into the vastus lateralis. The dorsogluteal site is not recommended for any age group, but it may be appropriate in the adult. The deltoid and the ventrogluteal are not appropriate because of lack of muscle mass.

6. **Answer: a, b, and e**
RATIONALE: Appropriate intravenous sites for infants include hands, feet, and scalp. The antecubital fossa and the jugular are appropriate in infants.

7. **Answer: c**
RATIONALE: Oral medications are best administered to infants with a dropper or oral syringe. The use of feeding nipples is controversial because some believe that infants may then refuse feedings if they associate food with the taste of medicine. Infants are not able to drink from a plastic medicine cup, and a calibrated teaspoon is difficult to fit into an infant's mouth.

8. **Answer: a**
RATIONALE: Many medications come in suppository form which makes administration easier. Toddlers and preschoolers have strong reactions to suppositories which may make it difficult to insert the medication. School age and adolescents are usually embarrassed by the insertion.

9. **Answer: a, b, and c**
RATIONALE: Adolescents need explanations about the use of acne medications and antibiotics, including adverse effects. The nurse should tell teenage girls who are taking birth control pills about the adverse effects and possible drug interactions. Adolescents must realize that they need to be protected from sun and that there is no safe use of alcohol in this age range.

10. **Answer: a**
RATIONALE: Total body water, fat stores, and protein amounts change throughout childhood and greatly influence the effectiveness of drugs in the pediatric population. Skin permeability and gastric emptying are examples of variables in drug absorption.

11. **Answer: b**
RATIONALE: The prescriber uses weight alone to calculate pediatric dosages. Total body water, height, and gastric acidity are not used in the exact calculation.

12. **Answer: c**
RATIONALE: The risk of CNS effects related to drugs is higher in infants than in adults because of the immature blood–brain barrier. Immature liver and renal function would affect effectiveness but is not directly related to CNS effects. The peripheral nervous system immaturity would not affect the central nervous system effects.

13. **Answer: a**
RATIONALE: Chewable tablets work well for children who cannot swallow other forms of tablets or capsules.

14. **Answer: a, b, and c**
RATIONALE: For toddlers, IV sites in the scalp are still occasionally appropriate, but for older toddlers and preschoolers, the feet, the hands, or antecubital are more often preferable.

15. **Answer: a**
RATIONALE: Neonates are especially prone to increased levels of drugs that are eliminated primarily by the kidneys. The prescriber should give smaller doses until renal function reaches that of an adult—between 1 and 2 years of age.

16. **Answer: c**
RATIONALE: In adults, total body water is approximately 60%, whereas in newborns, it is 80%.

17. **Answer: b, c, and d**
RATIONALE: During infancy, neonates have delayed, irregular gastric emptying and reduced gastric acidity that leads to increased gastric pH. Neonates do not normally have a constricted pyloric sphincter.

18. **Answer: a**
RATIONALE: Initially prescribers assumed that antidepressants could be safely used therapeutically in adolescents and children. However, it was found that they may play a causal role in inducing suicidality in pediatric patients. Antidepressants are not associated with schizophrenia, bulimia, and anorexia nervosa.

19. **Answer: b, c, and e**
RATIONALE: Causes of pharmacodynamic variability across the lifespan include difference in body composition, immature systems, and genetic makeup. Skin permeability and route of administration are variables associated with drug absorption.

20. **Answer: b**
RATIONALE: Body surface area is expressed in square meters.

CHAPTER 5

SECTION I: ASSESSING YOUR UNDERSTANDING

Activity A FILL IN THE BLANKS

1. Risk-to-benefit ratio
2. sensitive
3. decrease, receptors
4. Cardiovascular disease
5. Beers Criteria

Activity B MATCHING

1. c   **2.** a   **3.** d   **4.** e   **5.** b

Activity C SHORT ANSWERS

1. Aging results in body mass changes; the proportion of body fat increases while lean body mass decreases. Lipid-soluble drugs such as anesthetic agents stay in the fat tissue for a longer period of time. This places older adults at risk for respiratory depression following surgery.

2. Some older adults may have to choose between the cost of their medications and the ability to purchase food or pay for utilities.

3. The nurse should assess the patient's memory, ability to care for self, and the caregivers' ability to assist in care when assessing the patient's ability to maintain adherence to medications.

4. The nurse should educate the patient and family about all medications and possible drug–drug, drug–herb, and drug–diet interactions.

5. Some responses to drug therapy are genetically determined and may differ in various ethnic and racial populations. Caucasian Americans and African Americans are poor metabolizers of medication compared with Asian Americans. Asian Americans have the ability to metabolize and excrete medications more quickly than those of Caucasian and African descent. Beta-blockers are less effective in African Americans, and Asian Americans may require a smaller dose of the same medication.

SECTION II: APPLYING YOUR KNOWLEDGE

Activity D CASE STUDY

1. In older adults, the amount of body fluid decreases in proportion to total body weight. Water-soluble drugs such as antibiotics are distributed in smaller volumes due to the decrease in total body fluid volume. This increases the risk of toxicity because drug concentrations are greater.

2. Edward's mild congestive heart failure leads to decreased circulation and diminished cardiac output. This leads to inadequate distribution of medication.

3. The glomerular filtration rate is the most reliable measure for evaluation of renal function. This is very costly to obtain. The physician may order a creatinine clearance, which is an important indicator of the ability of the renal system to eliminate medication and prevent adverse drug effects.

SECTION III: PRACTICING FOR NCLEX

Activity E

1. Answer: b
RATIONALE: The most relevant physiologic change is the decreased function of vital organs needed for the pharmacokinetic process. Decreased affinity to receptor sites for medication, decreased function of the beta-receptor system, and decreased cellular biochemical reactions are all

changes related to the aging process, but they are related to the pharmacodynamics area.

2. Answer: d
RATIONALE: The more physically active older adults are, the less likely they are to experience altered drug responses.

3. Answer: b, c, and e
RATIONALE: In older adults, changes in the GI tract include decreased gastric acidity, with an increase in the gastric pH, and delayed absorption or lack of absorption of medications that require this decreased pH. Other changes in the GI tract affecting absorption in older adults are decreased blood flow and decreased surface area to support absorption. Diminished gastric emptying also plays a role by causing the medication to be in the stomach for a longer period.

4. Answer: b and c
RATIONALE: Diminished gastric emptying increases the risk of developing nausea and vomiting, thus causing elimination of the medication in emesis and promoting fluid volume deficit that may lead to dehydration. It does not cause edema of the stomach lining, constipation, or diarrhea.

5. Answer: a and d
RATIONALE: In older patients, decreased circulation means that parenteral medications are also slowly absorbed. Decreased muscle mass and altered circulation can result in abnormal blood concentrations of medication administered IM.

6. Answer: c
RATIONALE: A slow rate of absorption in older adults can result in changes in peak serum drug levels, which may require greater dosages to be administered to produce therapeutic results.

7. Answer: a, b, and d
RATIONALE: Physiological factors that contribute to alterations in distribution of medications include diminished cardiac output, increased body fat, decreased body mass and body fluid, and decreased serum albumin.

8. Answer: c
RATIONALE: Aging results in changes in body mass. The proportion of body fat increases while lean body mass decreases.

9. Answer: b
RATIONALE: The glomerular filtration rate is the most reliable measure for evaluation of renal function.

10. Answer: a
RATIONALE: With a decreased creatinine clearance, it is necessary to reduce the dosage of medication.

11. Answer: a, c, and d
RATIONALE: In older adults, physiologic changes associated with alterations in medication excretion include diminished renal blood flow, number of functioning nephrons, glomerular filtration rate, and tubular secretion. In most older adults, the serum creatinine remains within normal range due to decreasing creatinine levels in association with a decrease in muscle mass.

12. Answer: b
RATIONALE: The assessment of the patient's creatinine clearance is an important indicator of the ability of the renal system to eliminate a medication and prevent adverse drug effects.

13. Answer: a, c, d, and e
RATIONALE: Improper medication use may be influenced by altered mental status and diminished visual acuity. It is also often difficult to remember medications or maintain appropriate administration schedules. Economic factors also contribute to nonadherence.

14. Answer: b
RATIONALE: Starting slow and with low doses improves adherence to the medication regimen. Starting with smaller doses minimizes adverse effects.

15. Answer: d
RATIONALE: Being asymptomatic may contribute to nonadherence to a medication regimen. This is particularly true in patients being treated for hypertension. Arthritis and gout are both painful conditions. Patients with congestive heart failure often have edema and possibly trouble breathing.

16. Answer: c, d, and e
RATIONALE: To improve adherence, nurses should keep the care inexpensive, using generic preparations, and provide easy-to-follow directions, using the fewest number of doses required.

17. Answer: b, d, and e
RATIONALE: At approximately 60 years of age, the liver begins to decrease in size and mass. There is also a decrease in hepatic circulation, lowering the rate of metabolism. The hepatic enzymes of the liver are decreased, altering the ability to remove metabolic by-products.

18. Answer: a, b, and d
RATIONALE: Some of the most common medical problems seen in older adults include diabetes mellitus, arthritis, and heart disease. Systemic lupus erythematosus and ventral hernia may be seen in older adults, but they are seen in all adults.

19. Answer: b
RATIONALE: Older adults are more prone to antibiotic-resistant infections because they have been exposed to many different antibiotics over their lifetime.

20. Answer: c
RATIONALE: Thirty percent of elderly hospital admissions are linked to drug reactions.

CHAPTER 6

SECTION I: ASSESSING YOUR UNDERSTANDING

Activity A FILL IN THE BLANKS

1. teratogenic
2. Organogenesis
3. arterial blood pressure
4. tocolytics
5. third week

Activity B MATCHING

1. b   **2.** d   **3.** a   **4.** e   **5.** c

Activity C SHORT ANSWERS

1. During pregnancy, mother and fetus undergo physiologic changes that influence drug effects. In pregnant women, physiologic changes alter drug pharmacokinetics. In general, drug effects are less predictable because plasma volume expansion decreases plasma drug concentrations, and increased metabolism by the liver and increased elimination by the kidneys shorten the duration of drug actions and effects.

2. After drugs enter the fetal circulation, relatively large amounts are pharmacologically active, because the fetus has low levels of serum albumin and therefore low levels of drug binding. Most drug molecules are transported to the liver, where they are metabolized. Metabolism occurs slowly, because the fetal liver is immature in quantity and quality of drug-metabolizing enzymes. Drugs metabolized by the fetal liver are excreted by fetal kidneys into amniotic fluid. Excretion also is slow and inefficient due to immature development of fetal kidneys.

3. Drugs enter the brain easily because the blood–brain barrier is poorly developed in the fetus.

4. Approximately half of the drug-containing blood is transported through the umbilical arteries to the placenta, where it reenters the maternal circulation. Thus, the mother can metabolize and excrete some drug molecules for the fetus.

5. The fetus is sensitive to drug effects because it is small, has few plasma proteins that can bind drug molecules, and has a weak capacity for metabolizing and excreting drugs. In addition, the fetus is exposed to any drugs circulating in maternal blood. When drugs are taken on a regular schedule, fetal blood usually contains 50% to 100% of the amount in maternal blood. This means that any drug that stimulates or depresses the central nervous, cardiovascular, respiratory, or other body system in the mother has the potential to stimulate or depress those systems in the fetus. In some cases, fetotoxicity occurs.

SECTION II: APPLYING YOUR KNOWLEDGE

Activity D CASE STUDY

1. In women, the most common causes of infertility are ovulatory disorders, blocked fallopian tubes, endometriosis, and advanced maternal age, which affect egg quality and quantity. In men, causes include absence of sperm, declining sperm counts, testicular abnormalities, and ejaculatory dysfunction.

2. Menotropin is a gonadotropin given to women who have been diagnosed with anovulation. The drug stimulates FSA and LH to promote the development and maturation of ovarian follicles.

It should be administered subcutaneously on alternating sides of the abdomen or IM in large muscles.

3. During menotropin therapy, it is necessary to monitor both hCG and serum estradiol measurements.

4. Drugs that add in ovulation may cause ovarian hypersensitivity, which means an increased chance that more than one egg will be released from the ovary during ovulation. This could mean that more than one egg is fertilized which could lead to multiple births.

SECTION III: PRACTICING FOR NCLEX
Activity E

1. **Answer: b**
   RATIONALE: Some drugs should be avoided during lactation; all drugs should be used cautiously.

2. **Answer: d**
   RATIONALE: Drugs should be avoided during pregnancy when possible and used cautiously when required.

3. **Answer: a**
   RATIONALE: A folic acid supplement is recommended for women who may become pregnant and during pregnancy, to prevent neural tube defects.

4. **Answer: a**
   RATIONALE: Fetal organs are formed during the first trimester of pregnancy, possibly before a woman knows she is pregnant. The fetus' brain continues to develop throughout pregnancy and after birth.

5. **Answer: c, d, and e**
   RATIONALE: A few drugs are given to the mother for therapeutic effects on the fetus. These include digoxin for fetal tachycardia or heart failure, levothyroxine for hypothyroidism, penicillin for exposure to maternal syphilis and group B *Streptococcus*, and prenatal betamethasone to promote lung surfactant production. There are no medications that can be given to the mother that would be effective treatment for fetal skeletal or fetal chromosomal abnormalities.

6. **Answer: b**
   RATIONALE: Many obstetric patients with conditions such as preterm labor, hyperemesis, and elevated blood pressure are managed in the home. The home care nurse who assists in managing these patients should be an obstetric specialist who is knowledgeable about normal pregnancy and potential complications.

7. **Answer: a**
   RATIONALE: The American Academy of Pediatrics (AAP) supports breast-feeding as optimal nutrition for infants during the first year of life and does not recommend stopping maternal drug therapy unless necessary. In some instances, mothers may pump and discard breast milk while receiving therapeutic drugs, to maintain lactation.

8. **Answer: c**
   RATIONALE: Women with HIV infection should not breast-feed. The virus can be transmitted to the nursing infant.

9. **Answer: a**
   RATIONALE: Counsel pregnant women about the use of immunizations during pregnancy. Live-virus vaccines (e.g., measles, mumps, and rubella) should be avoided because of possible harmful effects to the fetus.

10. **Answer: d**
    RATIONALE: Regardless of the designated pregnancy risk category or presumed safety, no drug should be used during pregnancy unless it is clearly needed and the potential benefit to the mother outweighs the risk of potential harm to the fetus. The physician should be consulted.

11. **Answer: c**
    RATIONALE: When a health care provider is assessing the neonate, drugs received by the mother during pregnancy, labor and delivery, and lactation must be considered.

12. **Answer: d**
    RATIONALE: Hemorrhagic disease of the newborn occurs because the intestinal tract lacks the bacteria that normally synthesize vitamin K and there is little if any dietary intake of vitamin K. Vitamin K is required for liver production of several clotting factors, including prothrombin. Therefore, the neonate is at increased risk of bleeding during the first week of life. One dose of phytonadione 0.5 to 1 mg is injected at delivery or on admission to the nursery.

13. **Answer: a, d, and e**
    RATIONALE: Preferred treatment for constipation is to increase exercise and intake of fluids and high-fiber foods. If a laxative is required, the bulk-producing agent psyllium (Metamucil) is the most physiological for the mother and safest for the fetus because it is not absorbed systemically. A stool softener such as docusate or an occasional saline laxative (milk of magnesia) may also be used. Mineral oil should not be used because it interferes with absorption of fat-soluble vitamins. Castor oil and all strong laxatives should be avoided because they can cause uterine contractions and initiate labor.

14. **Answer: b**
    RATIONALE: Ophthalmia neonatorum is a form of bacterial conjunctivitis that can cause ulceration and blindness. It may be caused by several bacteria, most commonly *Chlamydia trachomatis*, a sexually transmitted organism.

15. **Answer: a**
    RATIONALE: With regional anesthesia, the mother is usually conscious and comfortable, and the neonate is rarely depressed.

16. Answer: b

RATIONALE: After a cesarean section, a long-acting form of morphine (e.g., Duramorph) may be injected into the epidural catheter to provide analgesia for up to 24 hours. Possible adverse effects include maternal urinary retention, but no significant effects on the fetus have been noted.

17. Answer: d

RATIONALE: Parenteral opioid analgesics (e.g., IV or IM meperidine, morphine, or fentanyl) are commonly used to control pain during labor and delivery. They may prolong labor and cause sedation and respiratory depression in the mother and neonate. Meperidine may cause less neonatal depression than other opioid analgesics. Butorphanol is also widely used. If neonatal respiratory depression occurs, it can be reversed by naloxone (Narcan).

18. Answer: b

RATIONALE: After delivery, Pitocin is the drug of choice for prevention or control of postpartum uterine bleeding. The drug reduces uterine bleeding by contracting uterine muscle. It also plays a role in letdown of breast milk to the nipples during lactation.

19. Answer: b, c, and e

RATIONALE: Medications used in the treatment of severe preeclampsia include labetalol, hydralazine, and magnesium sulfate. Nifedipine is an oral medication and is used to treat mild to moderate PIH. Terbutaline can be used to treat preterm labor though it is not used very frequently.

20. Answer: a

RATIONALE: Magnesium sulfate has long been given IV as a first-line agent. However, studies indicate that the drug is ineffective as a tocolytic, and some clinicians recommend stopping usage for this purpose. In addition, the drug if used, it requires special precautions for administration and monitoring due to potentially severe adverse effects. Safety measures include a unit protocol that standardizes drug concentration, flow rate, type of infusion pump, and frequency and type of assessment data to be documented (e.g., serum magnesium levels, respiratory status, reflexes, uterine activity, urine output). The antidote, calcium gluconate, should be readily available for use if hypermagnesemia occurs.

CHAPTER 7

SECTION I: ASSESSING YOUR UNDERSTANDING

Activity A   FILL IN THE BLANKS

1. thrombus
2. Blood clotting
3. embolus
4. macrophages
5. foam cells

Activity B   MATCHING

1. d   **2.** e   **3.** a   **4.** b   **5.** c

Activity C   SHORT ANSWERS

1. Hemostasis is prevention or stoppage of blood loss from an injured blood vessel and is the process that maintains the integrity of the vascular compartment. It involves activation of several mechanisms, including vasoconstriction, formation of a platelet plug (a cluster of aggregated platelets), sequential activation of clotting factors in the blood, and growth of fibrous tissue (fibrin) into the blood clot to make it more stable and to repair the tear (opening) in the damaged blood vessel.

2. When a blood clot is being formed, plasminogen (an inactive protein found in many body tissues and fluids) is bound to fibrin and becomes a component of the clot. After the outward blood flow is stopped and the tear in the blood vessel is repaired, plasminogen is activated by plasminogen activator (produced by endothelial cells or the coagulation cascade) to produce plasmin. Plasmin is an enzyme that breaks down the fibrin meshwork that stabilizes the clot; this fibrinolytic or thrombolytic action dissolves the clot.

3. Arterial thrombosis is usually associated with atherosclerotic plaque, hypertension, and turbulent blood flow. These conditions damage arterial endothelium and activate platelets to initiate the coagulation process. Arterial thrombi cause disease by obstructing blood flow. If the obstruction is incomplete or temporary, local tissue ischemia (deficient blood supply) occurs. If the obstruction is complete or prolonged, local tissue death (infarction) occurs.

4. Venous thrombosis is usually associated with venous stasis. When blood flows slowly, thrombin and other procoagulant substances present in the blood become concentrated in local areas and initiate the clotting process. With a normal rate of blood flow, these substances are rapidly removed from the blood, primarily by Kupffer's cells in the liver. A venous thrombus is less cohesive than an arterial thrombus, and an embolus can easily become detached and travel to other parts of the body.

5. Venous thrombi cause disease by two mechanisms. First, thrombosis causes local congestion, edema, and perhaps inflammation by impairing normal outflow of venous blood (e.g., thrombophlebitis, deep vein thrombosis). Second, embolization obstructs the blood supply when the embolus becomes lodged. The pulmonary arteries are common sites of embolization.

SECTION II: APPLYING YOUR KNOWLEDGE

Activity D   CASE STUDY

1. Heparin combines with antithrombin III (a natural anticoagulant in the blood) to inactivate clotting factors IX, X, XI, and XII; inhibit the conversion of prothrombin to thrombin; and prevent thrombus formation. After thrombosis has developed, heparin

can inhibit additional coagulation by inactivating thrombin, preventing the conversion of fibrinogen to fibrin, and inhibiting factor XIII (the fibrin-stabilizing factor). Other effects include inhibiting factors V and VIII and platelet aggregation.

2. Heparin acts immediately after intravenous (IV) injection and within 20 to 30 minutes after subcutaneous (Sub-Q) injection.

3. Heparin does not cross the placental barrier and is not secreted in breast milk, making it the anticoagulant of choice for use during pregnancy and lactation.

4. Heparin is prescribed for patients who are expected to be on bed rest or to have limited activity for longer than 5 days.

5. DIC is disseminated intravascular coagulation, a life-threatening condition characterized by widespread clotting, which depletes the blood of coagulation factors. Heparin is prescribed for DIC also. The goal of heparin therapy in DIC is to prevent blood coagulation long enough for clotting factors to be replenished and thus be able to control hemorrhage.

SECTION III: PRACTICING FOR NCLEX

Activity E

1. **Answer: b**
   RATIONALE: When the thrombolytic agents are used in acute myocardial infarction, cardiac dysrhythmias may occur when blood flow is reestablished; antidysrhythmic drugs should be readily available.

2. **Answer: a, b, and d**
   RATIONALE: The FDA has issued a black box warning for the use of protamine sulfate due to the risk of severe hypotension, cardiovascular collapse, noncardiogenic pulmonary edema, catastrophic pulmonary vasoconstriction, and pulmonary hypertension.

3. **Answer: b**
   RATIONALE: Alteplase is a thrombolytic, and its action is to lyse a clot, and it is indicated for use during an acute myocardial infarction. It is also used for pulmonary embolism. Heparin prevents the formation of other clots but is not intended for use to lyse a clot. Ticlopidine and clopidogrel are both adenosine diphosphate receptor antagonists and are used primarily for their antiplatelet activity.

4. **Answer: c**
   RATIONALE: Monitoring of aPTT is not necessary with low-dose standard heparin given Sub-Q for prophylaxis of thromboembolism or with the LMWHs.

5. **Answer: c**
   RATIONALE: Currently available LMWHs (dalteparin, enoxaparin) differ from standard heparin and each other and are not interchangeable.

6. **Answer: d**
   RATIONALE: The FDA has issued a black box warning for warfarin due to its risk of causing major or fatal bleeding.

7. **Answer: a, b, and d**
   RATIONALE: This drug is not suitable for long-term treatment because it must be given IV and no antidote is available in the event of an overdose or if bleeding occurs. Its duration of action is 24 hours. It requires frequent lab tests that might not be readily available. It may cause anxiety, not depression.

8. **Answer: a**
   RATIONALE: Herbs commonly used that may increase the effects of warfarin include alfalfa, celery, clove, feverfew, garlic, ginger, ginkgo biloba, ginseng, and licorice.

9. **Answer: c**
   RATIONALE: Warfarin dosage is regulated according to the INR (derived from the prothrombin [PT] time), for which a therapeutic value is between 2.0 to 3.0 in most conditions. A therapeutic PT value is approximately 1.5 times the control, or 18 seconds.

10. **Answer: b**
    RATIONALE: No antidote exists for the effects of aspirin or the adenosine diphosphate receptor antagonists, because both produce irreversible platelet effects; platelet transfusion may be required.

11. **Answer: a and b**
    RATIONALE: Thrombolytic agents are used to dissolve thrombi and limit tissue damage in selected thromboembolic disorders.

12. **Answer: c**
    RATIONALE: This drug is intended for the treatment of intermittent claudication, which is an arterial disorder. Pulmonary embolism, deep-vein thrombosis, and venous stasis are all venous disorders.

13. **Answer: d**
    RATIONALE: Anticoagulant drugs are given to prevent formation of new clots and extension of clots already present.

14. **Answer: d**
    RATIONALE: Many commonly used herbs and supplements have a profound effect on drugs used for anticoagulation. Multivitamin supplements may contain 25 to 28 µg of vitamin K and should be taken consistently to avoid fluctuating vitamin K levels.

15. **Answer: c**
    RATIONALE: Daily visits by a home care nurse may be needed if the patient or a family member is unable or unwilling to inject the medication. Platelet counts should be obtained before therapy and every 2 to 3 days during heparin therapy. Heparin should be discontinued if the platelet count falls to less than 100,000 or to less than half the baseline value.

16. **Answer: a**
    RATIONALE: Warfarin is more likely to cause bleeding in patients with liver disease because of decreased synthesis of vitamin K. In addition, warfarin is eliminated only by hepatic metabolism and may accumulate with liver impairment.

17. Answer: a
RATIONALE: Most anticoagulant, antiplatelet, and thrombolytic drugs may be used in patients with impaired renal function. For example, heparin and warfarin may be used in usual dosages, and thrombolytic agents (e.g., streptokinase, urokinase) may be used to dissolve clots in IV catheters or vascular access sites for hemodialysis.

18. Answer: c
RATIONALE: NSAIDs, which are commonly used by older adults, also have antiplatelet effects. Patients who take an NSAID daily may not need low-dose aspirin for antithrombotic effects.

19. Answer: a
RATIONALE: Thrombolytics are contraindicated when the patient has had a recent surgery or traumatic accident because the thrombolytic would disturb clots that have recently formed from the surgery. A history of a recent migraine headache, sprained ankle, or bronchitis would not contraindicate the use of a thrombolytic.

20. Answer: b
RATIONALE: When warfarin is started, PT and INR should be assessed daily until a stable daily dose is reached (the dose that maintains PT and INR within therapeutic ranges and does not cause bleeding).

CHAPTER 8

SECTION I: ASSESSING YOUR UNDERSTANDING

Activity A FILL IN THE BLANKS

1. Dyslipidemic
2. intestine
3. cell membranes
4. steroid
5. cholic acid

Activity B MATCHING

1. e   2. d   3. a   4. c   5. d

Activity C SHORT ANSWERS

1. Blood lipids are transported in plasma by specific proteins called lipoproteins. Each lipoprotein contains cholesterol, phospholipid, and triglyceride bound to protein.
2. The lipoproteins vary in density and in their amounts of lipid and protein. Density is determined mainly by the amount of protein, which is more dense than fat. Therefore, density increases as the proportion of protein increases.
3. Metabolic syndrome is a group of cardiovascular risk factors linked with obesity. *The Third Report of the National Cholesterol Education Program Expert Panel on Detection, Evaluation, and Treatment of High Blood Cholesterol in Adults* (NCEP III) clustered several elements of the metabolic syndrome: elevated waist circumference (central adiposity), elevated triglycerides, reduced high density lipoprotein

cholesterol, elevated blood pressure, and elevated fasting glucose.
4. These risk factors frequently produce an additive effect on cardiovascular, cerebrovascular, and peripheral vascular disease and are principal contributors to the significant morbidity and mortality of these conditions.
5. Improvements in insulin resistance and lipid profiles are essential lifestyle modifications and constitute first-line treatment of metabolic syndrome.

SECTION II: APPLYING YOUR KNOWLEDGE

Activity D CASE STUDY

1. Elevated total and LDL cholesterol and reduced HDL cholesterol are the abnormalities that are major risk factors for coronary artery disease. Triglycerides also play a role in cardiovascular disease. For example, high blood levels of triglycerides reflect excessive caloric intake (excessive dietary fats are stored in adipose tissue; excessive proteins and carbohydrates are converted to triglycerides and also stored in adipose tissue) and obesity.
2. For accurate interpretation of a patient's lipid profile, blood samples for laboratory testing of triglycerides should be drawn after the patient has fasted for 12 hours. Fasting is not required for cholesterol testing.
3. NCEP III recommends treatment of patients according to their blood levels of total and LDL cholesterol and their risk factors for cardiovascular disease. Therapeutic lifestyle changes (TLC), including exercise, smoking cessation, changes in diet, and drug therapy, are recommended at lower serum cholesterol levels in patients who already have cardiovascular disease or diabetes mellitus. Also, the target LDL serum level is lower in these patients. The so-called Mediterranean diet, which includes moderate amounts of monounsaturated fats (e.g., canola, olive oils) and polyunsaturated fats (e.g., safflower, corn, cottonseed, sesame, soybean, sunflower oils), also decreases risks of cardiovascular disease. Further, the patient should be encouraged to increase dietary intake of soluble fiber (e.g., psyllium preparations, oat bran, pectin, fruits, and vegetables). This diet lowers serum LDL cholesterol by 5% to 10%.

SECTION III: PRACTICING FOR NCLEX

Activity E

1. **Answer: a**
   RATIONALE: Fibrates are the most effective drugs for reducing serum triglyceride levels.
2. **Answer: c**
   RATIONALE: Skin flushing may occur with niacin.
3. **Answer: c**
   RATIONALE: Lovastatin should be taken with food; fluvastatin, pravastatin, or simvastatin should be taken in the evening, with or without food; atorvastatin may be taken with or without food and without regard to time of day.

4. Answer: a
RATIONALE: Lifestyle changes that can help improve cholesterol levels include a low-fat diet, regular aerobic exercise, losing weight, and not smoking.

5. Answer: a, b, and c
RATIONALE: Metabolic syndrome is a group of cardiovascular risk factors that are linked with obesity and include elevated waist circumference (central adiposity), elevated triglycerides, reduced high density lipoprotein cholesterol, elevated blood pressure, and elevated fasting glucose.

6. Answer: d
RATIONALE: For accurate interpretation of a patient's lipid profile, blood samples for laboratory testing of triglycerides should be drawn after the patient has fasted for 12 hours. Fasting is not required for cholesterol testing.

7. Answer: a
RATIONALE: Unless a person has a genetic disorder of lipid metabolism, the amount of cholesterol in the blood is strongly related to dietary intake of saturated fat.

8. Answer: b
RATIONALE: Flax or flax seed is used internally as a laxative and a dyslipidemic agent. Absorption of all medications may be decreased when taken with flax, resulting in a less than therapeutic effect.

9. Answer: a
RATIONALE: Niacin may cause hepatotoxicity, especially with doses greater than 2 g daily, with timed-release preparations, and if given in combination with a statin or a fibrate.

10. Answer: c
RATIONALE: Cholesterol absorption inhibitors as monotherapy (without statins) do not require dosage reduction in mild hepatic insufficiency.

11. Answer: b
RATIONALE: Statins are metabolized in the liver and may accumulate in patients with impaired hepatic function. They are contraindicated in patients with active liver disease or unexplained elevations of serum aspartate or alanine aminotransferase.

12. Answer: b
RATIONALE: Fluvastatin is cleared hepatically, and less than 6% of the dose is excreted in urine; therefore, dosage reduction for mild to moderate renal impairment is unnecessary. Use caution with severe impairment. Recent randomized, controlled clinical trials have demonstrated the drug's safety in kidney transplant recipients.

13. Answer: d
RATIONALE: In postmenopausal women, estrogen replacement therapy increases HDL cholesterol.

14. Answer: a
RATIONALE: Dyslipidemic drugs are not recommended for children younger than 10 years of age, except for pravastatin, which has dosing recommendations for children as young as 8 years.

15. Answer: c
RATIONALE: Despite an increased prevalence of diabetes and obesity, American Indians appear to have lower cholesterol levels than the United States population as a whole. This suggests that diet and exercise may be more useful than lipid-lowering drugs for this group.

16. Answer: a, b, and c
RATIONALE: To lower cholesterol and triglycerides, a statin (atorvastatin), a cholesterol absorption inhibitor (ezetimibe), gemfibrozil, or niacin may be used. A bile acid sequestrant agent (cholestyramine and colesevelam) is not recommended to lower both cholesterol and triglycerides.

17. Answer: a
RATIONALE: A fibrate–statin combination should be avoided because of increased risks of severe myopathy. A niacin–statin combination increases the risks of hepatotoxicity.

18. Answer: c
RATIONALE: The cholesterol absorption inhibitors (e.g., ezetimibe), the newest class of dyslipidemic drugs, act in the small intestine to inhibit absorption of cholesterol and decrease the delivery of intestinal cholesterol to the liver, resulting in reduced hepatic cholesterol stores and increased clearance of cholesterol from the blood. This distinct mechanism is complementary to that of HMG-CoA reductase inhibitors.

19. Answer: d
RATIONALE: Niacin (nicotinic acid) decreases both cholesterol and triglycerides. It inhibits mobilization of free fatty acids from peripheral tissues, thereby reducing hepatic synthesis of triglycerides and secretion of VLDL, which leads to decreased production of LDL cholesterol.

20. Answer: d
RATIONALE: In conjunction with an acceptable total cholesterol-to-HDL ratio, it is also important for the LDL reading to be between 80 and 100 mg/dL to further decrease the risk of coronary artery disease.

CHAPTER 9

SECTION I: ASSESSING YOUR UNDERSTANDING

Activity A FILL IN THE BLANKS
1. pluripotent
2. cytokines
3. hematopoiesis
4. Interferons
5. immunostimulants

Activity B MATCHING
1. d   2. a   3. e   4. b   5. c

Activity C SHORT ANSWERS

1. Clinical manifestations of inadequate erythropoiesis include anemia. This results in a decrease in the oxygen-carrying capacity of blood and consequently a decrease in oxygen availability to the tissues. A compensatory increase in heart rate and cardiac output initially increases cardiac output, offsetting the lower oxygen-carrying capacity of the blood. However, the oxygen demand becomes greater than the supply, and clinical manifestations are directly attributable to tissue hypoxia. Muscle weakness and easy fatigability are common.

2. Exogenous drug preparations have the same mechanisms of action as the endogenous products. CSF binds to receptors on the cell surfaces of immature blood cells in the bone marrow and increases the number, maturity, and functional ability of the cells. Interferons, called alfa, beta, or gamma according to specific characteristics, also bind to specific cell-surface receptors and alter intracellular activities. In viral infections, they induce enzymes that inhibit protein synthesis and degrade viral ribonucleic acid. As a result, viruses are less able to enter uninfected cells, reproduce, and release new viruses.

3. In addition to their antiviral effects, interferons also have antiproliferative and immunoregulatory activities. They can increase expression of major histocompatibility complex (MHC) molecules, augment the activity of natural killer (NK) cells, increase the effectiveness of antigen-presenting cells in inducing the proliferation of cytotoxic T cells, aid the attachment of cytotoxic T cells to target cells, and inhibit angiogenesis (formation of blood vessels). Because of these characteristics, the interferons are used mainly to treat viral infections and cancers.

4. Exogenous cytokines are given by subcutaneous (Sub-Q) or intravenous (IV) injection because they are proteins that would be destroyed by digestive enzymes if given orally.

5. Immunostimulants are drugs that enhance immune function; they help a person fight disease. Health care providers use these drugs to restore normal function or to increase the ability of the immune system to eliminate potentially harmful invaders.

SECTION II: APPLYING YOUR KNOWLEDGE

Activity D CASE STUDY

1. Epoetin alfa is a drug formulation of a hormone, erythropoiesis, from the kidneys that stimulates bone marrow production of red blood cells. Erythropoiesis-stimulating drugs have been used to raise the hemoglobin level and reduce the need for blood transfusions in many patients with anemia. Epoetin is prescribed at the lowest dose that is effective in raising hemoglobin levels just enough to avoid the need for blood transfusion. The hemoglobin levels must be regularly monitored until they stabilize.

2. Exogenous cytokines are given by subcutaneous (Sub-Q) or intravenous (IV) injection. Mrs. Cantos must be taught how to administer these injections for herself.

3. Studies indicated an increased risk of serious cardiovascular problems (e.g., hypertension, thrombo-embolic events) and death in patients with chronic renal failure and an increased risk of tumor progression and death in patients with cancer. These problems became evident when the drugs were used to achieve normal hemoglobin levels of 12 to 14 grams per deciliter (g/dL). A black box warning for this drug advises prescribers to avoid using Epogen in patients with hemoglobin values of 12 g/dL or greater.

SECTION III: PRACTICING FOR NCLEX

Activity E

1. **Answer: a**
   RATIONALE: All hematopoietic and immune blood cells are derived from stem cells in the bone marrow.

2. **Answer: c**
   RATIONALE: Cytokines regulate the immune response by stimulating or inhibiting the activation, proliferation, and differentiation of various cells and by regulating the secretion of antibodies or other cytokines.

3. **Answer: b**
   RATIONALE: Interferons are used mainly for viral hepatitis and certain types of cancer.

4. **Answer: a**
   RATIONALE: Filgrastim is used to increase white blood cells and decrease risks of infection in patients who have or are at high risk for severe neutropenia.

5. **Answer: c**
   RATIONALE: Adverse effects of epoetin and darbepoetin include increased risks of hypertension, myocardial infarction, and stroke, especially when used to increase hemoglobin above 12 g/dL.

6. **Answer: a**
   RATIONALE: Epoetin is not effective unless sufficient iron is present, and most patients need an iron supplement. When an iron preparation is prescribed, the home care nurse may need to emphasize the importance of taking it.

7. **Answer: d**
   RATIONALE: With filgrastim, the nurse may need to help the patient and family with techniques to reduce exposure to infection.

8. **Answer: a**
   RATIONALE: With preexisting hepatic impairment, sargramostim increases serum bilirubin and liver enzymes. Values decline to baseline levels when the drug is stopped or its dosage is reduced. Liver function tests are recommended every 2 weeks for patients with preexisting impairment.

9. **Answer: c**
   RATIONALE: Hepatitis B becomes chronic in 5% to 10% of patients. Interferon alfa and lamivudine or other antiviral drugs may be used for treatment. Drug resistance may develop, and active hepatitis may resume when the drugs are discontinued.

10. **Answer: a**
   RATIONALE: Interferon alfa has demonstrated antitumor effects in multiple myeloma, renal cell carcinoma, and others.

11. **Answer: b**
   RATIONALE: In hairy cell leukemia, interferons normalize WBC counts in 70% to 90% of patients. Drug therapy must be continued indefinitely to avoid relapse, which usually develops rapidly after the drug is discontinued.

12. **Answer: d**
   RATIONALE: When sargramostim is given to patients with cancer who have undergone bone marrow transplantation, the drug should be started 2 to 4 hours after the bone marrow infusion and at least 24 hours after the last dose of antineoplastic chemotherapy or 12 hours after the last radiotherapy treatment.

13. **Answer: b**
   RATIONALE: With darbepoetin and epoetin, iron stores (transferrin saturation and serum ferritin) should be measured before and periodically during treatment. Hemoglobin should be measured twice weekly until the level is stabilized and maintenance drug doses are established.

14. **Answer: b**
   RATIONALE: With darbepoetin and epoetin, dosage is adjusted to achieve and maintain a hemoglobin value of no more than 12 g/dL (serous adverse effects may occur with values higher than 12 g/dL). Dosage should be reduced if the hemoglobin level approaches 12 g/dL or increases by more than 1 g/dL in any 2-week period.

15. **Answer: c and e**
   RATIONALE: Patients who are neutropenic will have a history of frequent colds and flu and also opportunistic infections such as thrush. Shortness of breath while walking is a symptom of anemia. Easy bruising and bleeding from the gums are examples of thrombocytopenia.

16. **Answer: b**
   RATIONALE: The most important assessment is the blood pressure because epoetin can cause hypertension.

17. **Answer: a**
   RATIONALE: Filgrastim must be held for 24 hours prior to a patient receiving chemotherapy.

18. **Answer: d**
   RATIONALE: Interferon should not be administered to newborns or infant. A baby is considered an infant until 12 months of age.

19. **Answer: c**
   RATIONALE: The patient should return to the clinic as soon as possible for reevaluation. If the patient is depressed, the medication will need to be stopped because the patient can also develop psychiatric symptoms such as hallucinations.

20. **Answer: c**
   RATIONALE: A patient with a low WBC should avoid crowds to reduce the chance of coming into contact with a person who has an infection such as a cold, which could be very serious in a person who has little defense against infection.

CHAPTER 10

SECTION I: ASSESSING YOUR UNDERSTANDING

Activity A FILL IN THE BLANKS

1. Immunization
2. Vaccines
3. Attenuated
4. Toxoids
5. boosters

Activity B MATCHING

1. c   **2.** e   **3.** a   **4.** b   **5.** d

Activity C SHORT ANSWERS

1. Additional components of vaccines and toxoids may include aluminum phosphate, aluminum hydroxide, or calcium phosphate. Products containing aluminum should be given intramuscularly only, because they cannot be given intravenously and greater tissue irritation occurs with subcutaneous injections.
2. Additives are used to delay absorption and increase antigenicity.
3. Preparations used for immunization are biologic products prepared by pharmaceutical companies and regulated by the U.S. Food and Drug Administration (FDA). Widespread use of these products has dramatically decreased the incidence of many infectious diseases.
4. The single vaccines for measles, mumps, and rubella have been largely replaced by the combination product containing all three vaccines (MMR).
5. Immunization of prepubertal girls or women of childbearing age against rubella is important because rubella during the first trimester of pregnancy is associated with a high incidence of birth defects in the newborn.

SECTION II: APPLYING YOUR KNOWLEDGE

Activity D CASE STUDY

1. The immune globulin will give temporary immunity to people exposed to a particular disease. Immune serums are the biologic products used for passive immunity. They act rapidly to provide temporary (1–3 months) immunity in people who have been exposed to or are experiencing a particular disease. You can explain to the patient

that immune globulin products are made from the serum of people with high concentrations of the specific antibody or immunoglobulin (Ig) required and will not cause the disease.

2. The goal of therapy is to prevent or modify the disease process (i.e., decrease the incidence and severity of symptoms).

3. These products may consist of whole serum or of the immunoglobulin portion of serum in which the specific antibodies are concentrated. Immuno-globulin fractions are preferred over whole serum because they are more likely to be effective. Plasma used to prepare these products is negative for hepatitis B surface antigen (HB_sAg).

4. Hyperimmune serums are available for cytomegalovirus, hepatitis B, rabies, rubella, tetanus, varicella zoster (shingles), and respiratory syncytial virus infections.

SECTION III: PRACTICING FOR NCLEX
Activity E

1. **Answer: b**
   RATIONALE: Health care providers need to assess and inform patients about recommended immunizations.

2. **Answer: b**
   RATIONALE: For patients with active malignant disease, live vaccines should not be given. Although killed vaccines and toxoids may be given, antibody production may be inadequate to provide immunity. If possible, patients should receive needed immunizations 2 weeks before or 3 months after immunosuppressive radiation or chemotherapy treatments.

3. **Answer: c**
   RATIONALE: For children with HIV infection, most routine immunizations (DTaP, IPV, MMR, Hib, influenza) are recommended.

4. **Answer: c**
   RATIONALE: Patients with asymptomatic HIV who are exposed to chickenpox should receive the varicella-zoster immune globulin for passive immunizations. Vaccinations are not intended to provide the immediate immunity needed when exposed to a disease and may be appropriate for a patient with HIV.

5. **Answer: c**
   RATIONALE: Patients with HIV infection have less-than-optimal responses to immunizing agents because the disease produces major defects in cell-mediated and humoral immunity. Live bacterial (BCG, oral typhoid) or viral (MMR, varicella) vaccines should not be given, because the bacteria or viruses may be able to reproduce and cause active infection.

6. **Answer: d**
   RATIONALE: Persons with asymptomatic HIV infection should receive inactivated vaccines; those exposed to measles or varicella may be given immune globulin or varicella-zoster immune globulin for passive immunization.

7. **Answer: b**
   RATIONALE: Patients who have been on a systemic corticosteroid longer than 2 weeks should wait 3 months before receiving a live virus vaccine.

8. **Answer: d**
   RATIONALE: Long-term alternate-day therapy with short-acting corticosteroids; maintenance physiologic doses; and the use of topical, aerosol, or intra-articular injections are not contraindications to immunization.

9. **Answer: c**
   RATIONALE: Immunizations are not contraindicated with short-term use (less than 2 weeks) or low-to-moderate doses (less than 20 mg/d) of prednisone.

10. **Answer: d**
    RATIONALE: Patients with active malignant disease may be given killed vaccines or toxoids but should not be given live vaccines. (An exception is persons with leukemia who have not received chemotherapy for at least 3 months.)

11. **Answer: b**
    RATIONALE: When vaccines are used, they should be given at least 2 weeks before the start of chemotherapy or 3 months after chemotherapy is completed. Passive immunity with immunoglobulins may be used in place of active immunity.

12. **Answer: a, b, c, and e**
    RATIONALE: Patients diagnosed with diabetes mellitus or chronic pulmonary, renal, or hepatic disorders who are not receiving immunosuppressant drugs may be given both live attenuated and killed vaccines and toxoids to induce active immunity. They may also receive immune globulin serums if needed to provide passive immunity.

13. **Answer: b**
    RATIONALE: Vaccine to prevent shingles is available for adults aged 60 years and older.

14. **Answer: b**
    RATIONALE: The pneumococcal vaccine is recommended for children older than 2 years of age who have had a splenectomy. The quadrivalent human papillomavirus vaccine is recommended for adolescents. The Hib vaccine is recommended for infants, and the shingles vaccine is recommended for adults who previously have had chickenpox.

15. **Answer: d**
    RATIONALE: Patients who have diabetes mellitus may require increased dosage and more frequent administration of vaccines.

16. **Answer: a, c, and d**
    RATIONALE: Recommended immunizations for older adults have usually consisted of a tetanus–diphtheria (Td) booster every 10 years, annual influenza vaccine, and a one-time administration of pneumococcal vaccine at 65 years of age. Rotavirus vaccine is recommended for infants.

17. **Answer: a**
    RATIONALE: A second dose of pneumococcal vaccine may be given at age 65 years if the first dose was given 5 years previously.

18. Answer: a and b
RATIONALE: Adolescents who received all primary immunizations as infants and young children should have a second dose of varicella (chickenpox) vaccine, hepatitis A and hepatitis B vaccines (if not received earlier), a tetanus–diphtheria–pertussis booster (Tdap) between 11 and 18 years if 5 years has passed since a tetanus–diphtheria (Td) booster was given, and meningococcal vaccine at 11 or 12 years of age. The shingles vaccine is recommended for older adults who have had chickenpox as a child.

19. Answer: b
RATIONALE: MMR is administered to adolescent females if they are not pregnant and their rubella titer is inadequate or proof of immunization is unavailable.

20. Answer: d
RATIONALE: Recommendations regarding immunizations change periodically as additional information and new immunizing agents become available. Consequently, health care providers need to update their knowledge at least annually. The best source of information for current recommendations is the Centers for Disease Control and Prevention (http://www.cdc.gov).

CHAPTER 11

SECTION I: ASSESSING YOUR UNDERSTANDING

Activity A FILL IN THE BLANKS
1. cytokines
2. antigens
3. proteins
4. immunosuppressant
5. immunosuppression

Activity B MATCHING
1. d   **2.** a   **3.** c   **4.** b   **5.** e

Activity C SHORT ANSWERS
1. An appropriate but undesirable immune response occurs when foreign tissue is transplanted into the body. If the immune response is not suppressed, the body reacts as with other antigens and attempts to destroy the foreign tissue (graft rejection reaction). Although numerous advances have been made in transplantation technology, the immune response remains a major factor in determining the success or failure of transplantation.
2. Tumor necrosis factor (TNF)-alpha is a cytokine that plays a major role in the response to infection. Functions of TNF include activation of monocytes, macrophages, and cytotoxic T cells; enhancement of natural killer (NK) cell functions; increased leukocyte movement into areas of tissue injury; increased phagocytosis by neutrophils; and stimulation of B and T lymphocytes. Despite the beneficial effects of a "normal" amount of TNF, however, an excessive TNF response has been associated with the pathogenesis of autoimmune disorders such as RA and Crohn's disease.
3. Several factors prevent the immune system from "turning off" the abnormal immune or inflammatory process. One of these factors may be an inadequate number of suppressor T cells, which are thought to be a subpopulation of helper or cytotoxic T cells. Another factor may be inadequate amounts of anti-inflammatory cytokines (e.g., interleukin-10).
4. A rejection reaction occurs when the host's immune system is stimulated to destroy the transplanted organ. The immune cells of the transplant recipient attach to the donor cells of the transplanted organ and react against the antigens of the donor organ. The rejection process involves T and B lymphocytes, antibodies, multiple cytokines, and inflammatory mediators. In general, T-cell activation and proliferation are more important in the rejection reaction than B-cell activation and formation of antibodies. Cytotoxic and helper T cells are activated; activated helper T cells stimulate B cells to produce antibodies, leading to a delayed hypersensitivity reaction. The antibodies injure the transplanted organ by activating complement, producing antigen–antibody complexes, or causing antibody-mediated tissue breakdown.
5. Acute reactions may occur from 10 days to a few months after transplantation and mainly involve cellular immunity and proliferation of T lymphocytes. Characteristics include signs of organ failure and vasculitis lesions that often lead to arterial narrowing or obliteration. Treatment with immunosuppressant drugs is usually effective in ensuring short-term survival of the transplant but does not prevent chronic rejection.

SECTION II: APPLYING YOUR KNOWLEDGE
Activity D CASE STUDY
1. With bone marrow/stem cell transplantation, the donor cells mount an immune response (mainly by stimulating T lymphocytes) against antigens on the host's tissues, producing GVHD. Tissue damage is produced directly by the action of cytotoxic T cells or indirectly through the release of inflammatory mediators (e.g., complement) and cytokines (e.g., TNF-alpha, interleukins).
2. Acute GVHD occurs in 30% to 50% of patients, usually within 6 weeks after transplant. Signs and symptoms include delayed recovery of blood cell production in the bone marrow, skin rash, liver dysfunction (indicated by increased alkaline phosphatase, aminotransferases, and bilirubin), and diarrhea. The skin reaction is usually a pruritic maculopapular rash that begins on the palms and soles and may extend over the entire body. Liver

involvement can lead to bleeding disorders and coma. Chronic GVHD occurs when symptoms persist or occur 100 days or longer after transplantation. It is characterized by abnormal humoral and cellular immunity, severe skin disorders, and liver disease. Chronic GVHD appears to be an autoimmune disorder in which activated T cells perceive self-antigens as foreign antigens.

3. Methotrexate is used (with cyclosporine) to prevent GVHD after bone marrow transplantation. Lower doses are given for these conditions than for treatment of cancers, and adverse drug effects are fewer and less severe. When methotrexate is administered, CBC, platelet counts, and renal and liver function tests should be monitored.

SECTION III: PRACTICING FOR NCLEX
Activity E

1. **Answer: a**
RATIONALE: Newer immunosuppressants have more specific effects on the immune system and may cause fewer or less severe adverse effects than older drugs.

2. **Answer: a**
RATIONALE: Cyclosporine and tacrolimus are similar drugs that are effective immunosuppressants, are widely used in organ transplantation, cause nephrotoxicity, and are subject to numerous drug interactions (enzyme-inhibiting drugs increase blood levels and enzyme-inducing drugs decrease blood levels).

3. **Answer: c**
RATIONALE: Immunosuppressant drugs greatly increase risk of infection.

4. **Answer: d**
RATIONALE: With current treatments, most transplant patients must be maintained on immunosuppressive drug therapy for the rest of their lives.

5. **Answer: c**
RATIONALE: Psoriasis is an autoimmune disorder that causes a skin condition and may also cause arthritic changes in the joints, a condition called psoriatic arthritis. Rheumatoid arthritis, Crohn's disease, and graft versus host disease are all autoimmune disorders that do not have both skin and arthritic joint changes.

6. **Answer: b**
RATIONALE: With patients who are taking immunosuppressant drugs, a major role of the home care nurse is to assess the environment for potential sources of infection, assist patients and other members of the household to understand the patient's susceptibility to infection, and teach ways to decrease risks of infection. Although infections often develop from the patient's own body flora, other potential sources include people with infections, caregivers, water or soil around live plants, and raw fruits and vegetables.

7. **Answer: d**
RATIONALE: Leflunomide may be hepatotoxic in patients with normal liver function and is not recommended for use in patients with liver impairment or in patients with positive serology tests for hepatitis B or C.

8. **Answer: c**
RATIONALE: Tacrolimus is metabolized in the liver by the cytochrome P450 enzyme system. Impaired liver function may decrease presystemic (first-pass) metabolism of oral tacrolimus and produce higher blood levels. Also, the elimination half-life is significantly longer. As a result, dosage must be decreased in patients with impaired liver function.

9. **Answer: c**
RATIONALE: Sirolimus is extensively metabolized in the liver and may accumulate in the presence of hepatic impairment. The maintenance dose should be reduced by 35%; it is not necessary to reduce the loading dose.

10. **Answer: a**
RATIONALE: Cyclosporine is nephrotoxic but is commonly used in patients with renal and other transplants. Nephrotoxicity usually subsides with decreased dosage or stopping the drug. In renal transplant recipients, when serum creatinine and blood urea nitrogen levels remain elevated, a complete evaluation of the patient must be done to differentiate cyclosporine-induced nephrotoxicity from a transplant rejection reaction.

11. **Answer: b**
RATIONALE: Immunosuppressants are used for the same purposes and produce similar therapeutic and adverse effects in older adults as in younger adults. Because older adults often have multiple disorders and organ impairments, it is especially important that drug choices, dosages, and monitoring tests be individualized. In addition, infections occur more commonly in older adults, and this tendency is increased with immunosuppressant therapy.

12. **Answer: b and c**
RATIONALE: A patient who may be experiencing organ rejection may develop weight gain, edema, fever, decreased urine output, and flank tenderness over the graft organ site.

13. **Answer: b**
RATIONALE: Most immunosuppressants are used in children for the same disorders and with similar effects as in adults. Corticosteroids impair growth in children. As a result, some transplantation centers avoid prednisone therapy until a rejection episode occurs.

14. **Answer: a, c, and e**
RATIONALE: Patients who use long-term immunosuppressant agents are at risk for malignancies (especially lymphoma), hypertension, metabolic bone disease, and renal and hepatic dysfunction. Migraine headaches are not a complication of long-term immunosuppressant therapy.

15. Answer: d
RATIONALE: Opportunistic infections can occur as a result of using TNF-alpha blocking agents. Rheumatoid arthritis, systemic lupus erythematosus, and psoriasis are autoimmune disorders.

16. Answer: c
RATIONALE: A woman of childbearing age who is prescribed mycophenolate mofetil must have a negative pregnancy test and must agree to use contraception while taking this medication.

17. Answer: b
RATIONALE: Rheumatoid arthritis is an abnormal immune response that leads to inflammation and damage of joint cartilage and bone. It is thought to involve the activation of T lymphocytes, release of inflammatory cytokines, and formation of antibodies.

18. Answer: d
RATIONALE: Psoriatic arthritis is a type of arthritis associated with psoriasis that is similar to RA. It may be characterized by extensive and disabling joint damage, especially in hand and finger joints. Etanercept (Enbrel) is a TNF-alpha inhibitor approved for treatment of psoriatic arthritis.

19. Answer: d
RATIONALE: Crohn's disease is a chronic, recurrent, inflammatory bowel disorder that can affect any area of the GI tract.

20. Answer: c
RATIONALE: One of the most common adverse effects associated with methotrexate is stomatitis or oral mucositis. This may cause nutritional impairment. The patient doesn't commonly develop fever, severe nausea, or constipation.

CHAPTER 12

SECTION I: ASSESSING YOUR UNDERSTANDING
Activity A FILL IN THE BLANKS
1. Oncology
2. Chemotherapy
3. cancer
4. Normal
5. cell cycle

Activity B MATCHING
1. b   2. d   3. a   4. e   5. c

Activity C SHORT ANSWERS
1. Antimetabolites are diverse drugs that are allowed to enter cancer cells because they are similar to metabolites or nutrients needed by the cells for reproduction. Inside the cell, the drugs replace normal metabolites or inhibit essential enzymes. These actions deprive the cell of substances needed for formation of DNA or cause formation of abnormal DNA.

2. Antimetabolites are cell cycle–specific because they exert their cytotoxic effects only during the S phase of the cell's reproductive cycle, when DNA is being synthesized.

3. The nitrosoureas (e.g., carmustine, lomustine) are unique in being lipid soluble and able to cross the blood–brain barrier; hence, they are widely used in the treatment of brain tumors. Carmustine is also formulated as a dissolving wafer, which can be implanted in the brain tissue at the time of surgical tumor resection.

4. The toxic effects of folic acid antagonists include bone marrow depression, mucositis and ulceration of the GI tract, and hair loss.

5. Folic acid antagonists (e.g., methotrexate [prototype]), purine antagonists (e.g., mercaptopurine), and pyrimidine antagonists (e.g., fluorouracil) are most effective against rapidly growing tumors, and individual drugs vary in their effectiveness with different kinds of cancer.

SECTION II: APPLYING YOUR KNOWLEDGE
Activity D CASE STUDY
1. Most cytotoxic antineoplastic drugs kill malignant cells by interfering with cell replication, with the supply and use of nutrients (e.g., amino acids, purines, pyrimidines), or with the genetic materials in the cell nucleus (DNA or RNA). Each drug dose kills a specific percentage of cells. To achieve a cure, all malignant cells must be killed or reduced to a small number that can be killed by the person's immune system.

2. Doxorubicin and daunorubicin are available in conventional and liposomal preparations. The liposomal preparations increase drug concentration in malignant tissues and decrease concentration in normal tissues, thereby increasing effectiveness while decreasing toxicity (e.g., cardiotoxicity). With treatment of leukemias and lymphomas, a serious, life-threatening adverse effect called tumor lysis syndrome may occur. This syndrome occurs when large numbers of cancer cells are killed or damaged and release their contents into the bloodstream.

3. This patient needs more teaching, because he has not demonstrated accurate understanding of his condition. With tumor lysis syndrome, hyperkalemia, hyperphosphatemia, hyperuricemia, hypomagnesemia, hypocalcemia, and acidosis develop. Signs and symptoms depend on the severity of the metabolic imbalances but may include GI upset, fatigue, altered mental status, hypertension, muscle cramps, paresthesias (numbness and tingling), tetany, seizures, electrocardiographic changes (e.g., dysrhythmias), cardiac arrest, reduced urine output, and acute renal failure.

4. Tumor lysis syndrome can be prevented or minimized by aggressive hydration with IV normal saline, alkalinization with IV sodium bicarbonate, and administration of allopurinol (e.g., 300 mg daily

for adults, 10 mg/kg/d for children) to reduce uric acid levels. Maintaining a urine pH of 7 or higher prevents renal failure from precipitation of uric acid crystals in the kidneys. Treatment of hyperkalemia may include IV dextrose and regular insulin (to drive potassium into cells) or Kayexalate to eliminate potassium in feces. Treatment of hyperphosphatemia may include administration of aluminum hydroxide or another phosphate-binding agent.

SECTION III: PRACTICING FOR NCLEX

Activity E

1. Answer: d
RATIONALE: Cancer in older adults presents a unique challenge, due in part to the presence of comorbidities and the physical, biologic, and physiologic changes that occur with normal aging. Until recently, older adults were excluded from participating in clinical trials.

2. Answer: c
RATIONALE: Hormonal therapies that block the effects of estrogen (in an estrogen-responsive tumor) and androgen (in an androgen-responsive tumor), respectively, are essential in the treatment of breast and prostate cancers.

3. Answer: a, c, and d
RATIONALE: The most common adverse effects of chemotherapy include alopecia, neutropenia, thrombocytopenia, and anemia as well or oral mucositis. Stomach ulcers may occur in some patients, but it is not a common adverse effect.

4. Answer: a
RATIONALE: Traditional cytotoxic antineoplastic drugs are nonselective in their effect on proliferating cells; therefore, bone marrow toxicity is a common adverse effect of many cytotoxic drugs. These drugs kill the same fraction of cells with each cycle of chemotherapy treatment; repeated cycles of cytotoxic drugs potentially lower the number of cancer cells to a level where a person's immune responses are able to take over and destroy the remaining cancer cells.

5. Answer: a
RATIONALE: Patients may receive parenteral cytotoxic drugs as outpatients and return home, or these and other antineoplastic drugs may be administered at home by the patient or a caregiver. If a patient is receiving erythropoietin or oprelvekin subcutaneously, the patient or a caregiver may need to be taught injection technique.

6. Answer: c
RATIONALE: Some antineoplastic drugs are hepatotoxic, and many are metabolized in the liver. With impaired hepatic function, risks of further impairment or accumulation of toxic drug levels are increased. However, abnormal values for the usual liver function tests (e.g., aspartate aminotransferase [AST], alanine aminotransferase [ALT], bilirubin, alkaline phosphatase) may indicate liver injury but do not indicate decreased ability to metabolize drugs. Patients with metastatic cancer often have impaired liver function.

7. Answer: c
RATIONALE: L-Asparaginase is hepatotoxic in most patients; it may increase preexisting hepatic impairment and hepatotoxicity of other medications. Signs of liver impairment, which usually subsides when the drug is discontinued, include increased AST, ALT, alkaline phosphatase, and bilirubin and decreased serum albumin, cholesterol, and plasma fibrinogen.

8. Answer: d
RATIONALE: Capecitabine blood levels are significantly increased with hepatic impairment, and patients with liver metastases should be monitored closely.

9. Answer: d
RATIONALE: Some antineoplastic drugs are nephrotoxic (e.g., cisplatin, MTX), and many are excreted through the kidneys. In the presence of impaired renal function, risks of further impairment or accumulation of toxic drug levels are increased. Therefore, renal function should be monitored carefully during therapy, and drug dosages are often reduced based on CrCl levels.

10. Answer: b, c, and d
RATIONALE: Symptoms of tumor lysis syndrome include decreased urine output, numbness and tingling of the extremities, GI disturbances, altered mental status, and hypertension.

11. Answer: a, c, d, and e
RATIONALE: In addition to comorbidities, issues that affect treatment for older adults include access to care, financial and transportation issues, functional status, need for independence, social support, and physiologic age-related changes.

12. Answer: d
RATIONALE: Creatinine clearance (CrCl) should be monitored; serum creatinine level is not a reliable indicator of renal function in older adults because of their decreased muscle mass.

13. Answer: c
RATIONALE: In recent years, there have been rapid advances in cancer care for children and high cure rates for many pediatric malignancies. Many of these advances have resulted from the systematic enrollment of children in well-designed clinical trials.

14. Answer: b
RATIONALE: Many chemotherapeutic drugs must be administered IV because the enzymes in the stomach deactivate the medication.

15. Answer: b
RATIONALE: Dosage of cytotoxic drugs for children should be based on body surface area, because this measurement takes size into account.

16. Answer: a
RATIONALE: Children who receive an anthracycline drug (e.g., doxorubicin) are at increased risk of developing cardiotoxic effects (e.g., heart failure) during treatment or after receiving the drug.

Efforts to reduce cardiotoxicity include using alternative drugs when effective, giving smaller cumulative doses of anthracycline drug, and observing patients closely so that early manifestations can be recognized and treated before heart failure occurs.

17. Answer: a, b, and c
RATIONALE: Most cytotoxic antineoplastic drugs are carcinogenic, mutagenic, and teratogenic. Exposure during pregnancy increases risks of fetal abnormalities, ectopic pregnancy, and spontaneous abortion.

18. Answer: a
RATIONALE: When handling cytotoxic antineoplastic drugs, the nurse should avoid direct contact with solutions for injection by wearing gloves, face shields, and protective clothing (e.g., disposable, liquid-impermeable gowns).

19. Answer: d
RATIONALE: When caring for patients receiving cytotoxic antineoplastic drugs, wear gloves when handling patients' clothing, bed linens, or excreta. Blood and body fluids are contaminated with drugs or metabolites for about 48 hours after a dose.

20. Answer: b
RATIONALE: When both hormone inhibitor and cytotoxic drug therapies are needed, they are not given concurrently, because hormone antagonists decrease malignant cell growth and cytotoxic agents are most effective when the cells are actively dividing.

CHAPTER 13

SECTION I: ASSESSING YOUR UNDERSTANDING

Activity A FILL IN THE BLANKS
1. Antimicrobial
2. microorganisms
3. Viruses
4. adenoviruses
5. Fungi

Activity B MATCHING
1. b   2. e   3. a   4. c   5. d

Activity C SHORT ANSWERS
1. The human body and the environment contain many microorganisms, most of which do not cause disease and live in a state of balance with the human host. When the balance is upset and infection occurs, the characteristics of the infecting microorganisms and the adequacy of host defense mechanisms are major factors in the severity of the infection and the person's ability to recover. Conditions that impair defense mechanisms increase the incidence and severity of infections and impede recovery. In addition, use of antimicrobial drugs may lead to serious infections caused by drug-resistant microorganisms.
2. Normal flora protects the human host by occupying space and consuming nutrients. This interferes with the ability of potential pathogens to establish residence and proliferate. If the normal flora is suppressed by antimicrobial drug therapy, potential pathogens may thrive. For example, the yeast *Candida albicans* is a normal resident of the vagina and the intestinal tract. An antibacterial drug may destroy the normal bacterial flora without affecting the fungal organism. As a result, *C. albicans* can proliferate and cause infection. Much of the normal flora can cause disease under certain conditions, especially in elderly, debilitated, or immune-suppressed people. Normal bowel flora also synthesizes vitamin K and vitamin B complex.
3. Colonization involves the presence of normal microbial flora or transient environmental organisms that do not harm the host. Infectious disease involves the presence of a pathogen plus clinical signs and symptoms indicative of an infection. These microorganisms are usually spread by direct contact with an infected person or contaminated hands, food, water, or objects.
4. Opportunistic infections are likely to occur in people with severe burns, cancer, human immunodeficiency virus (HIV) infection, indwelling intravenous (IV) or urinary catheters, and antibiotic or corticosteroid drug therapy.
5. Broad-spectrum antibiotics affect the bacteria for which they are prescribed, transient organisms, other pathogens, and normal flora.

SECTION II: APPLYING YOUR KNOWLEDGE

Activity D CASE STUDY
1. The human body normally has areas that are sterile and areas that are colonized with microorganisms. Sterile areas are body fluids and cavities, the lower respiratory tract (trachea, bronchi, lungs), much of the gastrointestinal (GI) and genitourinary tracts, and the musculoskeletal system. Colonized areas include the skin, upper respiratory tract, and colon.
2. Microorganisms that are part of the normal flora and nonpathogenic in one area of the body may be pathogenic in other parts of the body; for example, *Escherichia coli* often causes urinary tract infections. Normal flora protects the human host by occupying space and consuming nutrients. This interferes with the ability of potential pathogens to establish residence and proliferate. Normal bowel flora synthesizes vitamin K and vitamin B complex.
3. If the normal flora is suppressed by antimicrobial drug therapy, pathogens may thrive. Normal flora may cause disease when antibiotics are used. For example, *Candida albicans* is a normal resident of the vagina and the intestinal tract. An antibacterial drug may destroy the normal bacterial flora without affecting the fungal organism. As a result, *C. albicans* can proliferate and cause infection. Much of the normal flora can cause disease under certain conditions, especially in elderly, debilitated, or immunosuppressed people.

SECTION III: PRACTICING FOR NCLEX

Activity E

1. Answer: a
RATIONALE: Patient education related to antibiotic therapy should stress the importance of completing a full course of antibiotics as prescribed.

2. Answer: a and b
RATIONALE: Inappropriate use of antibiotics increases adverse drug effects, infections with drug-resistant microorganisms, and health care costs as well as reduce the number of available effective drugs for serious or antibiotic-resistant infections. It causes increased resistance to antibiotics, not increased sensitivity to them.

3. Answer: a
RATIONALE: Check specific recommendations with regard to the administration of the antibiotic with food and other medications to decrease binding to food and drugs and prevent inactivation.

4. Answer: b
RATIONALE: When a patient hasn't responded to an antibiotic after 24 to 36 hours, it is a possible sign that the infectious agent is resistant to the antibiotic. Though it is possible the patient isn't taking the medication, or that the patient's infection is viral, not bacterial, they are not the most likely reason. Lack of improvement does not signify an allergic reaction.

5. Answer: a
RATIONALE: Antimicrobial drug therapy requires close monitoring in patients with renal impairment, because many drugs are excreted primarily by the kidneys and some are nephrotoxic and may further damage the kidneys.

6. Answer: d
RATIONALE: For most surgeries involving an incision through the skin, a first-generation cephalosporin such as cefazolin (Kefzol) with activity against *Staphylococcus aureus* or *Streptococcus* species is commonly used.

7. Answer: a
RATIONALE: The amount and frequency of anti-infective and antimicrobial agents should be individualized according to characteristics of the causative organism, the chosen drug, and the patient's size and condition (e.g., type and severity of infection, ability to use and excrete the chosen drug).

8. Answer: b, c, and d
RATIONALE: Certain areas of the body are difficult to treat with antibiotics because antibacterials don't reach adequate levels of concentration in these areas such as the prostate gland, gall bladder, brain, and eyes. Certain antibacterials will concentrate in the bladder. There are certain antibacterials that work well to treat infections in the stomach.

9. Answer: b
RATIONALE: Some infections that require relatively long-term IV antibiotic therapy include endocarditis, osteomyelitis, and some surgical-wound infections.

10. Answer: a, b, and e
RATIONALE: The patient should report a skin rash, any sign of a new infection, vomiting, and diarrhea. Bad breath and a metallic taste in the mouth are unpleasant side effects but do not need to be reported to the physician.

11. Answer: c
RATIONALE: General infection-control practices include frequent and thorough hand hygiene, use of gloves when indicated, and appropriate handling and disposal of body substances (e.g., blood, urine, feces, sputum, vomitus, wound drainage).

12. Answer: c
RATIONALE: Measurement of plasma drug levels and dosage adjustment are often necessary to accommodate the changing physiology of a critically ill patient. Drug levels are usually measured after four or five doses are given so that steady-state concentrations have been reached.

13. Answer: d
RATIONALE: Patients in critical care units are at high risk for acquiring nosocomial pneumonia because of the severity of their illness, duration of hospitalization, and antimicrobial drug therapy. The strongest predisposing factor is mechanical ventilation, which bypasses airway defenses against movement of microorganisms from the upper to the lower respiratory tract. Organisms often associated with nosocomial pneumonia are *Staphylococcus aureus* and gram-negative bacilli.

14. Answer: a
RATIONALE: Bacterial pneumonia is usually treated with a broad-spectrum antibiotic until culture and susceptibility reports become available.

15. Answer: a
RATIONALE: Selection of antibacterial drugs may be difficult because of frequent changes in antibiotic resistance patterns. Antibiotic rotation (i.e., switching preferred antibiotic or antibiotic classes used to treat infections, on a scheduled basis) has been successful in reducing rates of ventilator-associated pneumonia and mortality.

16. Answer: a, b, and d
RATIONALE: Risk factors for infection include malnutrition, presence of chronic illness such as diabetes mellitus and renal disease, or a depressed immune system because of chemotherapy or HIV infection. Factors that help prevent disease include good personal hygiene and a normal WBC count.

17. Answer: c
RATIONALE: A laboratory value that indicates severe renal impairment is CrCl less than 15 to 30 mL/min.

18. **Answer: a, b, and e**
    RATIONALE: Normal body defenses against infection include coughing, sneezing, swallowing, and normal amounts of stomach acid. Risk factors include an impaired blood supply and any impairment or possible impairment to skin integrity such as the use of a prosthetic device that may chronically irritate the skin.

19. **Answer: b**
    RATIONALE: Dosing of antibiotics is important in patients with acute or chronic renal failure who are receiving hemodialysis or peritoneal dialysis. Some drugs are removed by dialysis, and an extra dose may be needed during or after dialysis.

20. **Answer: a**
    RATIONALE: The patient most at risk for an opportunistic infection is the one with the HIV infection because the immune system is compromised with this disease.

CHAPTER 14

SECTION I: ASSESSING YOUR UNDERSTANDING

Activity A FILL IN THE BLANKS

1. antiprostaglandin drugs
2. Prostaglandins
3. hypothalamus
4. Inflammation
5. -itis

Activity B MATCHING

1. c   **2.** e   **3.** a   **4.** b   **5.** d

Activity C SEQUENCING

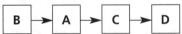

Activity D SHORT ANSWERS

1. Prostaglandins are chemical mediators found in most body tissues; they help regulate many cell functions and participate in the inflammatory response. They are formed when cellular injury occurs and phospholipids in cell membranes release *arachidonic acid*. Arachidonic acid is metabolized by *cyclooxygenase* (*COX*) enzymes to produce prostaglandins, which act briefly in the area where they are produced and are then inactivated. Prostaglandins exert various and opposing effects in different body tissues.

2. Fever occurs when the set point of the hypothalamus is raised in response to the presence of *pyrogens* (fever-producing agents). Endogenous pyrogenes include cytokines such as interleukin-1, interleukin-6, and tumor necrosis factor. Exogenous pyrogens include bacteria and their toxins or other by-products. The upward adjustment of the hypothalamic set point in response to the pres-

ence of a pyrogen is mediated by prostaglandin E_2. The body responds to the higher hypothalamic set point by vasoconstriction of blood vessels and shivering, raising the core body temperature to the higher set point. Fever may accompany conditions such as dehydration, inflammation, infectious processes, brain injury, or diseases involving the hypothalamus.

3. Systemic manifestations include leukocytosis, increased erythrocyte sedimentation rate, fever, headache, loss of appetite, lethargy or malaise, and weakness. Both local and systemic manifestations vary according to the cause and extent of tissue damage.

4. To relieve fever, aspirin and other NSAIDs act on the hypothalamus to decrease its response to pyrogens and reset the "thermostat" at a lower level. For inflammation, the drugs prevent prostaglandins from increasing the pain and edema produced by other substances released by damaged cells. Although these drugs relieve symptoms and contribute greatly to the patient's comfort and quality of life, they do not cure the underlying disorders that cause the symptoms.

5. Aspirin and nonselective NSAIDs also have antiplatelet effects that differ in mechanism and extent. When aspirin is absorbed into the bloodstream, the acetyl portion dissociates and then binds irreversibly to platelet COX-1. This action prevents synthesis of thromboxane A_2, a prostaglandin derivative, thereby inhibiting platelet aggregation. A small, single dose (325 mg) of aspirin irreversibly acetylates circulating platelets within a few minutes, and effects last for the lifespan of the platelets (7–10 days). Most other NSAIDs bind reversibly with platelet COX-1, so that antiplatelet effects occur only while the drug is present in the blood. Therefore, aspirin has greater effects, but all of these drugs except acetaminophen and the COX-2 inhibitors inhibit platelet aggregation, interfere with blood coagulation, and increase the risk of bleeding.

SECTION II: APPLYING YOUR KNOWLEDGE

Activity E CASE STUDY

1. Degenerative joint disease (DJD), also known as osteoarthritis (OA), is a disease that affects the articular cartilage, subchondral bone, and synovium of weight-bearing joints. The joints of the fingers may also be affected by OA. Signs and symptoms of OA include pain, stiffness, and functional impairment. As joint cartilage deteriorates over time, there is less padding and lubricating fluid; underlying bone is exposed; and friction and abrasion lead to inflammation of the synovial membrane lining of the joint. Deformity of the joint occurs as the disease advances.

2. COX-2 is also normally present in several tissues (e.g., brain, bone, kidneys, GI tract, and female reproductive system). However, it is thought to occur in small amounts or to be inactive until

stimulated by pain and inflammation. In inflamed tissues, COX-2 is induced by inflammatory chemical mediators such as interleukin-1 and tumor necrosis factor-alpha. In the GI tract, COX-2 is also induced by trauma and by *Helicobacter pylori* infection, a common cause of peptic ulcer disease. Overall, prostaglandins produced by COX-2 are associated with pain and other signs of inflammation. Inhibition of COX-2 results in the therapeutic effects of analgesia and anti-inflammatory activity. The COX-2 inhibitor drugs are NSAIDs designed to selectively inhibit COX-2 and relieve pain and inflammation with fewer adverse effects, especially stomach damage; however, with long-term use, adverse effects still occur in the GI, renal, and cardiovascular systems.

SECTION III: PRACTICING FOR NCLEX

Activity F

1. Answer: b
RATIONALE: When colchicine is taken for acute gout, pain is usually relieved in 4 to 12 hours with IV administration or in 24 to 48 hours with oral administration. Inflammation and edema may not decrease for several days.

2. Answer: a
RATIONALE: With colchicine for chronic gout, carry the drug and take as directed when pain begins until relief is obtained or nausea, vomiting, and diarrhea occur.

3. Answer: d
RATIONALE: Drink 2 to 3 quarts of fluid daily with antigout drugs. An adequate fluid intake helps prevent formation of uric acid kidney stones. Fluid intake is especially important initially, when uric acid levels in the blood are high and large amounts of uric acid are being excreted in the urine.

4. Answer: c
RATIONALE: Acetaminophen is often the initial drug of choice for relieving mild to moderate pain and fever, because it does not cause gastric irritation or bleeding. It may be taken on an empty stomach.

5. Answer: a
RATIONALE: Acetaminophen is an effective aspirin substitute for pain or fever but not for inflammation or prevention of heart attack or stroke.

6. Answer: b
RATIONALE: Do not exceed recommended doses of acetaminophen due to risk of life-threatening liver damage. People with liver disorders such as hepatitis or those who ingest alcoholic beverages frequently should use it with extreme caution.

7. Answer: a
RATIONALE: If a patient has a history of taking aspirin, including the low doses prescribed for antithrombotic effects, there is a risk of bleeding from common therapeutic procedures (e.g., intramuscular injections, venipuncture, insertion of urinary catheters or GI tubes) or diagnostic procedures (e.g., drawing blood, angiography).

8. Answer: c
RATIONALE: Older patients on long-term NSAIDs therapy should be evaluated for GI blood loss, renal dysfunction, edema, hypertension, and drug–drug or drug–disease interactions (level A). Use of gastroprotective agents is recommended for people at risk of upper GI bleeding events (level B). COX-2 inhibitors may be preferred in older adults, because they are less likely to cause gastric ulceration and bleeding; however, this benefit must be weighed against the increased risk of cardiovascular events.

9. Answer: c
RATIONALE: Age is the most significant risk factor for the development of osteoarthritis. Occupation can have an effect especially if it is one that causes "wear and tear" motions, but age remains the most significant.

10. Answer: b
RATIONALE: Ibuprofen also may be given for fever. Alternating acetaminophen and ibuprofen every 4 hours over a 3-day period to control fever in young children (aged 6–36 months) has been shown to be more effective than monotherapy with either agent.

11. Answer: d
RATIONALE: There is a risk of overdose and hepatotoxicity, because acetaminophen is a very common ingredient in OTC cold, flu, fever, and pain remedies. An overdose can occur with large doses of one product or smaller amounts of several different products. In addition, toxicity has occurred when parents or caregivers have given the liquid concentration intended for children to infants.

12. Answer: a
RATIONALE: Cancer often produces chronic pain from tumor invasion of tissues or complications of treatment (chemotherapy, surgery, or radiation). As with acute pain, acetaminophen, aspirin, or other NSAIDs prevent sensitization of peripheral pain receptors by inhibiting prostaglandin formation. NSAIDs are especially effective for pain associated with bone metastases.

13. Answer: b
RATIONALE: Aspirin should generally be avoided for 1 to 2 weeks before and after surgery, because it increases the risk of bleeding. Most other NSAIDs should be discontinued approximately 3 days before surgery; nabumetone and piroxicam have long half-lives and must be discontinued approximately 1 week before surgery. NSAIDs, administered intraoperatively, have been shown to reduce postoperative pain and use of opioids after abdominal surgery.

14. Answer: a
RATIONALE: Acetaminophen is not an anti-inflammatory medication. It is an analgesic and an antipyretic. Aspirin, naproxen sodium, and ibuprofen decrease pain and inflammation.

15. Answer: c
RATIONALE: Both categories of migraine abortive drugs (e.g., ergot alkaloids and serotonin agonists) exert powerful vasoconstrictive effects and have the potential to raise blood pressure.

16. Answer: c
RATIONALE: Severe pain and swelling in the great toe that is worse at night and lasts longer than 10 days is most likely gout.

17. Answer: a
RATIONALE: If an ergot preparation is used, it should be given at the onset of headache, and the patient should lie down in a quiet, darkened room.

18. Answer: c
RATIONALE: Preparations containing sedatives such as butalbital should be limited due to the possibility of overuse headaches and withdrawal issues (level C).

19. Answer: a, b, and e
RATIONALE: Symptoms of Reye's syndrome are related to liver toxicity (jaundice and elevated liver enzymes and encephalopathy).

20. Answer: d
RATIONALE: The nurse will administer aspirin 625 mg at 6 hours after coronary bypass surgery. The patient will take it daily for the next year.

CHAPTER 15

SECTION I: ASSESSING YOUR UNDERSTANDING

Activity A FILL IN THE BLANKS
1. Corticosteroids
2. Exogenous
3. slows, stops
4. negative feedback mechanism
5. Corticosteroids

Activity B MATCHING
1. c   2. d   3. a   4. b   5. e

Activity C SHORT ANSWERS
1. Corticosteroid secretion is controlled by the hypothalamus, the anterior pituitary, and adrenal cortex (the hypothalamic–pituitary–adrenal, or HPA, axis). Various stimuli (e.g., low plasma levels of corticosteroids, pain, anxiety, trauma, illness, anesthesia) activate the system. These stimuli cause the hypothalamus of the brain to secrete corticotropin-releasing hormone or factor (CRH or CRF), which stimulates the anterior pituitary gland to secrete corticotropin, and corticotropin then stimulates the adrenal cortex to secrete corticosteroids.
2. The stress response activates the sympathetic nervous system (SNS) to produce more epinephrine and norepinephrine and the adrenal cortex to produce as much as 10 times the normal amount of cortisol. The synergistic interaction of these hormones increases the person's ability to respond to stress. However, the increased SNS activity continues to stimulate cortisol production (the main glucocorticoids secreted as part of the body's response to stress) and overrules the negative feedback mechanism. Excessive and prolonged corticosteroid secretion damages body tissues.
3. Glucocorticoids are important in metabolic, inflammatory, and immune processes. Glucocorticoids include cortisol, corticosterone, and cortisone. Cortisol accounts for at least 95% of glucocorticoid activity; corticosterone and cortisone account for a small amount of activity. Glucocorticoids are secreted cyclically, with the largest amount being produced in the early morning and the smallest amount during the evening hours (in people with a normal day–night schedule). At the cellular level, glucocorticoids account for most of the characteristics and physiologic effects of the corticosteroids.
4. Mineralocorticoids are a class of steroids that play a vital role in the maintenance of fluid and electrolyte balance through their influence on salt and water metabolism. Aldosterone is the main mineralocorticoid and is responsible for approximately 90% of mineralocorticoid activity.
5. The adrenal cortex secretes male (androgens) and female (estrogens and progesterone) sex hormones. Compared with the effect of hormones produced by the testes and ovaries, the adrenal sex hormones have an insignificant effect on normal body function. Adrenal androgens, secreted continuously in small quantities by both sexes, are responsible for most of the physiologic effects exerted by the adrenal sex hormones. They increase protein synthesis (anabolism), which increases the mass and strength of muscle and bone tissue; they affect development of male secondary sex characteristics; and they increase hair growth and libido in women.

SECTION II: APPLYING YOUR KNOWLEDGE

Activity D CASE STUDY
1. Systemic lupus erythematosus is a collagen disorder, as are scleroderma and periarteritis nodosa. Collagen is the basic structural protein of connective tissue, tendons, cartilage, and bone, and it is therefore present in almost all body tissues and organ systems. The collagen disorders are characterized by inflammation of various body tissues, particularly tendons, cartilage, and connective tissues. Signs and symptoms depend on which body tissues or organs are affected and the severity of the inflammatory process.
2. Dermatologic disorders that may be treated with systemic corticosteroids include acute contact dermatitis, erythema multiforme, herpes zoster (prophylaxis of postherpetic neuralgia), lichen planus, pemphigus, skin rashes caused by drugs, and toxic epidermal necrolysis.

3. The effectiveness of corticosteroids in neoplastic diseases, such as acute and chronic leukemias, Hodgkin's disease, other lymphomas, and multiple myelomas, probably stems from their ability to suppress lymphocytes and other lymphoid tissue.

4. Corticosteroids suppress cellular and humoral immune responses and help prevent rejection of transplanted tissue. Drug therapy is usually continued as long as the transplanted tissue is in place.

5. In patients with asthma, corticosteroids increase the number of beta-adrenergic receptors and increase or restore the responsiveness of beta receptors to beta-adrenergic bronchodilating drugs. In cases of asthma, COPD, and rhinitis, the drugs decrease mucus secretion and inflammation. In anaphylactic shock resulting from an allergic reaction, corticosteroids may increase or restore cardiovascular responsiveness to adrenergic drugs.

SECTION III: PRACTICING FOR NCLEX

Activity E

1. **Answer: d**
   RATIONALE: A black box warning has been issued by the FDA for people who are transferred from systemically active corticosteroids to flunisolide inhaler; deaths from adrenal insufficiency have been reported.

2. **Answer: b and c**
   RATIONALE: Adverse effects of systemic corticosteroids may include infections, hypertension, glucose intolerance, obesity, cosmetic changes, bone loss, growth retardation in children, cataracts, pancreatitis, peptic ulcerations, and psychiatric disturbances. Patients also develop cervicodorsal fat pad or buffalo hump, which exists between the shoulder blades, not on the buttocks.

3. **Answer: b**
   RATIONALE: Strategies to minimize HPA suppression and risks of acute adrenal insufficiency include administering a systemic corticosteroid during high-stress situations in patients who are on long-term systemic therapy (i.e., are steroid dependent).

4. **Answer: a**
   RATIONALE: Strategies to minimize HPA suppression and risks of acute adrenal insufficiency include giving short courses of systemic therapy for acute disorders.

5. **Answer: c**
   RATIONALE: Strategies to minimize HPA suppression and risks of acute adrenal insufficiency include gradually tapering the dose of any systemic corticosteroid.

6. **Answer: d**
   RATIONALE: Strategies to minimize HPA suppression and risks of acute adrenal insufficiency include using local rather than systemic therapy when possible, alone or in combination with low doses of systemic drugs.

7. **Answer: c**
   RATIONALE: The mother will need further instruction if she believes that a corticosteroid will cure the asthma. This class of drugs is intended to control symptoms, not cure illness.

8. **Answer: d**
   RATIONALE: Daily administration of corticosteroids and mineralocorticoids is required in cases of chronic adrenocortical insufficiency (Addison's disease).

9. **Answer: c**
   RATIONALE: The patient's thinning skin may make IV insertion more difficult because the skin is so much more fragile and it bruises so easily due to capillary fragility.

10. **Answer: a, b, and d**
    RATIONALE: The most frequently desired pharmacologic effects of exogenous corticosteroids are anti-inflammatory, immunosuppressive, antiallergic, and antistress effects. Corticosteroids have been shown to decrease pain as they decrease inflammation, but they are not usually prescribed for their analgesic properties.

11. **Answer: a**
    RATIONALE: Because of potentially serious adverse effects, especially with oral drugs, it is extremely important that corticosteroids be used as prescribed. A major responsibility of home care nurses is to teach, demonstrate, supervise, monitor, or do whatever is needed to facilitate correct use.

12. **Answer: b**
    RATIONALE: Corticosteroids improve survival and decrease the risk of respiratory failure with pneumocystosis, a common cause of death in patients with AIDS.

13. **Answer: b**
    RATIONALE: Sepsis may be complicated by impaired corticosteroid production. There is sufficient evidence to support the idea that giving a long course of low-dose corticosteroids in patients with septic shock can improve survival without causing harm. However, overall, corticosteroids do not affect mortality.

14. **Answer: d**
    RATIONALE: Although corticosteroids have been widely used, several well-controlled studies demonstrated that the drugs are not beneficial in early treatment or in prevention of adult respiratory distress syndrome (ARDS).

15. **Answer: a**
    RATIONALE: Some studies support the use of IV methylprednisolone. So, if other medications do not produce adequate bronchodilation, it seems reasonable to try an IV corticosteroid during the first 72 hours of the illness. However, corticosteroid therapy increases the risks of pulmonary infection.

16. **Answer: b**
    RATIONALE: In adrenal insufficiency, hypotension is a common symptom in critically ill patients, and hypotension caused by adrenal insufficiency

may mimic either hypovolemic or septic shock. If adrenal insufficiency is the cause of the hypotension, administration of corticosteroids can eliminate the need for vasopressor drugs to maintain adequate tissue perfusion.

17. **Answer: a, c, and e**
    RATIONALE: Long-term corticosteroid therapy may cause a patient to develop diabetes due to the increase in glucose tolerance, peptic ulcer disease due to the gastric erosion, and tuberculosis because of the decreased immunity. It is used as a treatment for rheumatoid arthritis and COPD.

18. **Answer: c**
    RATIONALE: An adverse effect in women who take corticosteroids is acne and hair on the face. This side effect usually resolves after the medication is discontinued. The drug should never be stopped abruptly but weaned gradually.

19. **Answer: a, c, and d**
    RATIONALE: Corticosteroids are used for the same conditions in older adults as in younger ones. Older adults are especially likely to have conditions that are aggravated by the drugs (e.g., congestive heart failure, hypertension, diabetes mellitus, arthritis, osteoporosis, increased susceptibility to infection, concomitant drug therapy that increases risks of gastrointestinal ulceration and bleeding). Consequently, risk–benefit ratios of systemic corticosteroid therapy should be carefully considered, especially for long-term therapy. It is used as a treatment for contact dermatitis.

20. **Answer: a**
    RATIONALE: After a craniotomy, the drug of choice is either IV or PO dexamethasone.

CHAPTER 16

SECTION I: ASSESSING YOUR UNDERSTANDING

Activity A FILL IN THE BLANKS

1. penicillin
2. penicillins
3. cross-allergenicity
4. Dicloxacillin, nafcillin, oxacillin
5. Carbenicillin (Geocillin), ticarcillin, piperacillin

Activity B MATCHING

1. d   2. a   3. b   4. c   5. e

Activity C SHORT ANSWERS

1. Patients on hemodialysis usually require an additional dose of penicillin after treatment, because hemodialysis removes substantial amounts and produces subtherapeutic serum drug levels.
2. Amoxicillin–clavulanate (Augmentin) should be used with caution in patients with hepatic impairment. It is contraindicated in patients who have had cholestatic jaundice and hepatic dysfunction

with previous use of the drug. Cholestatic liver impairment usually subsides when the drug is stopped. Hepatotoxicity is attributed to the clavulanate component and has also occurred with ticarcillin–clavulanate (Timentin).

3. Many beta-lactam antibiotics are given in the home setting. With oral agents, the role of the home care nurse is mainly to teach accurate administration and observation for therapeutic and adverse effects. With liquid suspensions for children, shaking to resuspend the medication and measuring with a measuring spoon or calibrated device are required for safe dosing. Household spoons should not be used, because they vary widely in capacity.
4. Metabolic and electrolyte imbalances may occur in patients receiving penicillins who have renal impairment or congestive heart failure. Hypernatremia and hypokalemic metabolic acidosis are most likely to occur with ticarcillin, and hyperkalemia with large IV doses of penicillin G potassium.
5. Beta-lactam antimicrobials are commonly used in critical care units to treat pneumonia, bloodstream infections, wound infections, and other infections.

SECTION II: APPLYING YOUR KNOWLEDGE
Activity D CASE STUDIES

Case Study 1
1. Central nervous system toxicity, including seizures, has been reported. Seizures are more likely in patients with a seizure disorder or when recommended doses are exceeded; however, they have occurred in other patients as well.
2. Lidocaine is mixed in preparation of the solution for IM injection to decrease pain with administration, and the same cautions should be used as with imipenem. Unlike imipenem and meropenem, ertapenem does not have in vitro activity against *Pseudomonas aeruginosa* or *Acinetobacter baumannii*. The drug would be discontinued.

Case Study 2
1. "The physician orders aztreonam because it is effective against *Pseudomonas aeruginosa*, which caused your infection." Aztreonam (Azactam) is active against gram-negative bacteria, including Enterobacteriaceae and *P. aeruginosa*, and many strains that are resistant to multiple antibiotics.
2. Activity of aztreonam against gram-negative bacteria is similar to that of the aminoglycosides, but the drug does not cause kidney damage or hearing loss.

SECTION III: PRACTICING FOR NCLEX
Activity E

1. **Answer: a**
   RATIONALE: Probenecid (Benemid) blocks renal excretion of the penicillins and can be given concurrently with penicillins to increase serum drug levels.

2. Answer: c
RATIONALE: In the rare instance in which penicillin is considered essential, a skin test may be helpful in assessing hypersensitivity.

3. Answer: b
RATIONALE: As a class, penicillins usually are more effective in infections caused by gram-positive bacteria than those caused by gram-negative bacteria.

4. Answer: a, b, and e
RATIONALE: Choice of a beta-lactam antibacterial depends on the organism causing the infection, the severity of the infection, and other factors including a history of other chronic illnesses such as liver and kidney diseases. These conditions may contraindicate the use of a beta-lactam antibiotic.

5. Answer: a, b, and c
RATIONALE: Beta-lactam antibiotics include penicillins, cephalosporins, carbapenems, and monobactams. Sulfonamides and fluoroquinolones are not considered beta-lactam antibiotics.

6. Answer: c
RATIONALE: Beta-lactam antimicrobials are commonly used in critical care units to treat pneumonia, bloodstream infections, wound infections, and other infections. Renal, hepatic, and other organ functions should be monitored in critically ill patients, and drug dosages should be reduced when indicated.

7. Answer: d
RATIONALE: The beta-lactam drugs are frequently given concomitantly with other antimicrobial drugs because critically ill patients often have multiorganism or nosocomial infections.

8. Answer: d
RATIONALE: Aztreonam, imipenem, meropenem, and ertapenem may cause abnormalities in liver function test results (i.e., elevated alanine and aspartate aminotransferases [ALT and AST] and alkaline phosphatase), but hepatitis and jaundice rarely occur.

9. Answer: a
RATIONALE: For serious or life-threatening infections in patients on hemodialysis, give 12.5% of the initial dose after each hemodialysis session, in addition to maintenance doses.

10. Answer: b
RATIONALE: After an initial loading dose, the dosage of aztreonam should be reduced by 50% or more in patients with CrCl of 30 mL/min or less. Give at the usual intervals of 6, 8, or 12 hours.

11. Answer: d
RATIONALE: Dosage of imipenem should be reduced in most patients with renal impairment, and the drug is contraindicated in patients with severe renal impairment (CrCl of 5 mL/min or less) unless hemodialysis is started within 48 hours. For patients already on hemodialysis, the drug may cause seizures and should be used very cautiously, if at all.

12. Answer: c
RATIONALE: Penicillins and cephalosporins are widely used to treat infections in children and are generally safe. They should be used cautiously in neonates, because immature kidney function slows their elimination. Dosages should be based on age, weight, severity of the infection being treated, and renal function.

13. Answer: c
RATIONALE: Some cephalosporins are used in surgical prophylaxis. The particular drug depends largely on the type of organism likely to be encountered in the operative area. First-generation drugs, mainly cefazolin, are used for procedures associated with gram-positive postoperative infections, such as prosthetic implant surgery.

14. Answer: b
RATIONALE: Aminoglycosides are often given concomitantly with penicillins for serious infections, such as those caused by *Pseudomonas aeruginosa*. The drugs should not be admixed in a syringe or in an IV solution, because the penicillin inactivates the aminoglycoside.

15. Answer: b
RATIONALE: A patient who developed cholestatic jaundice with a previous use of ampicillin should not be given this medication again to prevent permanent liver damage. Vaginal yeast infections, nausea, and diarrhea are common adverse effects and would not preclude the use of this medication again.

16. Answer: a, c, and d
RATIONALE: Because anaphylactic shock may occur with administration of the penicillins, especially by parenteral routes, emergency drugs and equipment must be readily available. Treatment may require parenteral epinephrine, oxygen, and insertion of an endotracheal or tracheostomy tube if laryngeal edema occurs. A nasogastric tube would not be necessary at this time.

17. Answer: c
RATIONALE: Penicillin G benzathine is for IM use and may cause death in a patient if it is given IV. Ampicillin, oxacillin, and ampicillin–sulbactam may all be given IV.

18. Answer: b
RATIONALE: Patients with decreased renal function may develop seizure activity if given imipenem–cilastatin. Elevated liver function tests may occur in any patient who takes this medication, but they usually return to normal after the drug is discontinued. Rash and respiratory distress are symptoms of a hypersensitivity reaction and are not associated with decreased renal function.

19. Answer: c and e
RATIONALE: The most important adverse effects for the nurse to observe for in a patient receiving cefazolin or any other cephalosporin are superinfections and hypersensitivity reactions.

20. **Answer: a**

   RATIONALE: Imipenem is formulated with cilastatin, which inhibits the destruction of imipenem by the enzyme. The addition of cilastatin increases the urinary concentration of imipenem and reduces the potential renal toxicity of the antibacterial agent. Recommended doses indicate the amount of imipenem; the solution contains an equivalent amount of cilastatin.

CHAPTER 17

SECTION I: ASSESSING YOUR UNDERSTANDING

Activity A   FILL IN THE BLANKS

1. aminoglycosides
2. quinolones
3. fluoroquinolones
4. bactericidal
5. parenteral

Activity B   MATCHING

1. d   **2.** a   **3.** c   **4.** e   **5.** d

Activity C   SHORT ANSWERS

1. The fluoroquinolones are synthesized by adding a fluorine molecule to the quinolone structure. This addition increases drug activity against gram-negative microorganisms, broadens the antimicrobial spectrum to include several other microorganisms, and allows use of the drugs in treating systemic infections.
2. Aminoglycosides are bactericidal agents with similar pharmacologic, antimicrobial, and toxicologic characteristics. They are used to treat infections caused by gram-negative microorganisms such as *Pseudomonas* and *Proteus* species, *Escherichia coli*, and *Klebsiella*, *Enterobacter*, and *Serratia* species.
3. Aminoglycoside drugs are poorly absorbed from the gastrointestinal (GI) tract. When given orally, they exert local effects in the GI tract. They are well absorbed from intramuscular injection sites and reach peak effects in 30 to 90 minutes if circulatory status is good. After intravenous (IV) administration, peak effects occur within 30 to 60 minutes. Plasma half-life is 2 to 4 hours with normal renal function.
4. After parenteral administration, aminoglycosides are widely distributed in extracellular fluid and reach therapeutic levels in blood, urine, bone, inflamed joints, and pleural and ascitic fluids. They accumulate in high concentrations in the proximal renal tubules of the kidney leading to acute tubular necrosis. This damage to the kidney is termed *nephrotoxicity*. They also accumulate in high concentrations in the inner ear, damaging sensory cells in the cochlea (disrupting hearing) and the vestibular apparatus (disturbing balance). This damage to the inner ear is termed *ototoxicity*. They are poorly distributed to the central nervous system, intraocular fluids, and respiratory tract secretions.
5. Injected aminoglycosides are not metabolized; they are excreted unchanged in the urine, primarily by glomerular filtration. Oral aminoglycosides are excreted in feces.

SECTION II: APPLYING YOUR KNOWLEDGE

Activity D   CASE STUDY

1. Infections involving the respiratory and genitourinary tracts, skin, wounds, bowel, and bloodstream are commonly due to gram-negative organisms, although gram-negative infections can occur anywhere. Any infection with gram-negative organisms may be serious and potentially life threatening.
2. Radical surgery, such as in Ms. Blanchard's case, can lower a patient's resistance to infection. Nosocomial infections have become more common with control of other types of infections, widespread use of antimicrobial drugs, and diseases (e.g., acquired immunodeficiency syndrome [AIDS]) or treatments (e.g., radical surgery, therapy with antineoplastic or immunosuppressive drugs) that lower host resistance. Management is difficult, because the organisms are, in general, less susceptible to antibacterial drugs and drug-resistant strains develop rapidly.
3. The combination of an aminoglycoside and piperacillin has synergistic therapeutic effects. Management of nosocomial infection is difficult, because the organisms are, in general, less susceptible to antibacterial drugs and drug-resistant strains develop rapidly. In pseudomonal infections, an aminoglycoside is often given concurrently with an antipseudomonal penicillin (e.g., piperacillin). The penicillin-induced breakdown of the bacterial cell wall makes it easier for the aminoglycoside to reach its site of action inside the bacterial cell.
4. Decreased mortality has been demonstrated from combination antibiotic therapy in the treatment of infections due to *Pseudomonas aeruginosa* and other multidrug-resistant gram-negative bacilli. Routine use of combination antibiotic therapy containing an aminoglycoside has not been associated with decreased mortality in cases of other gram-negative infections.

SECTION III: PRACTICING FOR NCLEX

Activity E

1. **Answer: a**

   RATIONALE: Fluoroquinolones are associated with hyperglycemia and hypoglycemia, and older patients may be more at risk for these glucose disturbances.

2. **Answer: a and b**

   RATIONALE: Aminoglycosides reach higher concentrations in the kidneys and inner ears than in other body tissues; this is a major factor in nephrotoxicity and ototoxicity. There is low concentration in the central nervous system.

3. Answer: a
RATIONALE: Multiple-dose regimens (conventional dosing) of aminoglycosides must be carefully monitored with evaluation of peak and trough serum levels. Once-daily regimens are monitored with random level (12-hour) serum evaluation.

4. Answer: c
RATIONALE: Gentamicin and penicillin should never be administered in the same syringe or the same solution. When both antibiotics are prescribed for the patient, they must be administered at separate times using Y tubing.

5. Answer: c
RATIONALE: One of the first symptoms to occur in a patient who is developing ototoxicity is tinnitus or ringing in the ears. Fatigue, anorexia, and rash are other adverse effects but are not related to ototoxicity.

6. Answer: d
RATIONALE: The choice of aminoglycoside depends on local susceptibility patterns and specific organisms causing an infection.

7. Answer: b
RATIONALE: An increasing number of people with CAP are being treated at home for a number of reasons, including increased availability and cost considerations of oral antibiotics. Oral drugs have demonstrated effectiveness and are the preferred route for individuals and family members, but management with oral drugs has widely varied. The American College of Chest Physicians' position statement, cosponsored by the American Academy of Home Care Physicians, outlines recommendations for home care for patients with CAP and follow-up. Recommendations in the position statement take into consideration the best plan of care incorporating the best available evidence with clinician judgment and patient preferences.

8. Answer: c
RATIONALE: Fluoroquinolones are associated with hyperglycemia and hypoglycemia. Older patients may be more at risk for these glucose disturbances. Severe hypoglycemia has occurred in patients receiving concomitant glyburide and fluoroquinolones.

9. Answer: c
RATIONALE: Gatifloxacin has been associated with hypoglycemic and hyperglycemic events more commonly than other fluoroquinolones. The explanation for an increased association with gatifloxacin is not currently known.

10. Answer: d
RATIONALE: Fluoroquinolones are usually infused IV in critically ill patients. However, administration orally or by GI tube (e.g., nasogastric, gastrostomy, jejunostomy) may be feasible in some patients. Concomitant administration of antacids or enteral feedings decreases absorption.

11. Answer: b
RATIONALE: Because critically ill patients are at high risk for development of nephrotoxicity and ototoxicity with aminoglycosides, guidelines for safe drug use should be strictly followed. Renal function should be monitored to assess for needed dosage reductions in patients with renal dysfunction who are receiving aminoglycosides or fluoroquinolones. Because fluoroquinolones may be hepatotoxic, hepatic function should be monitored during therapy.

12. Answer: a
RATIONALE: Ciprofloxacin should be avoided in children and adolescents under the age of 18 unless the urinary tract infection is extremely severe. Ciprofloxacin may be used in other age groups.

13. Answer: d
RATIONALE: Ciprofloxacin in the older adult should be taken with extra fluid to prevent the development of crystalluria. It may be taken with food or on an empty stomach, and it should not be taken with an antacid.

14. Answer: c
RATIONALE: With aminoglycosides, hepatic impairment is not a significant factor, because the drugs are excreted through the kidneys.

15. Answer: b, c, and d
RATIONALE: With fluoroquinolones, reported renal effects include azotemia, crystalluria, hematuria, interstitial nephritis, nephropathy, and renal failure. Pyuria (pus in the urine) is one of the reasons a fluoroquinolone is prescribed.

16. Answer: b
RATIONALE: The trough should be drawn immediately before a dose of the gentamicin. The peak should be drawn 1 hour after the medication is infused.

17. Answer: a
RATIONALE: Aminoglycosides must be used cautiously in children as in adults. Dosage must be accurately calculated according to weight and renal function.

18. Answer: b
RATIONALE: Guidelines to decrease the incidence and severity of adverse effects when administering aminoglycosides include the following: Keep patients well hydrated to decrease drug concentration in serum and body tissues.

19. Answer: c
RATIONALE: When diphenhydramine is given with gentamicin, it may mask the symptoms of ototoxicity.

20. Answer: c
RATIONALE: Patients taking oral ciprofloxacin should avoid dairy products while taking this medication.

CHAPTER 18

SECTION I: ASSESSING YOUR UNDERSTANDING

Activity A FILL IN THE BLANKS
1. antiseptics
2. renal tubules
3. passive
4. renal failure
5. time

Activity B MATCHING
1. a **2.** c **3.** d **4.** b **5.** e

Activity C SHORT ANSWERS
1. The tetracyclines are similar in pharmacologic properties and antimicrobial activity. They are effective against a wide range of gram-positive and gram-negative organisms, although they are usually not drugs of choice. Bacterial infections caused by *Brucella* or by *Vibrio cholerae* are still treated with tetracyclines. The drugs also remain effective against rickettsiae, chlamydiae, some protozoans, spirochetes, and others. Doxycycline (Vibramycin) is one of the drugs of choice for *Bacillus anthracis* (anthrax) and *Chlamydia trachomatis*, and it is used in respiratory tract infections caused by *Mycoplasma pneumoniae*.
2. Tetracyclines are widely distributed into most body tissues and fluids. The older tetracyclines are excreted mainly in urine; doxycycline is eliminated in urine and feces; and minocycline is eliminated mainly by the liver.
3. Sulfonamides may be active against *Streptococcus pyogenes*, some staphylococcal strains, *Haemophilus influenzae*, *Nocardia*, *Chlamydia trachomatis*, and toxoplasmosis.
4. Tetracyclines penetrate microbial cells by passive diffusion and via an active transport system. Inside the cell, they bind to 30S ribosomes, like the aminoglycosides, and inhibit microbial protein synthesis. Sulfonamides act as antimetabolites of para-aminobenzoic acid (PABA); microorganisms require PABA to produce folic acid, which they need for the production of bacterial intracellular proteins. Sulfonamides enter into the reaction instead of PABA, compete for the enzyme involved, and cause formation of nonfunctional derivatives of folic acid.
5. Sulfonamides are commonly used to treat UTIs (e.g., acute and chronic cystitis, asymptomatic bacteriuria) caused by *Escherichia coli* and *Proteus* or *Klebsiella* organisms. In acute pyelonephritis, other agents are preferred.

SECTION II: APPLYING YOUR KNOWLEDGE

Activity D CASE STUDY
1. If a urinary tract infection is suspected, it is necessary to obtain urine culture and susceptibility tests before prescription of medication because of wide variability in possible pathogens and their susceptibility to antibacterial drugs. The best results are obtained with drug therapy indicated by the microorganisms isolated from each patient.
2. With systemically absorbed sulfonamides, an initial loading dose may be given, which is usually twice the maintenance dose. The purpose is to achieve therapeutic blood levels more rapidly.
3. Urine pH is important in drug therapy with sulfonamides and urinary antiseptics. With sulfonamide therapy, alkaline urine increases drug solubility and helps prevent crystalluria. It also increases the rate of sulfonamide excretion and the concentration of sulfonamide in the urine. The urine can be alkalinized by giving sodium bicarbonate. Alkalinization is not needed with sulfisoxazole (because the drug is highly soluble) or with sulfonamides used to treat intestinal infections or burn wounds (because there is little systemic absorption).

SECTION III: PRACTICING FOR NCLEX

Activity E
1. **Answer: a**
   RATIONALE: Urinary antiseptics may be bactericidal for sensitive organisms in the urinary tract because these drugs are concentrated in renal tubules and reach high levels in urine.
2. **Answer: b**
   RATIONALE: Urinary antiseptics are not used in systemic infections because they do not attain therapeutic plasma levels.
3. **Answer: a**
   RATIONALE: Sulfasalazine (Azulfidine) is contraindicated in people who are allergic to salicylates.
4. **Answer: d**
   RATIONALE: Sulfonamides are bacteriostatic against a wide range of gram-positive and gram-negative bacteria, although increasing resistance is making them less useful.
5. **Answer: c**
   RATIONALE: The tetracyclines are effective against a wide range of gram-positive and gram-negative organisms, although they are usually not drugs of choice.
6. **Answer: d**
   RATIONALE: Sulfonamides are rarely used in critical care settings, except that topical silver sulfadiazine (Silvadene) is used to treat burn wounds.
7. **Answer: a**
   RATIONALE: Trimethoprim–sulfamethoxazole is used to treat *Pneumocystis jiroveci* pneumonia.
8. **Answer: b**
   RATIONALE: Tetracyclines decrease the effectiveness of oral contraceptives, so the patient should use alternative means of contraception while taking tetracycline.
9. **Answer: a and d**
   RATIONALE: Tetracyclines are generally contraindicated in pregnant women because they may cause

fatal hepatic necrosis in the mother (as well as interfere with bone and tooth development in the fetus). They do not cause renal impairment in the mother or fetus or decrease brain development in the fetus.

10. **Answer: a**
    RATIONALE: Because tetracyclines are metabolized in the liver, hepatic impairment or biliary obstruction slows drug elimination.

11. **Answer: b**
    RATIONALE: In patients with renal impairment, high IV doses of tetracycline (greater than 2 g/d) have been associated with death from liver failure.

12. **Answer: a, d, and e**
    RATIONALE: A patient with renal failure who receives tetracycline may develop azotemia, increased BUN, hyperphosphatemia, hyperkalemia, and acidosis.

13. **Answer: b**
    RATIONALE: The patient who is taking tetracycline should take enough fluid in each day to produce at least 1500 mL of urine per day to prevent crystalluria. This requires the patient to drink at least 2 L of fluid per day.

14. **Answer: d**
    RATIONALE: Trimethoprim–sulfamethoxazole may only be mixed with 5% dextrose and water for IV infusion.

15. **Answer: b and c**
    RATIONALE: The nurse should not disconnect the catheter system or irrigate the Foley catheter unless there is evidence of an obstruction. The Foley catheter should be removed as soon as possible. The drainage bag should be kept below the level of the patient's bladder, and perineal care should be performed frequently.

16. **Answer: a**
    RATIONALE: Tetracyclines should not be used in children younger than 8 years of age because of their effects on teeth and bones.

17. **Answer: a and d**
    RATIONALE: If a fetus or young infant receives a sulfonamide by placental transfer, in breast milk, or by direct administration, the drug displaces bilirubin from binding sites on albumin. As a result, bilirubin may accumulate in the bloodstream (hyperbilirubinemia) and in the central nervous system (kernicterus) and may cause life-threatening toxicity.

18. **Answer: b**
    RATIONALE: Patients who take sulfasalazine should expect for their urine to turn yellow-orange while on the medication.

19. **Answer: c**
    RATIONALE: Sulfonamides are often used to treat UTI in children older than 2 months of age.

20. **Answer: b and d**
    RATIONALE: Tetracyclines must be used cautiously in the presence of liver or kidney impairment.

CHAPTER 19

SECTION I: ASSESSING YOUR UNDERSTANDING

Activity A FILL IN THE BLANKS

1. bacteriostatic
2. human immunodeficiency virus
3. azithromycin
4. liver
5. ribosomes

Activity B MATCHING

1. c   2. a   3. b   4. e   5. d

Activity C SHORT ANSWERS

1. Erythromycin is metabolized in the liver and excreted mainly in bile; approximately 20% is excreted in urine. Depending on the specific salt formulation used, food can have a variable effect on the absorption of oral erythromycin.

2. The macrolides and ketolides enter microbial cells and reversibly bind to the 50S subunits of ribosomes, thereby inhibiting microbial protein synthesis. Ketolides have a greater affinity for ribosomal RNA, expanding their antimicrobial spectrum compared to macrolides.

3. Macrolides and ketolides are contraindicated in people who have had hypersensitivity reactions. Telithromycin is contraindicated in people who have had hypersensitivity reactions to macrolides. All macrolides and telithromycin must be used with caution in patients with preexisting liver disease. A black box warning for erythromycin estolate and an FDA alert for telithromycin emphasize the liver toxicity associated with these drugs. Use of erythromycin and telithromycin concurrently with drugs highly dependent on CYP 3A4 liver enzymes for metabolism (e.g., pimozide) is contraindicated. The FDA has issued a black box warning alerting health care professionals that telithromycin is contraindicated in patients with myasthenia gravis due to the potential for life-threatening or fatal respiratory failure.

4. Clinical indications for the use of metronidazole include prevention or treatment of anaerobic bacterial infections (e.g., in colorectal surgery, intra-abdominal infections) and treatment of *Clostridium difficile* infections associated with pseudomembranous colitis. As part of a combination regimen, it is also useful in the treatment of infections due to *Helicobacter pylori*. It is contraindicated during the first trimester of pregnancy and must be used with caution in patients with CNS or blood disorders.

5. Quinupristin–dalfopristin is a strong inhibitor of cytochrome P450 3A4 enzymes and therefore interferes with the metabolism of drugs such as cyclosporine, antiretrovirals, carbamazepine, and many others. Toxicity may occur with the inhibited drugs.

SECTION II: APPLYING YOUR KNOWLEDGE
Activity D CASE STUDY

1. Vancomycin (Vancocin) is active only against gram-positive microorganisms. It acts by inhibiting cell wall synthesis.
2. Oral vancomycin is used only to treat staphylococcal enterocolitis and pseudomembranous colitis caused by *Clostridium difficile*. In initial treatment for *C. difficile* colitis, metronidazole is preferred.
3. Partly because of the widespread use of vancomycin, vancomycin-resistant enterococci (VRE) are being encountered more often, especially in critical care units, and treatment options for infections caused by these organisms are limited. To decrease the spread of VRE, the Centers for Disease Control and Prevention (CDC) recommend limiting the use of vancomycin.
4. "Red man syndrome" is an adverse reaction characterized by hypotension, flushing, and skin rash. It is caused by giving an IV infusion too quickly and is attributed to histamine release. It is very important to give IV infusions slowly, over 1 to 2 hours, to avoid this reaction.
5. Vancomycin is excreted through the kidneys; dosage should be reduced in the presence of renal impairment.

SECTION III: PRACTICING FOR NCLEX
Activity E

1. **Answer: d**
   RATIONALE: Metronidazole is effective against infections with anaerobic bacteria and some protozoa.
2. **Answer: a**
   RATIONALE: Spectinomycin is an alternative treatment for gonococcal infection when patients are unable to comply with the preferred regimen.
3. **Answer: b**
   RATIONALE: Rifaximin is prescribed for traveler's diarrhea caused by *Escherichia coli* infection.
4. **Answer: b**
   RATIONALE: Patients who are receiving metronidazole should not drink alcohol because the patient will develop a disulfiram-type reaction if alcohol is consumed while the patient is receiving metronidazole.
5. **Answer: c**
   RATIONALE: Quinupristin–dalfopristin belongs to the streptogramin class of antibiotics. It is indicated for VREF and MSSA.
6. **Answer: c**
   RATIONALE: Tigecycline belongs to the glycylcycline class of antibiotics. It is similar to tetracycline in structure and properties and can be used to treat skin infections caused by MRSA.
7. **Answer: a**
   RATIONALE: Daptomycin belongs to the lipopeptide class of antibiotics that kills gram-positive bacteria by inhibiting synthesis of bacterial proteins, DNA, and RNA.

8. **Answer: d**
   RATIONALE: Clindamycin belongs to the lincosamide class of antimicrobials, similar to macrolides in its mechanism of action and antimicrobial spectrum. A life-threatening adverse effect of clindamycin is the development of pseudomembranous colitis.
9. **Answer: b**
   RATIONALE: Chloramphenicol (Chloromycetin) is rarely used due to the possible development of serious and fatal blood dyscrasias with its use. It is effective against some strains of VRE.
10. **Answer: a**
    RATIONALE: Telithromycin is contraindicated in patients with myasthenia gravis because of the potential for life-threatening or fatal respiratory failure.
11. **Answer: a**
    RATIONALE: The presence of muscle pain or weakness is an indication that the patient is developing a severe musculoskeletal reaction, and the medication must be discontinued immediately.
12. **Answer: d**
    RATIONALE: The ketolide, telithromycin, is approved only for community-acquired pneumonia. Its mechanism of action is inhibition of microbial protein synthesis.
13. **Answer: b**
    RATIONALE: Erythromycin shares a similar antibacterial spectrum with penicillin, making it a good choice for patients with penicillin allergy.
14. **Answer: d**
    RATIONALE: For acute bacterial sinusitis, azithromycin is approved for an abbreviated 3-day treatment duration.
15. **Answer: b**
    RATIONALE: With the drug linezolid, myelosuppression (anemia, leukopenia, pancytopenia, and thrombocytopenia) is a serious adverse effect that may occur with prolonged therapy lasting longer than 2 weeks. The patient's complete blood count should be monitored; if myelosuppression occurs, linezolid should be discontinued. Myelosuppression usually improves with drug discontinuation.
16. **Answer: a**
    RATIONALE: Patients receiving linezolid and selective serotonin reuptake inhibitors (SSRIs) may be at risk for serotonin syndrome, which is characterized by fever and cognitive dysfunction.
17. **Answer: a, c, and d**
    RATIONALE: Because linezolid is a weak monoamine oxidase (MAO) inhibitor, patients should avoid foods high in tyramine content (aged cheeses, fermented or air-dried meats, sauerkraut, soy sauce, tap beers, red wine) while taking the drug.
18. **Answer: a**
    RATIONALE: Erythromycin is generally considered safe. Because it is metabolized in the liver and excreted in bile, it may be an alternative in patients with impaired renal function.

19. Answer: b
RATIONALE: The nurse must be careful to infuse vancomycin at the prescribed rate to prevent the occurrence of red man syndrome. With this syndrome, the patient's face and upper trunk becomes bright red, and it has led to cardiovascular collapse.

20. Answer: c
RATIONALE: The patient who is receiving chloramphenicol is at risk for blood dyscrasias. That is one reason why this medication is not prescribed very often.

CHAPTER 20

SECTION I: ASSESSING YOUR UNDERSTANDING

Activity A FILL IN THE BLANKS

1. kidneys
2. *Mycobacterium tuberculosis*
3. phagocytosis
4. antitubercular
5. one-third

Activity B MATCHING

1. d   2. a   3. b   4. e   5. c

Activity C SHORT ANSWERS

1. Transmission of tuberculosis occurs when an un-infected person inhales infected airborne particles that are exhaled by an infected person. Major factors affecting transmission are the number of bacteria expelled by the infected person and the closeness and duration of the contact between the infected and the uninfected person.

2. It is estimated that 30% of persons exposed to tuberculosis bacilli become infected and develop a mild, pneumonia-like illness that is often undiagnosed; this is the *primary infection*. About 6 to 8 weeks after exposure, those infected have positive reactions to tuberculin skin tests. Within approximately 6 months after exposure, spontaneous healing occurs as the bacilli are encapsulated into calcified tubercles.

3. The immune system is able to stop bacterial growth in most people who become infected with TB bacteria. The bacteria become inactive, although they remain alive in the body and can become active later. People with inactive or latent TB infection have no symptoms, do not feel sick, do not spread TB to others, usually have a positive skin-test reaction, and can develop active TB disease years later if the latent infection is not effectively treated. In many people with LTBI, the infection remains inactive throughout their lives. In others, the TB bacteria become active and cause tuberculosis, usually when the person's immune system becomes weak as a result of disease, immunosuppressive drugs, or aging.

4. Active tuberculosis has long been thought to result almost exclusively from reactivation of latent infection, with only a few cases from new primary infections. However, more recent studies indicate that almost half of new TB cases may result from new infections or reinfections from exogenous sources.

5. Signs and symptoms of active disease (e.g., cough that is persistent and often productive of sputum, chest pain, chills, fever, hemoptysis, night sweats, weight loss, weakness, lack of appetite, positive skin test, abnormal chest radiograph, positive sputum smear or culture) are estimated to develop in 5% of people with LTBI within 2 years and in another 5% after 2 years.

SECTION II: APPLYING YOUR KNOWLEDGE

Activity D CASE STUDY

1. "The resistant bacteria may always have been present in your system." In addition to LTBI, a major concern among public health and infectious-disease authorities is an increase in drug-resistant infections. Drug-resistant mutants of *Mycobacterium tuberculosis* microorganisms are present in any infected person. When infected people receive antitubercular drugs, drug-resistant mutants are not killed or weakened by the drugs. Instead, they are able to reproduce in the presence of the drugs and to transmit the property of drug resistance to newly produced bacteria. Eventually, the majority of TB bacilli in the body are drug resistant.

2. Once a drug-resistant strain of TB develops, it can be transmitted to other people just like a drug-susceptible strain.

3. Multidrug-resistant tuberculosis (MDR-TB) organisms are resistant to isoniazid (INH) and rifampin, the most effective drugs available. They may or may not be resistant to other antitubercular drugs. Factors contributing to the development of drug-resistant disease, whether acquired or new infection, include delayed diagnosis and delayed determination of drug susceptibility, which may take several weeks.

4. Delay in effective treatment allows rapid disease progression and rapid transmission to others, especially to those with impaired immune systems.

SECTION III: PRACTICING FOR NCLEX

Activity E

1. **Answer: c**
RATIONALE: In drug-resistant TB, there is no standardized treatment regimen; treatment must be individualized for each patient according to drug susceptibility reports.

2. **Answer: a, b, and e**
RATIONALE: Patients with HIV, diabetes mellitus, and cancer are at highest risk for developing TB after exposure because of a compromised immune system.

3. **Answer: c**
RATIONALE: INH is the treatment of choice for LTBI.
4. **Answer: b**
RATIONALE: Directly observed therapy (DOT) is recommended to prevent inadequate drug therapy and the development of drug-resistant TB organisms.
5. **Answer: d**
RATIONALE: Patients who are diagnosed with XDR-TB have already demonstrated the disease is resistant to medications that fight TB, therefore there is no effective treatment left.
6. **Answer: d**
RATIONALE: TB is a worldwide problem. Although TB is not as extensive in the United States as in many other countries, the public health infrastructure for diagnosing and treating TB needs to be maintained.
7. **Answer: a, b, and d**
RATIONALE: With individual patients receiving antitubercular drugs for latent or active infection, the home care nurse needs to assist the patient in taking the drugs as directed. Specific interventions vary widely and may include administering the drugs (DOT); teaching about the importance of taking the drugs and the possible consequences of not taking them (i.e., more severe disease, longer treatment regimens with more toxic drugs, spreading the disease to others); monitoring for adverse drug effects and assisting the patient to manage them or reporting them to the drug prescriber; and assisting the patient in obtaining the drugs and keeping follow-up appointments for blood tests and chest radiographs. Also there is increased adherence with short-course drug regimens.
8. **Answer: a, b, and d**
RATIONALE: In relation to community needs, the nurse needs to be active in identifying cases, investigating contacts of newly diagnosed cases, and promoting efforts to manage tuberculosis effectively. Family members will need special TB masks while in contact with the infected person until the TB medication has been effective.
9. **Answer: a**
RATIONALE: For patients at risk of developing hepatotoxicity, serum ALT and AST should be measured before starting and periodically during drug therapy. If hepatitis occurs, these enzyme levels usually increase before other signs and symptoms develop.
10. **Answer: b**
RATIONALE: Rifampin is mainly eliminated by the liver. However, up to 30% of a dose is excreted by the kidneys, and dose reduction may be needed in patients with renal impairment.
11. **Answer: c**
RATIONALE: Although INH is the drug of choice for treatment of LTBI, its use is controversial in older adults. Because risks of drug-induced hepatotoxicity are higher in this population, some clinicians believe that those patients with positive skin tests should have additional risk factors (e.g., recent

skin-test conversion, immunosuppression, previous gastrectomy) before receiving INH.
12. **Answer: b**
RATIONALE: For treatment of LTBI, only one of the four regimens currently recommended for adults (INH for 9 months) is recommended for those younger than 18 years of age.
13. **Answer: a**
RATIONALE: A major difficulty with treatment of TB in patients with HIV infection is that rifampin interacts with many PIs and NNRTIs. If the drugs are given concurrently, rifampin decreases blood levels and therapeutic effects of the anti-HIV drugs.
14. **Answer: b**
RATIONALE: Treatment of active TB disease in HIV-positive patients is similar to that in persons who do not have HIV infection. Those with HIV infection who adhere to standard treatment regimens do not have an increased risk of treatment failure.
15. **Answer: d**
RATIONALE: Pyrazinamide may decrease the effects of allopurinol and cyclosporine.
16. **Answer: c**
RATIONALE: The rifamycins (rifampin, rifabutin, rifapentine) induce cytochrome P450 drug-metabolizing enzymes and therefore accelerate the metabolism and decrease the effectiveness of many drugs. Rifampin is the strongest inducer and may decrease the effects of angiotensin-converting enzyme (ACE) inhibitors, anticoagulants, antidysrhythmics, some antifungals (e.g., fluconazole), anti-HIV protease inhibitors (e.g., amprenavir, indinavir), anti-HIV NNRTIs (e.g., efavirenz, nevirapine), benzodiazepines, beta-blockers, corticosteroids, cyclosporine, digoxin, and diltiazem, as well as estrogens and oral contraceptives.
17. **Answer: a**
RATIONALE: Isoniazid (INH) increases risks of toxicity with several drugs by inhibiting their metabolism and increasing their blood levels. These drugs include carbamazepine, fluconazole, haloperidol, phenytoin (effects of rifampin are opposite to those of INH and tend to predominate if both drugs are given with phenytoin), and vincristine.
18. **Answer: b, c, and e**
RATIONALE: Older adults with TB demonstrate fever, hemoptysis, night sweats, increased sputum production, and mental status changes.
19. **Answer: c**
RATIONALE: Individualizing treatment regimens is used, when possible, to increase patient convenience and minimize disruption of usual activities of daily living. Short-course regimens, intermittent dosing (e.g., two or three times weekly rather than daily), and fixed-dose combinations of drugs (e.g., Rifater, Rifamate) reduce the number of pills and the duration of therapy.
20. **Answer: c**
RATIONALE: Patients taking INH are most at risk for hepatotoxicity.

CHAPTER 21

SECTION I: ASSESSING YOUR UNDERSTANDING

Activity A   FILL IN THE BLANKS

1. pneumonia
2. breaks
3. intracellular
4. numbers
5. human immunodeficiency virus (HIV)

Activity B   MATCHING

1. e   **2.** c   **3.** a   **4.** b   **5.** d

Activity C   SHORT ANSWERS

1. Inside host cells, viruses use cellular metabolic activities for their own survival and replication. Viral replication involves dissolution of the protein coating and exposure of the genetic material—deoxyribonucleic acid (DNA) or ribonucleic acid (RNA). With DNA viruses, the viral DNA enters the host cell's nucleus, where it becomes incorporated into the host cell's chromosomal DNA. Then, host cell genes are coded to produce new viruses. In addition, the viral DNA incorporated with host DNA is transmitted to the host's daughter cells during host cell mitosis and becomes part of the inherited genetic information of the host cell and its progeny. With RNA viruses (e.g., HIV), viral RNA must be converted to DNA by an enzyme called reverse transcriptase before replication can occur.
2. After new viruses are formed, they are released from the infected cell either by budding out and breaking off from the cell membrane (leaving the host cell intact) or by causing lysis of the cell. When the cell is destroyed, the viruses are released into the blood and surrounding tissues, from which they can transmit the viral infection to other host cells.
3. Symptoms usually associated with acute viral infections include fever, headache, cough, malaise, muscle pain, nausea and vomiting, diarrhea, insomnia, and photophobia. White blood cell counts usually remain normal. Other signs and symptoms vary with the type of virus and body organs involved.
4. Some viruses (e.g., herpesviruses) can survive in host cells for many years and cause a chronic, latent infection that periodically becomes reactivated.
5. Antibodies are proteins that defend against microbial or viral invasion. They are very specific (i.e., an antibody protects only against a specific virus or other antigen). The protein coat of the virus allows the immune system of the host to recognize the virus as a "foreign invader" and to produce antibodies against it. Antibodies against infecting viruses can prevent the viruses from reaching the bloodstream or, if they are already in the bloodstream, prevent their invasion of host cells. After the virus has penetrated the cell, it is protected from antibody action, and the host depends on cell-mediated immunity (lymphocytes and macrophages) to eradicate the virus along with the cell harboring it.

SECTION II: APPLYING YOUR KNOWLEDGE

Activity D   CASE STUDY

1. Acyclovir, famciclovir, and valacyclovir penetrate virus-infected cells, become activated by an enzyme, and inhibit viral DNA reproduction. Acyclovir is used to treat genital herpes; it decreases viral shedding and the duration of skin lesions and pain. It does not eliminate inactive virus in the body and therefore does not prevent recurrence of the disease unless oral drug therapy is continued. Prolonged or repeated courses of acyclovir therapy may result in the emergence of acyclovir-resistant viral strains, especially in immunocompromised patients.
2. The disease will reoccur. Acyclovir does not prevent recurrence of the disease unless oral drug therapy is continued.
3. Acyclovir does not eliminate inactive virus in the body and therefore does not prevent recurrence of the disease unless oral drug therapy is continued.
4. Acyclovir may be given orally, intravenously (IV), or applied topically to lesions.

SECTION III: PRACTICING FOR NCLEX

Activity E

1. **Answer: a**
   RATIONALE: Antiretroviral drugs are given in combination to increase effectiveness and decrease emergence of drug-resistant viruses.
2. **Answer: a**
   RATIONALE: Because viruses are intracellular parasites, antiviral drugs are relatively toxic to human cells.
3. **Answer: b, c, d, and e**
   RATIONALE: Viral infections for which drug therapy is available include genital herpes, hepatitis B and C, HIV infection, influenza, and cytomegalovirus.
4. **Answer: b**
   RATIONALE: Vaccinations, avoiding contact with people who have viral infections, and thorough hand hygiene are effective ways to prevent viral infections.
5. **Answer: c**
   RATIONALE: Viral infections commonly occur in all age groups.
6. **Answer: b**
   RATIONALE: The CD4 count is the laboratory test used to determine a patient's ability to fight against infections in a patient with HIV. A BUN measures kidney function, an AST monitors liver function, and RBCs monitor the number of red blood cells that a patient has. None of these measures will give information about the patient's ability to fight infection.

7. **Answer: c**
   RATIONALE: When antiviral agents are prescribed, all patients with hepatic impairment should be monitored closely for abnormal liver function tests (LFTs) and drug-related toxicity.

8. **Answer: a**
   RATIONALE: Nevirapine may cause abnormal LFTs, and a few cases of fatal hepatitis have been reported. If moderate or severe LFT abnormalities occur, nevirapine administration should be discontinued until LFTs return to baseline. If liver dysfunction recurs when the drug is resumed, nevirapine should be discontinued permanently.

9. **Answer: d**
   RATIONALE: Zidovudine is eliminated slowly and has a longer half-life in patients with moderate to severe liver disease. Therefore, daily doses should be reduced by 50% in patients with hepatic impairment.

10. **Answer: c**
    RATIONALE: Amantadine, emtricitabine, entecavir, famciclovir, ganciclovir, lamivudine, telbivudine, and valacyclovir are eliminated mainly through the kidneys. In patients with renal impairment, they may accumulate, produce higher blood levels, have longer half-lives, and cause toxicity. For all of these drugs except famciclovir and emtricitabine, dosage should be reduced with creatinine clearance (CrCl) rates lower than 50 mL/min.

11. **Answer: c**
    RATIONALE: Foscarnet may cause or worsen renal impairment and should be used with caution in all patients. Manifestations of renal impairment are most likely to occur during the second week of induction therapy, but they may occur any time during treatment.

12. **Answer: a**
    RATIONALE: When foscarnet is administered, renal impairment may be minimized by monitoring renal function (e.g., at baseline; two or three times weekly during induction; at least every 1 or 2 weeks during maintenance therapy) and reducing dosage accordingly. The drug should be stopped if creatinine clearance drops to less than 0.4 mL/min/kg. Adequate hydration should also be maintained throughout the course of drug therapy.

13. **Answer: c**
    RATIONALE: Indinavir may cause nephrolithiasis, flank pain, and hematuria. Symptoms usually subside with increased hydration and drug discontinuation. To avoid nephrolithiasis, patients taking indinavir should consume 48 to 64 ounces of water or other fluids daily.

14. **Answer: a and c**
    RATIONALE: When amantadine is given to prevent or treat influenza A, adverse effects include CNS effects (e.g., hallucinations, depression, confusion, dizziness) and cardiovascular effects (e.g., congestive heart failure, orthostatic hypotension, peripheral edema). Other adverse effects include dry nose and GI distress and mottling of the hands and arms.

15. **Answer: b**
    RATIONALE: Oseltamivir may be used in children 1 year of age and older. However, some serious adverse effects have been reported in children 16 years and younger who were taking oseltamivir. The adverse effects include neurologic and psychiatric problems (e.g., delirium, hallucinations, confusion, abnormal behavior, seizures, encephalitis) and a few severe skin reactions.

16. **Answer: d**
    RATIONALE: HIV-seropositive pregnant women should receive zidovudine to prevent perinatal transmission. At 14 to 34 weeks of gestation, zidovudine should be administered at a dose of 100 mg PO five times a day until delivery.

17. **Answer: c**
    RATIONALE: Viral load is a measure of the number of HIV RNA particles within the blood; it does not measure viral levels in tissues, where viral reproduction may be continuing.

18. **Answer: b**
    RATIONALE: Ganciclovir is the antiviral drug that is prescribed for cytomegalovirus. Ribavirin is prescribed for RSV, and amantadine and oseltamivir are prescribed for influenza.

19. **Answer: a**
    RATIONALE: Efavirenz should be given at bedtime to minimize the CNS effects.

20. **Answer: b**
    RATIONALE: Using diaphragm will prevent pregnancy but won't prevent transmission of genital herpes because it still allows contact with the genitalia.

CHAPTER 22

SECTION I: ASSESSING YOUR UNDERSTANDING

Activity A   FILL IN THE BLANKS

1. Fungi
2. multicellular
3. dermatophytes
4. Dimorphic
5. coccidioidomycosis

Activity B   MATCHING

1. c   **2.** a   **3.** d   **4.** b   **5.** e

Activity C   SHORT ANSWERS

1. *Candida albicans* organisms are part of the normal microbial flora of the skin, mouth, gastrointestinal tract, and vagina. Growth of *Candida* organisms is normally restrained by intact immune mechanisms and bacterial competition for nutrients.
2. When the body's natural restraining forces are altered, such as by suppression of the immune system

or antibacterial drug therapy, fungal overgrowth and opportunistic infection can occur.

3. *Aspergillus* organisms produce protease, an enzyme that allows them to destroy structural proteins and penetrate body tissues.

4. *Cryptococcus neoformans* organisms can become encapsulated, which allows them to evade the normal immune defense mechanism of phagocytosis.

SECTION II: APPLYING YOUR KNOWLEDGE
Activity D CASE STUDY

1. Amphotericin B is active against most types of pathogenic fungi and is fungicidal or fungistatic, depending on the concentration in body fluids and the susceptibility of the causative fungus. Because of its toxicity, the drug is used only for serious fungal infections. It is usually given for 4 to 12 weeks.

2. Lipid formulations of amphotericin B (Abelcet, AmBisome, and Amphotec) reach higher concentrations in diseased tissues than in normal tissues, so that larger doses can be given to increase therapeutic effects. At the same time, they cause less damage to normal tissues and decrease adverse effects. These products are much more expensive than the deoxycholate formulation (Fungizone). They are most likely to be used for patients with preexisting renal impairment or conditions in which other nephrotoxic drugs are routinely given (e.g., bone marrow transplantation) and when high doses are needed for difficult-to-treat infections.

3. "The formulations cannot be interchanged." The lipid preparations differ in their characteristics and cannot be used interchangeably.

4. Amphotericin B drug concentrations in most body fluids are higher in the presence of inflammation. Amphotericin B must be given intravenously for systemic infections. After infusion, the drug is rapidly taken up by the liver and other organs. It is then slowly released back into the bloodstream. Despite its long-term use, little is known about its distribution and metabolic pathways.

5. Nephrotoxicity is the most common and the most serious long-term adverse effect of amphotericin B use. The drug constricts afferent renal arterioles and reduces blood flow to the kidneys. Several strategies may decrease nephrotoxicity, such as keeping the patient well hydrated, giving 0.9% sodium chloride IV prior to drug administration, and avoiding the concomitant administration of other nephrotoxic drugs (e.g., aminoglycoside antibiotics).

6. Peripheral lines can become phlebitic. Hypokalemia and hypomagnesemia also occur and may require oral or IV mineral replacement. Additional adverse effects include anorexia, nausea, vomiting, anemia, and phlebitis at peripheral infusion sites. A central vein is preferred for administration.

SECTION III: PRACTICING FOR NCLEX
Activity E

1. **Answer: d**
   RATIONALE: Liver function should be monitored with all systemic antifungal drugs; both hepatic and renal function should be monitored with amphotericin B.

2. **Answer: a**
   RATIONALE: Systemic antifungal drugs may cause serious adverse effects. Nephrotoxicity is associated with amphotericin B; hepatotoxicity is associated with azole drugs.

3. **Answer: c**
   RATIONALE: Fungal infections often require long-term drug therapy.

4. **Answer: d**
   RATIONALE: Patients whose immune systems are suppressed are at high risk of serious fungal infections.

5. **Answer: c**
   RATIONALE: Lipid formulations of amphotericin B are used in patients with diminished renal function because these formulations are less nephrotoxic.

6. **Answer: b, c, and e**
   RATIONALE: With IV antifungal drugs for serious infections, the home care nurse needs to teach the patient and family to keep fresh flowers and potted plants from the house. The bathroom should be cleaned daily with bleach and ensure that the air conditioning filters are clean. It is not necessary to remove all rugs and curtains from the house.

7. **Answer: b**
   RATIONALE: Because the immune function of these patients is often severely suppressed, protective interventions are needed. These may include teaching about frequent and thorough hand hygiene by patients, all members of the household, and visitors; safe food preparation and storage; removal of potted plants and fresh flowers; and avoiding activities that generate dust in the patient's environment. In addition, air conditioning and air filtering systems should be kept meticulously clean, and any plans for renovations should be postponed or canceled.

8. **Answer: a**
   RATIONALE: When itraconazole is used in critically ill patients, a loading dose of 200 mg three times daily may be given for the first 3 days.

9. **Answer: c**
   RATIONALE: Amphotericin B penetrates tissues well, except for CSF, and only small amounts are excreted in urine. With prolonged administration, the half-life increases from 1 to 15 days. Hemodialysis does not remove the drug.

10. **Answer: b**
    RATIONALE: Amphotericin B penetrates tissues well, except for CSF, and only small amounts are

excreted in urine. Fluconazole penetrates tissues well, including CSF.

11. Answer: d

RATIONALE: The azole antifungals are relatively contraindicated in patients with increased liver enzymes, active liver disease, or a history of liver damage from other drugs. They should be given only if expected benefits outweigh risks of liver injury.

12. Answer: b

RATIONALE: Caspofungin is prescribed for patients with a suspected fungal infection who are neutropenic.

13. Answer: a, b, and d

RATIONALE: Digoxin, antibiotics, and antineoplastic and cortisone drugs will increase the effects of amphotericin B.

14. Answer: a

RATIONALE: Nystatin is a topical and oral preparation that has the same mechanism of action as amphotericin B and is used only in the treatment of candidiasis.

15. Answer: c

RATIONALE: There are several recommendations for reducing toxicity of IV amphotericin B, but most have not been tested in controlled studies. The treatment to decrease fever and chills includes premedication with acetaminophen, diphenhydramine, and a corticosteroid.

16. Answer: a, b, d, and e

RATIONALE: There are several recommendations for reducing toxicity of IV amphotericin B, but most have not been tested in controlled studies. Recommendations to decrease phlebitis at injection sites include administering on alternate days, adding 500 to 2000 units of heparin to the infusion, rotating infusion sites, administering through a central vein, removing the needle after infusion, using a pediatric scalp vein needle, and administering the medication through a separate IV line.

17. Answer: a

RATIONALE: Maintenance doses of Fungizone may be doubled and infused on alternate days. However, a single daily dose of Fungizone should not exceed 1.5 mg/kg; overdoses can result in cardiorespiratory arrest.

18. Answer: d

RATIONALE: Itraconazole, for 3 to 6 months, is the drug of choice for localized lymphocutaneous infection.

19. Answer: a

RATIONALE: Use of antihistamines is a predisposing factor for fungal infections. In addition, some candidal infections respond to the removal of predisposing factors such as antibacterial drugs, corticosteroids or other immunosuppressant drugs, and indwelling IV or bladder catheters.

20. Answer: d

RATIONALE: Candidiasis occurs in warm moist places, so it is important for the nurse to ensure that all of the patient's skin folds are dry.

CHAPTER 23

SECTION I: ASSESSING YOUR UNDERSTANDING

Activity A FILL IN THE BLANKS

1. parasite
2. *Entamoeba histolytica*
3. amebic cysts
4. Trophozoites
5. enzyme

Activity B MATCHING

1. d **2.** a **3.** b **4.** e **5.** c

Activity C SHORT ANSWERS

1. Amebiasis is a common disease in Africa, Asia, and Latin America, but it can occur in any geographic region. In the United States, it is most likely to occur among residents of institutions for the mentally challenged, among men who have sex with men, and among residents or travelers in countries with poor sanitation.
2. Toxoplasmosis is caused by *Toxoplasma gondii*, a parasite that is spread by ingestion of undercooked meat or other food containing encysted forms of the organism, by contact with feces from infected cats, and by congenital spread from mothers with acute infection.
3. The most common form of trichomoniasis is a vaginal infection caused by *Trichomonas vaginalis*. The disease is usually spread by sexual intercourse.
4. Scabies is caused by the "itch mite" (*Sarcoptes scabiei*), which burrows into the skin and lays eggs that hatch in 4 to 8 days. The burrows may produce visible skin lesions, most often between the fingers and on the wrists.
5. Pediculosis capitis (head lice) is the most common type of lice infestation in the United States. It is diagnosed by finding louse eggs (nits) attached to hair shafts close to the scalp.

SECTION II: APPLYING YOUR KNOWLEDGE

Activity D CASE STUDY

1. Eating locally grown food and drinking fruit juice reconstituted at a local restaurant are possible sources of the patient's infection. Giardiasis is caused by *Giardia lamblia*, a common intestinal parasite. It is spread by food or water contaminated with human feces containing encysted forms of the organism or by contact with infected people or animals.
2. Giardial infections usually occur 1 to 2 weeks after ingestion of the cysts, so symptoms often do not appear until travelers are back home. Giardial infections may be asymptomatic, or they may produce diarrhea, abdominal cramping, and abdominal distention.
3. If giardiasis is left untreated, it may resolve spontaneously, or it may progress to a chronic disease with anorexia, nausea, malaise, weight loss, and continued

diarrhea with large, foul-smelling stools. Malaise and fatigue can develop, which are attributable to deficiencies of vitamin B$_{12}$ and fat-soluble vitamins that are a consequence of untreated giardiasis.
4. Adults and children older than 8 years of age with symptomatic giardiasis are usually treated with oral metronidazole.

SECTION III: PRACTICING FOR NCLEX
Activity E
1. **Answer: a**
   RATIONALE: Antiparasitic drugs are usually given for local effects in the GI tract or on the skin.
2. **Answer: b**
   RATIONALE: Personal and public health hygienic practices can prevent many parasitic infections and should be followed diligently.
3. **Answer: d**
   RATIONALE: Travelers to malarious regions should generally receive chloroquine to prevent malaria and take precautions to avoid or minimize exposure to the causative mosquito.
4. **Answer: b**
   RATIONALE: The nurse checks for the presence of ova (nits) sticking to the hair shafts when checking the school child for head lice.
5. **Answer: b**
   RATIONALE: When children have parasitic infections, the home care nurse may need to collaborate with day care centers and schools to prevent or control outbreaks.
6. **Answer: a, b, d, and e**
   RATIONALE: The home care nurse may need to examine close contacts of the infected person and assess their need for treatment; assist parents and patients so that drugs are used appropriately; and teach personal and environmental hygiene measures to prevent reinfection. The nurse should also ensure that follow-up measures such as repeat stool samples are completed.
7. **Answer: a**
   RATIONALE: Children often receive an antiparasitic drug for head lice or worm infestations. These products should be used exactly as directed and with appropriate precautions to prevent reinfection.
8. **Answer: a**
   RATIONALE: Malaria is usually more severe in children than in adults, and children should be protected from exposure whenever possible. If chemoprophylaxis or treatment for malaria is indicated, the same drugs are used for children as for adults, with appropriate dosage adjustments. The tetracyclines are an exception and should not be given to children younger than 8 years of age.
9. **Answer: a**
   RATIONALE: The nurse suspects that the child has pinworms, which come out of the anus at night and cause severe itching.

10. **Answer: b**
    RATIONALE: Malathion (Ovide) is a pediculicide used in the treatment of resistant head lice infestations, and pyrethrin preparations (e.g., RID) are available over the counter for treatment of pediculosis. These preparations require two applications approximately 10 days apart.
11. **Answer: b**
    RATIONALE: Mebendazole is a PO medication that must be chewed and swallowed or crushed in food. It is not given IM or IV or swallowed whole.
12. **Answer: d**
    RATIONALE: Permethrin is used to treat both pediculosis and scabies. Malathion and Spinosad are used to treat pediculosis, and metronidazole is used for intestinal amebae.
13. **Answer: b**
    RATIONALE: Metronidazole commonly causes a patient's urine to turn dark. It is a temporary side effect. The color of the urine goes back to normal after the medication has been completed.
14. **Answer: a**
    RATIONALE: Nitazoxanide (Alinia) is approved for treatment of diarrhea caused by giardiasis or cryptosporidiosis in children. It is the first drug approved for treatment of cryptosporidiosis, which may be life threatening in immunocompromised hosts.
15. **Answer: d**
    RATIONALE: Quinine also relaxes skeletal muscles and has been used for prevention and treatment of nocturnal leg cramps.
16. **Answer: c**
    RATIONALE: When used to prevent initial occurrence of malaria (causal prophylaxis), primaquine is given concurrently with a suppressive agent (e.g., chloroquine, hydroxychloroquine) after the patient has returned from a malarious area.
17. **Answer: d**
    RATIONALE: Chloroquine is a widely used antimalarial agent. It acts against erythrocytic forms of plasmodial parasites to prevent or treat malarial attacks.
18. **Answer: a and c**
    RATIONALE: Tetracycline and doxycycline are antibacterial drugs that act against amebae in the intestinal lumen by altering the bacterial flora required for amebic viability. One of these drugs may be used with other amebicides in the treatment of all forms of amebiasis except asymptomatic intestinal amebiasis.
19. **Answer: a**
    RATIONALE: Metronidazole is contraindicated during the first trimester of pregnancy and must be used with caution in patients with central nervous system (CNS) or blood disorders. Patients should also avoid all forms of ethanol while taking this medication.
20. **Answer: d**
    RATIONALE: Hydroxychloroquine is used as a prophylaxis for malaria and also as a treatment for rheumatoid arthritis and systemic lupus erythematosus.

CHAPTER 24

SECTION I: ASSESSING YOUR UNDERSTANDING

Activity A FILL IN THE BLANKS

1. Heart failure
2. systolic dysfunction
3. diastolic dysfunction
4. fluid accumulation
5. heart failure

Activity B MATCHING

1. d   **2.** a   **3.** b   **4.** e   **5.** c

Activity C SHORT ANSWERS

1. At the cellular level, HF stems from dysfunction of contractile myocardial cells and the endothelial cells that line the heart and blood vessels (see Chap. 47). Vital functions of the endothelium include maintaining equilibrium between vasodilation and vasoconstriction, coagulation and anticoagulation, and cellular growth promotion and inhibition. Endothelial dysfunction allows processes that narrow the blood vessel lumen (e.g., buildup of atherosclerotic plaque, growth of cells, inflammation, activation of platelets) and leads to blood-clot formation and vasoconstriction that further narrow the blood vessel lumen. These are major factors in coronary artery disease and hypertension, the most common conditions leading to HF.

2. As the heart fails, the low cardiac output and inadequately filled arteries activate the neurohormonal system by several feedback mechanisms. One mechanism is increased sympathetic activity and circulating *catecholamines* (neurohormones), which increases the force of myocardial contraction, increases heart rate, and causes vasoconstriction. The effects of the baroreceptors in the aortic arch and carotid sinus that normally inhibit undue sympathetic stimulation are blunted in patients with HF, and the effects of the high levels of circulating catecholamines are intensified. Endothelin, a neurohormone secreted primarily by endothelial cells, is the most potent endogenous vasoconstrictor and may exert direct toxic effects on the heart and result in myocardial cell proliferation.

3. Cardinal manifestations of HF are dyspnea and fatigue, which can lead to exercise intolerance and fluid retention resulting in pulmonary congestion and peripheral edema. Patients with compensated (asymptomatic) HF usually have no symptoms at rest and no edema; dyspnea and fatigue occur only with activities involving moderate or higher levels of exertion. Symptoms that occur with minimal exertion or at rest and are accompanied by ankle edema and distention of the jugular vein (from congestion of veins and leakage of fluid into tissues) reflect decompensation (symptomatic HF). Acute, severe cardiac decompensation is manifested by pulmonary edema, a medical emergency that requires immediate treatment. Two models currently exist for classification of HF. The New York Heart Association (NYHA) classifies HF based on functional limitations. A newer system of staging HF, proposed by the American College of Cardiology (ACC) and the American Heart Association (AHA), is based on the progression of HF.

4. Renin is an enzyme produced in the kidneys in response to impaired blood flow and tissue perfusion. When released into the bloodstream, renin stimulates the production of angiotensin II, a powerful vasoconstrictor. Arterial vasoconstriction impairs cardiac function by increasing the resistance (afterload) against which the ventricle ejects blood. This raises filling pressures inside the heart, increases stretch and stress on the myocardial wall, and predisposes to subendocardial ischemia. In addition, patients with severe HF have constricted arterioles in cerebral, myocardial, renal, hepatic, and mesenteric vascular beds. This results in increased organ hypoperfusion and dysfunction. Venous vasoconstriction limits venous capacitance, resulting in venous congestion and increased diastolic ventricular filling pressures (preload). Angiotensin II also promotes sodium and water retention by stimulating aldosterone release from the adrenal cortex and the release of vasopressin (antidiuretic hormone) from the posterior pituitary gland.

5. Increased blood volume and pressure in the heart chambers; stretching of muscle fibers; and dilation, hypertrophy, and changes in the shape of the heart (a process called *cardiac or ventricular remodeling*) make it contract less efficiently.

SECTION II: APPLYING YOUR KNOWLEDGE

Activity D CASE STUDY

1. Food may decrease digoxin absorption, so she should take it on an empty stomach. In addition to drug dosage forms, other factors that may decrease digoxin absorption include the presence of food in the GI tract, delayed gastric emptying, malabsorption syndromes, and concurrent administration of some drugs (e.g., antacids, cholestyramine).

2. When digoxin is given orally, absorption varies among available preparations. Lanoxicaps, which are liquid-filled capsules, and the elixir used for children are better absorbed than tablets. With tablets, the most frequently used formulation, differences in bioavailability are also important, because a person who is stabilized on one formulation may be underdosed or overdosed if another formulation is taken. Differences are attributed to the rate and extent of tablet dissolution rather than amounts of digoxin.

3. The physician will decrease the digoxin dose. Therapeutic serum levels of digoxin are 0.5 to 2 nanograms per milliliter (ng/mL); serum levels greater than 2 ng/mL are toxic. In elderly patients

and in the presence of renal failure, therapeutic serum levels are 0.5 to 1.3 ng/mL. Research in the past decade has suggested that serum levels of 1.0 ng/mL or less are more appropriate in those with HF (see "Bridging the Gap with EBP"). However, toxicity may occur at virtually any serum level. Dosage must be reduced in the presence of renal failure to prevent drug accumulation and toxicity, because most of the digoxin (60%–70%) is excreted unchanged by the kidneys. The remainder is metabolized or excreted by nonrenal routes.

4. In patients with atrial dysrhythmias, digoxin slows the rate of ventricular contraction (negative chronotropic effect). With IV digoxin, the onset of action occurs within 10 to 30 minutes, and peak effects occur in 1 to 5 hours. Digoxin is given orally or intravenously. Although it can be given intramuscularly, this route is not recommended, because pain and muscle necrosis may occur at injection sites. When digoxin is given orally, the onset of action occurs in 30 minutes to 2 hours, and peak effects occur in approximately 6 hours.

SECTION III: PRACTICING FOR NCLEX
Activity E

1. **Answer: d**
RATIONALE: The normal digoxin level is 0.5 to 2.0 ng/mL. Serum levels greater than 2 ng/mL are toxic; however, toxicity may occur at any serum level.

2. **Answer: b**
RATIONALE: The patient with renal dysfunction is at an increased risk for digoxin toxicity.

3. **Answer: b**
RATIONALE: For acute HF, the first drugs of choice may include an IV loop diuretic, a cardiotonic–inotropic agent (e.g., digoxin, dobutamine, milrinone), and vasodilators (e.g., nitroglycerin and hydralazine or nitroprusside).

4. **Answer: c**
RATIONALE: Beta-blockers are not recommended for patients in acute HF because of the potential for an initial decrease in myocardial contractility.

5. **Answer: c**
RATIONALE: Cardinal manifestations of HF are dyspnea and fatigue, which can lead to exercise intolerance and fluid retention resulting in pulmonary congestion and peripheral edema.

6. **Answer: d**
RATIONALE: The nurse must assess the patient's apical pulse before administering digoxin because it has a narrow therapeutic index and can cause the heart rate to go too low, so the nurse takes the apical pulse and holds the medication if it is below a certain level (depending upon age of the patient.)

7. **Answer: a, b, c, and e**
RATIONALE: Heart failure may result from impaired myocardial contraction during systole (systolic dysfunction), impaired relaxation and filling of ventricles during diastole (diastolic dysfunction), or a combination of systolic and diastolic dysfunction. Cardiomyopathy (weakened and enlarged heart muscle) also increases the risk for the development of heart failure.

8. **Answer: a**
RATIONALE: Natural licorice blocks the effects of spironolactone and causes sodium retention and potassium loss, effects that may worsen HF and potentiate the effects of digoxin.

9. **Answer: a**
RATIONALE: When patients are receiving a combination of drugs for management of HF, the nurse needs to assist them in understanding that the different types of drugs have different actions and produce different responses. As a result, they work together to be more effective and maintain a more balanced state of cardiovascular function. Changing drugs or dosages can upset the balance and lead to acute and severe symptoms that may require hospitalization or may even cause death from HF. Therefore, it is extremely important that patients take all their medications as prescribed. If they are unable to take the medications for any reason, patients or caregivers should notify the prescribing health care provider. They should be instructed not to wait until symptoms become severe before seeking care.

10. **Answer: d**
RATIONALE: Hepatic impairment has little effect on digoxin clearance, and no dosage adjustments are needed.

11. **Answer: c**
RATIONALE: Digoxin should be used cautiously, in reduced dosages, because renal impairment delays its excretion. Both loading and maintenance doses should be reduced. Patients with advanced renal impairment can achieve therapeutic serum concentrations with a dosage of 0.125 mg three to five times per week.

12. **Answer: b**
RATIONALE: Digoxin is commonly used in children for the same indications as for adults and should be prescribed or supervised by a pediatric cardiologist when possible. The response to a given dose varies with age, size, and renal and hepatic function. There may be little difference between a therapeutic dose and a toxic dose. Very small amounts are often given to children. These factors increase the risks of dosage errors in children. In a hospital setting, institutional policies may require that each dose be verified by another nurse before it is administered. Liquid digoxin must be precisely measured in a syringe, and the dose should not be rounded. ECG monitoring is desirable when digoxin therapy is started.

13. **Answer: b**
RATIONALE: An ECG is obtained prior to the beginning of digoxin therapy to obtain a baseline so that early changes in the ECG can be seen that may indicate early digoxin toxicity.

14. Answer: a
RATIONALE: Atropine or isoproterenol, used in the management of bradycardia or conduction defects, may be administered to patients with digoxin toxicity.

15. Answer: c
RATIONALE: Digoxin dosages must be interpreted with consideration of specific patient characteristics, including age, weight, gender, renal function, general health state, and concurrent drug therapy. Loading or digitalizing doses are necessary for initiating therapy, because digoxin's long half-life makes therapeutic serum levels difficult to obtain without loading. Loading doses should be used cautiously in patients who have taken digoxin within the previous 2 or 3 weeks.

16. Answer: b
RATIONALE: In chronic HF, hypokalemia may be less likely to occur because lower doses of potassium-losing diuretics are usually being given. In addition, there may be more extensive use of potassium-sparing diuretics (e.g., amiloride, triamterene) and the aldosterone antagonist, spironolactone.

17. Answer: a, c, and d
RATIONALE: The nurse is aware that the nurse will monitor the patient's serum electrolytes, renal function, and serum digoxin level.

18. Answer: b and d
RATIONALE: The nurse teaches the patient to avoid salt, so added salt should not be used. The patient should lose weight if needed and avoid saturated fats. The patient should also be encouraged to eat a balanced diet and to avoid high-sodium foods.

19. Answer: b
RATIONALE: For patients who are obese, weight loss is desirable to decrease systemic vascular resistance and myocardial oxygen demand.

20. Answer: a, c, d, and e
RATIONALE: Administer oxygen, if needed, to relieve dyspnea, improve oxygen delivery, reduce the work of breathing, and decrease constriction of pulmonary blood vessels (which is a compensatory measure in patients with hypoxemia).

CHAPTER 25

SECTION I: ASSESSING YOUR UNDERSTANDING

Activity A FILL IN THE BLANKS

1. Dysrhythmias
2. contractile
3. Automaticity
4. calcium
5. excitability

Activity B MATCHING

1. d   **2.** a   **3.** e   **4.** b   **5.** c

Activity C SHORT ANSWERS

1. The heart is an electrical pump. Its "electrical" activity resides primarily in the specialized tissues that can generate and conduct an electrical impulse. Although impulses are also conducted through muscle cells, the rate is much slower. The mechanical or "pump" activity resides in contractile tissue. Normally, these activities result in effective cardiac contraction and distribution of blood throughout the body. Heart beats occur at regular intervals and consist of four events: *stimulation* from an electrical impulse, *transmission* of the electrical impulse to adjacent conductive or contractile tissue, *contraction* of atria and then ventricles, and *relaxation* of atria and then ventricles.

2. Automaticity is the heart's ability to generate an electrical impulse. Any part of the conduction system can spontaneously start an impulse, but the sinoatrial (SA) node normally has the fastest rate of automaticity and therefore the fastest rate of spontaneous impulse formation. Because it has a faster rate of electrical discharge or depolarization than other parts of the conduction system, the SA node serves as the pacemaker site.

3. The ability of a cardiac muscle cell to respond to an electrical stimulus is called *excitability*. The stimulus must reach a certain threshold to cause contraction. After contraction, sodium and calcium ions return to the extracellular space, potassium ions return to the intracellular space, muscle relaxation occurs, and the cell prepares for the next electrical stimulus followed by contraction.

4. After a contraction, there is also a period of decreased excitability (called the *absolute refractory period*) during which the cell cannot respond to a new stimulus. Before the resting membrane potential is reached, a stimulus greater than normal can evoke a response in the cell. This period is called the *relative refractory period*.

5. Conductivity is the ability of cardiac tissue to transmit electrical impulses. The orderly, rhythmic transmission of impulses to all cells is needed for effective myocardial contraction.

SECTION II: APPLYING YOUR KNOWLEDGE

Activity D CASE STUDY

1. Lidocaine decreases myocardial irritability (automaticity) in the ventricles. Lidocaine has little effect on atrial tissue and therefore is not useful in treating atrial dysrhythmias.

2. A bolus dose has a rapid onset and a short duration of action. After intravenous (IV) administration of a bolus dose of lidocaine, therapeutic effects occur within 1 to 2 minutes and last approximately 10 to 20 minutes. This characteristic is advantageous in emergency management but limits lidocaine use to intensive care settings.

3. The physician would decrease the dosage of the lidocaine in an alcoholic patient or in a patient with liver damage. Lidocaine is metabolized in the liver, so the dosage must be reduced in patients with hepatic insufficiency or right-sided heart failure to avoid drug accumulation and toxicity. Hives, as well as shortness of breath, are signs of an allergic reaction. Lidocaine is contraindicated for such a patient.

4. With a lidocaine serum level of 0.75 mcg/mL, the patient has achieved a subtherapeutic level of the drug. Therapeutic serum levels of lidocaine are 1.5 to 6 mcg/mL. Toxic serum levels are those greater than 6 mcg/mL.

SECTION III: PRACTICING FOR NCLEX
Activity E

1. **Answer: d**
   RATIONALE: The FDA has issued a black box warning for amiodarone recommending that it be used only in patients with life-threatening dysrhythmias due to the risk of developing potentially fatal pulmonary toxicity.

2. **Answer: a and d**
   RATIONALE: Amiodarone is a potassium channel blocker that prolongs conduction in all cardiac tissues and decreases heart rate; it also decreases contractility of the left ventricle. It has a vasodilation effect, not a vasoconstrictive effect.

3. **Answer: d**
   RATIONALE: Quinidine is administered at a rate of 1 mL/min.

4. **Answer: a and c**
   RATIONALE: Lidocaine dosages are reduced when a patient also has a liver disorder or right-sided heart failure. It would not be reduced when the patient has Alzheimer's disease, ventricular dysrhythmia, or rheumatoid arthritis.

5. **Answer: a**
   RATIONALE: Class II beta-adrenergic blockers are being used more extensively because of their effectiveness in reducing mortality after myocardial infarction and in patients with heart failure.

6. **Answer: d**
   RATIONALE: Flecainide, propafenone, and moricizine are class IC drugs that have no effect on the repolarization phase but greatly decrease conduction in the ventricles.

7. **Answer: a, b, and c**
   RATIONALE: Lidocaine is the prototype of class IB antidysrhythmics used for treating serious ventricular dysrhythmias associated with acute myocardial infarction, cardiac catheterization, or cardiac surgery and digitalis-induced ventricular dysrhythmias. It is not intended for use with patients experiencing cardiac arrest.

8. **Answer: a and c**
   RATIONALE: Quinidine, the prototype of class IA antidysrhythmics, reduces automaticity, slows conduction, and prolongs the refractory period. It doesn't increase contractility of the heart muscle.

9. **Answer: a**
   RATIONALE: If quinidine is ordered for a child, it may only be administered orally. It is not intended for IV use. It is not available as IM or SC.

10. **Answer: b**
    RATIONALE: The nurse would assess this patient for digoxin toxicity because quinidine and digoxin interact, leading to an increased digoxin level.

11. **Answer: c**
    RATIONALE: Patients receiving chronic antidysrhythmic drug therapy are likely to have significant cardiovascular disease. With each visit, the home care nurse needs to assess the patient's physical, mental, and functional status and evaluate pulse and blood pressure. In addition, patients and caregivers should be taught to report symptoms (e.g., dizziness or fainting, chest pain) and to avoid over-the-counter agents unless discussed with a health care provider.

12. **Answer: c**
    RATIONALE: Because serious problems may stem from either dysrhythmias or their treatment, health care providers should be adept in preventing, recognizing, and treating conditions that predispose to the development of serious dysrhythmias (e.g., electrolyte imbalances, hypoxia). If dysrhythmias cannot be prevented, early recognition and treatment are needed.

13. **Answer: c**
    RATIONALE: Dosages of digoxin, disopyramide, propafenone, and quinidine should be reduced in patients with impairment of hepatic function.

14. **Answer: a, b, and c**
    RATIONALE: Antidysrhythmic drug therapy in patients with renal impairment should be very cautious, with close monitoring of drug effects (e.g., plasma drug levels, ECG changes, symptoms that may indicate drug toxicity). Allergy/antigen testing is not indicated with the use of antidysrhythmic drug therapy.

15. **Answer: a**
    RATIONALE: Cardiac dysrhythmias are common in older adults, but in general only those causing symptoms of circulatory impairment should be treated with antidysrhythmic drugs.

16. **Answer: b, c, and d**
    RATIONALE: Patients who are experiencing a dysrhythmia often experience oliguria, hypotension, mental confusion or syncope, or shortness of breath. Leg pain is not a symptom of dysrhythmia.

17. **Answer: c**
    RATIONALE: Sotalol is the only beta-blocker that may be used in children over the age of 2.

18. **Answer: d**
    RATIONALE: Adenosine is administered like the adult dosing for children over 50 kg. For children weighing less than 50 kg, initially 0.1 mg/kg IV push is given, with a maximum dose

administration of 6 mg. If this initial dose is ineffective, a repeat dose of 0.2 mg/kg up to the maximum of 12 mg may be administered by IV push.

19. Answer: c
RATIONALE: Low-dose amiodarone is a pharmacologic choice for preventing recurrent A-Fib after electrical or pharmacologic conversion. The low doses cause fewer adverse effects than the higher ones used for life-threatening ventricular dysrhythmias.

20. Answer: a and b
RATIONALE: Nonpharmacologic management is preferred, at least initially, for several dysrhythmias. For example, sinus tachycardia usually results from such disorders as dehydration, fever, infection, or hypotension, and intervention and management should attempt to relieve the underlying cause. For PSVT with mild or moderate symptoms, Valsalva's maneuver, carotid sinus massage, or other measures to increase vagal tone are preferred. A cup of hot decaffeinated tea will not help with the management of PSVT.

CHAPTER 26

SECTION I: ASSESSING YOUR UNDERSTANDING

Activity A FILL IN THE BLANKS

1. Angina pectoris
2. myocardial
3. artery spasm
4. coronary artery disease (CAD)
5. variant

Activity B MATCHING

1. c   2. a   3. e   4. b   5. c

Activity C SHORT ANSWERS

1. Classic anginal pain is usually described as substernal chest pain of a constricting, squeezing, or suffocating nature. It may radiate to the jaw, neck, or shoulder; down the left or both arms; or to the back. The discomfort is sometimes mistaken for arthritis or for indigestion, because the pain may be associated with nausea, vomiting, dizziness, diaphoresis, shortness of breath, or fear of impending doom. The discomfort is usually brief, typically lasting 5 minutes or less until the balance of oxygen supply and demand is restored.
2. Current research indicates that gender differences exist in the type and quality of cardiac symptoms, with women reporting epigastric or back discomfort.
3. Older adults may have atypical symptoms of CAD and may experience "silent" ischemia that may delay them from seeking professional help.
4. Atherosclerosis begins with accumulation of lipid-filled macrophages (i.e., foam cells) on the inner lining of coronary arteries. Foam cells, which promote growth of atherosclerotic plaque, develop in response to elevated blood cholesterol levels. These early lesions progress to fibrous plaques containing foam cells covered by smooth muscle cells and connective tissue. Advanced lesions also contain hemorrhages, ulcerations, and scar tissue. Factors contributing to plaque development and growth include endothelial injury, lipid infiltration (i.e., cholesterol), recruitment of inflammatory cells (mainly monocytes and T lymphocytes), and smooth muscle cell proliferation. Endothelial injury may be the initiating factor in plaque formation, because it allows monocytes, platelets, cholesterol, and other blood components to come in contact with and stimulate abnormal growth of smooth muscle cells and connective tissue in the arterial wall.
5. Myocardial ischemia occurs when the coronary arteries are unable to provide sufficient blood and oxygen for normal cardiac functions. Also known as *ischemic heart disease*, *CAD*, or *coronary heart disease*, myocardial ischemia may manifest as an acute coronary syndrome with three main consequences. One consequence is unstable angina, with the occurrence of pain (symptomatic myocardial ischemia).

SECTION II: APPLYING YOUR KNOWLEDGE

Activity D CASE STUDIES

Case Study 1

1. Mrs. Smith is at risk for metabolic syndrome. *The Third Report of the National Cholesterol Education Program Expert Panel on Detection, Evaluation, and Treatment of High Blood Cholesterol in Adults* (NCEP III) defines metabolic syndrome as a cluster of several cardiovascular risk factors linked with obesity: elevated waist circumference, elevated triglycerides, reduced high density lipoprotein cholesterol, elevated blood pressure, and elevated fasting glucose.
2. Smoking cessation is a good place for this patient to start. Patients should avoid circumstances known to precipitate acute attacks, and those who smoke should stop.

Case Study 2

1. Organic nitrates relax smooth muscle in blood vessel walls. This action produces vasodilation, which relieves anginal pain by several mechanisms. First, dilation of veins reduces venous pressure and venous return to the heart. This decreases blood volume and pressure within the heart (preload), which in turn decreases cardiac workload and oxygen demand. Second, nitrates dilate coronary arteries at higher doses and can increase blood flow to ischemic areas of the myocardium. Third, nitrates dilate the arterioles, which lowers peripheral vascular resistance (afterload). This results in lower systolic blood pressure and, consequently, reduced cardiac workload.

2. When given sublingually, nitroglycerin is absorbed directly into the systemic circulation. It acts within 1 to 3 minutes, and its effects last for 30 to 60 minutes. Contraindications include hypersensitivity reactions, severe anemia, hypotension, and hypovolemia. The drugs should be used cautiously in the presence of head injury or cerebral hemorrhage because they may increase intracranial pressure.

3. Males taking nitroglycerin or any other nitrate should not take phosphodiesterase enzyme type 5 inhibitors such as sildenafil (Viagra) and vardenafil (Levitra) for erectile dysfunction. Nitrates and phosphodiesterase enzyme type 5 inhibitors decrease blood pressure, and the combined effect can produce profound, life-threatening hypotension.

SECTION III: PRACTICING FOR NCLEX
Activity E
1. **Answer: b**
   RATIONALE: Starting with relatively small doses of antianginal drugs and increasing them at appropriate intervals as necessary should achieve optimal benefit and minimal adverse effects.
2. **Answer: c**
   RATIONALE: Aspirin, antilipemics, and antihypertensives are used in conjunction with antianginal drugs to prevent progression of myocardial ischemia to MI.
3. **Answer: c**
   RATIONALE: In angina pectoris, calcium channel blockers improve blood supply to the myocardium by dilating coronary arteries and decrease the workload of the heart by dilating peripheral arteries; in variant angina, the drugs reduce coronary artery vasospasm.
4. **Answer: b**
   RATIONALE: Patients who take long-acting dosage forms of nitrates on a regular schedule develop tolerance to the vasodilating (antianginal) effects of the drug.
5. **Answer: a**
   RATIONALE: Traditional antianginal drugs that act via hemodynamic mechanisms (e.g., beta-blockers, calcium antagonists, nitrates) can pose a problem in older adults because of the associated higher risk of drug interactions and greater incidence of adverse drug effects.
6. **Answer: d**
   RATIONALE: Beta-blockers are more effective than nitrates or calcium channel blockers in decreasing the likelihood of silent ischemia and improving the mortality rate after transmural MI.
7. **Answer: c**
   RATIONALE: Ranolazine is contraindicated in patients who have a condition called QT-interval prolongation.

8. **Answer: b, c, and d**
   RATIONALE: Because oral nitroglycerin is rapidly metabolized in the liver, relatively small proportions reach systemic circulation; transmucosal, transdermal, and IV preparations are more effective. Nitroglycerin is not administered intrathecally.
9. **Answer: a, c, and d**
   RATIONALE: The goals of antianginal drug therapy are to relieve acute anginal pain, to reduce the number and severity of acute anginal attacks, to improve exercise tolerance and quality of life, to delay progression of CAD, to prevent MI, and to prevent sudden cardiac death. Antianginal drug therapy does not increase the vascularity of the heart.
10. **Answer: a**
    RATIONALE: Angina pectoris results from deficit in myocardial oxygen supply (myocardial ischemia) in relation to myocardial oxygen demand, most often caused by atherosclerotic plaque in the coronary arteries.
11. **Answer: a, b, d, and e**
    RATIONALE: The home care nurse's responsibilities may include monitoring the patient's response to antianginal medications; teaching patients and caregivers how to use, store, and replace medications to ensure a constant supply; and discussing circumstances in which the patient should seek emergency care. The patient should also be instructed in factors that contribute to angina such as smoking and obesity.
12. **Answer: a**
    RATIONALE: In addition to reduced effectiveness, absorption of oral drugs or topical forms of nitroglycerin may be impaired in patients with extensive edema, heart failure, hypotension, or other conditions that impair blood flow to the gastrointestinal tract or skin.
13. **Answer: a, c, and d**
    RATIONALE: Antianginal drugs have multiple cardiovascular effects and may be used alone or in combination with other cardiovascular drugs in patients with critical illness. They are probably used most often to manage severe angina, severe hypertension, or serious cardiac dysrhythmias. They are not indicated for treatment of serious heart failure.
14. **Answer: c**
    RATIONALE: The patient should take 1 pill as soon as chest pain occurs. Burning indicates the medication is active, and it often causes a headache because of the vasodilation. The pills are only good for approximately 6 months. If chest pain is not relieved after the first pill, the patient may take the second pill 5 minutes after the first and then may take a third pill 5 minutes later. At this point, if the patient still has chest pain, the patient should call 911.

15. Answer: a
RATIONALE: Nitroglycerin has been given IV for heart failure and intraoperative control of blood pressure, with the initial dose adjusted for weight and later doses titrated to response.

16. Answer: a
RATIONALE: For relief of acute angina and for prophylaxis before events that cause acute angina, nitroglycerin (sublingual tablets or translingual spray) is usually the primary drug of choice.

17. Answer: a
RATIONALE: Ranolazine (Ranexa) represents a new classification of antianginal medication, metabolic modulators, used in people with chronic angina. The drug is labeled for use in combination with amlodipine, beta-blockers, or nitrates. After oral administration, peak plasma concentrations are reached within 2 to 5 hours. The drug is rapidly and extensively metabolized in the liver. Because of a risk of dose-dependent QT prolongation on electrocardiogram, ranolazine is reserved for the treatment of patients with chronic angina who have not achieved a satisfactory antianginal response with traditional drugs.

18. Answer: c
RATIONALE: Propranolol, the prototype beta-blocker, is used to reduce the frequency and severity of acute attacks of angina. It is usually added to the antianginal drug regimen when nitrates do not prevent anginal episodes. It is especially useful in preventing exercise-induced tachycardia, which can precipitate anginal attacks.

19. Answer: d
RATIONALE: Vitamin E increases the effects of nitroglycerin.

20. Answer: a
RATIONALE: Isosorbide dinitrate (Isordil) is used to reduce the frequency and severity of acute anginal episodes. When given sublingually or in chewable tablets, it acts in about 2 minutes, and its effects last 2 to 3 hours. When higher doses are given orally, more drug escapes metabolism in the liver and produces systemic effects in approximately 30 minutes. Therapeutic effects last about 4 hours after oral administration. The effective oral dose is usually determined by increasing the dose until headache occurs, indicating the maximum tolerable dose. Sustained-release capsules also are available.

CHAPTER 27

SECTION I: ASSESSING YOUR UNDERSTANDING

Activity A FILL IN THE BLANKS

1. Adrenergic
2. isoproterenol
3. receptor
4. exogenous
5. heart

Activity B MATCHING

1. e   **2.** a   **3.** b   **4.** c   **5.** d

Activity C SHORT ANSWERS

1. Clinical indications for the use of adrenergic drugs stem mainly from their effects on the heart, blood vessels, and bronchi. They are often used as emergency drugs in the treatment of acute cardiovascular, respiratory, and allergic disorders.

2. In cardiac arrest, Stokes-Adams syndrome (sudden attacks of unconsciousness caused by heart block), and profound bradycardia, adrenergic drugs may be used as cardiac stimulants. In hypotension and shock, they may be used to increase blood pressure. In hemorrhagic or hypovolemic shock, the drugs are second-line agents that may be used if adequate fluid volume replacement does not restore sufficient blood pressure and circulation to maintain organ perfusion.

3. In bronchial asthma and other obstructive pulmonary diseases, the drugs are used as bronchodilators to relieve bronchoconstriction and bronchospasm. In upper respiratory infections, including the common cold and sinusitis, they may be given orally or applied topically to the nasal mucosa to reduce nasal congestion (decongestant effect).

4. Adrenergic drugs are useful in treating a variety of symptoms of allergic disorders. Severe allergic reactions are characterized by hypotension, bronchoconstriction, and laryngoedema. As vasoconstrictors, the drugs are useful in correcting the hypotension that often accompanies severe allergic reactions. The drug-induced vasoconstriction of blood vessels in mucous membranes produces a decongestant effect to relieve edema in the respiratory tract, skin, and other tissues. As bronchodilators, the drugs also help relieve the bronchospasm of severe allergic reactions. Adrenergic drugs may be used to treat allergic rhinitis, acute hypersensitivity (anaphylactoid reactions to drugs, animal serums, insect stings, and other allergens), serum sickness, urticaria, and angioneurotic edema.

5. Other clinical uses of adrenergic drugs include relaxation of uterine musculature and inhibition of uterine contractions in preterm labor. They also may be added to local anesthetics for their vasoconstrictive effect, thus preventing unwanted systemic absorption of the anesthetic, prolonging anesthesia, and reducing bleeding. Topical uses include application to skin and mucous membranes for vasoconstriction and hemostatic effects and to the eyes for vasoconstriction and mydriasis.

SECTION II: APPLYING YOUR KNOWLEDGE

Activity D CASE STUDY

1. The physician's treatment of choice to reduce bronchospasm would be epinephrine. In bronchial asthma and other obstructive pulmonary diseases, epinephrine is used as a bronchodilator to relieve bronchoconstriction and bronchospasm.

2. Over-the-counter epinephrine preparations have a short duration of action, which promotes frequent and excessive use. Prolonged use may cause adverse effects and result in the development of tolerance to the therapeutic effects of the drug. There is also concern by some health professionals that reliance on OTC medications may delay the patient who is asthmatic from seeking medical care. Supporters point out that OTC bronchodilators are much less costly than prescription medications and are an affordable "rescue treatment" option for patients who do not have insurance coverage for prescription medications.

3. Treatment guidelines for asthma recommend use of anti-inflammatory medications (e.g., corticosteroids) and prescription bronchodilators (e.g., beta$_2$-adrenergic agonists) for the optimal treatment of asthma.

4. Another area of concern is the ozone-depleting propellants used in OTC inhalation products such as Primatene Mist. At this time, however, these medications have "essential use designation" by the FDA, because they constitute the only over-the-counter inhalation products available to people with asthma.

5. Ephedrine is a common ingredient in OTC antiasthma tablets (e.g., Bronkaid, Primatene). The tablets contain 12.5 to 25 mg of ephedrine and 100 to 130 mg of theophylline, a xanthine bronchodilator.

6. People who have heart disease or are elderly should not use over-the-counter asthma treatments on a regular basis.

SECTION III: PRACTICING FOR NCLEX

Activity E

1. **Answer: a, b, and e**
   RATIONALE: The primary clinical manifestation of this adrenergic drug toxicity is severe hypertension, which may lead to headache, confusion, seizures, and intracranial hemorrhage. Other conditions associated with phenylephrine toxicity include reflex bradycardia and atrioventricular block. Pulmonary edema would not be expected in a phenylephrine overdose.

2. **Answer: d**
   RATIONALE: Phenylephrine stimulates alpha$_1$ receptors.

3. **Answer: a, b, and c**
   RATIONALE: Contraindications to adrenergic drugs include cardiac dysrhythmias, angina, hypertension, hyperthyroidism, cerebrovascular disease, narrow-angle glaucoma, and hypersensitivity to sulfites.

4. **Answer: d**
   RATIONALE: Local anesthetics containing adrenergics should not be used in any area of the body with a single blood supply (fingers, toes, nose, and ears).

5. **Answer: b**
   RATIONALE: A benefit of epinephrine in arrest situations due to asystole or pulseless electrical activity is the added ability to stimulate electrical and mechanical activity and produce myocardial contraction.

6. **Answer: b**
   RATIONALE: Adrenergic drugs are contraindicated in patients taking MAO inhibitors. It is essential not to give MAO inhibitors with adrenergic drugs because the combination may cause death. Concurrent use of MAO inhibitors and adrenergic drugs may lead to a danger of cardiac dysrhythmias, respiratory depression, and acute hypertensive crisis, with possible intracranial hemorrhage, convulsions, coma, and death.

7. **Answer: c**
   RATIONALE: Use of beta-adrenergic blocking drugs (e.g., propranolol) may decrease the effectiveness of epinephrine in cases of anaphylaxis.

8. **Answer: a**
   RATIONALE: Higher doses of epinephrine and use of intravenous fluids may be required to maintain a patent airway and restore blood pressure.

9. **Answer: a, b, and d**
   RATIONALE: The nurse obtains the patient's weight and assesses skin color, temperature, and turgor. Orientation status, reflexes, pulse, blood pressure, respiratory rate, and auscultation of lung sounds are also important to obtain. Required laboratory data include urinalysis, renal function, blood and urine glucose, serum electrolytes, and thyroid function. In addition, an electrocardiogram may be necessary. A hearing screen and arterial blood gases would not be needed.

10. **Answer: b, c, and d**
    RATIONALE: Administration of epinephrine is by inhalation, injection, or topical application. (Oral and sublingual administration of the drug is not effective because enzymes in the GI tract and liver destroy it.)

11. **Answer: a**
    RATIONALE: Adrenergic drugs are used as cardiac stimulants, vasopressors, bronchodilators, nasal decongestants, uterine relaxants, adjuncts to local anesthetics, and topically for hemostatic and mydriatic effects.

12. **Answer: d**
    RATIONALE: A major function of the home care nurse is to teach patients to use the drugs correctly (especially metered-dose inhalers), to report excessive CNS or cardiac stimulation to a health care provider, and not to take OTC drugs or herbal preparations with the same or similar ingredients as prescription drugs.

13. **Answer: b**
    RATIONALE: The liver is rich in the enzymes MAO and COMT, which are responsible for metabolism of circulating epinephrine and other adrenergic drugs (e.g., norepinephrine, dopamine, isoproterenol). However, other tissues in the body also possess these enzymes and are capable of metabolizing natural and synthetic

catecholamines. Any unchanged drug can be excreted in the urine. Many noncatecholamine adrenergic drugs are excreted largely unchanged in the urine. Therefore, liver disease is not usually considered a contraindication to administration of adrenergic drugs.

14. **Answer: c**
    RATIONALE: Adrenergic drugs exert effects on the renal system that may cause problems for patients with renal impairment. For example, adrenergic drugs with alpha1 activity cause constriction of renal arteries, thereby diminishing renal blood flow and urine production. These drugs also constrict urinary sphincters, causing urinary retention and painful urination, especially in men with prostatic hyperplasia.

15. **Answer: d**
    RATIONALE: Ophthalmic preparations of adrenergic drugs should be used cautiously. For example, phenylephrine is used as a vasoconstrictor and mydriatic. Applying larger-than-recommended doses to the normal eye or usual doses to the traumatized, inflamed, or diseased eye may result in systemic absorption of the drug sufficient to cause increased blood pressure and other adverse effects.

16. **Answer: c**
    RATIONALE: Prolonged use may cause adverse effects and result in the development of tolerance to the therapeutic effects of the drug. Increased body temperature, pruritus, and weight gain would not be expected with prolonged use of OTC epinephrine.

17. **Answer: c**
    RATIONALE: Epinephrine is mainly used in children for treatment of bronchospasm due to asthma or allergic reactions. Parenteral epinephrine may cause syncope when given to children with asthma.

18. **Answer: a and b**
    RATIONALE: Ephedrine and ephedra-containing herbal preparations (e.g., ma huang, herbal ecstasy) are often abused as an alternative to amphetamines.

19. **Answer: a**
    RATIONALE: Adrenergic drugs are given topically and systemically to constrict blood vessels in nasal mucosa and decrease the nasal congestion associated with the common cold, allergic rhinitis, and sinusitis. Topical agents are effective, undergo little systemic absorption, are available OTC, and are widely used. However, overuse leads to decreased effectiveness (tolerance); irritation and ischemic changes in the nasal mucosa; and rebound congestion. These effects can be minimized by using small doses only when necessary and for no longer than 3 to 5 days.

20. **Answer: d**
    RATIONALE: The usual goal of vasopressor drug therapy is to maintain tissue perfusion and a mean arterial blood pressure of at least 80 to 100 mm Hg.

CHAPTER 28

SECTION I: ASSESSING YOUR UNDERSTANDING

Activity A FILL IN THE BLANKS
1. Arterial
2. homeostatic
3. cardiac output
4. Cardiac output
5. Stroke volume

Activity B MATCHING
1. d   2. a   3. e   4. b   5. c

Activity C SHORT ANSWERS
1. Autoregulation is the ability of body tissues to regulate their own blood flow. Local blood flow is regulated primarily by nutritional needs of the tissue, such as lack of oxygen or accumulation of products of cellular metabolism (e.g., carbon dioxide, lactic acid). Local tissues produce vasodilating and vasoconstricting substances to regulate local blood flow. Important tissue factors include histamine, bradykinin, serotonin, and prostaglandins.
2. Histamine is found mainly in mast cells surrounding blood vessels and is released when these tissues are injured. In some tissues, such as skeletal muscle, mast cell activity is mediated by the sympathetic nervous system (SNS), and histamine is released when SNS stimulation is blocked or withdrawn.
3. Bradykinin is released from a protein in body fluids. Kinins dilate arterioles, increase capillary permeability, and constrict venules.
4. Serotonin is released from aggregating platelets during the blood clotting process. It causes vasoconstriction and plays a major role in control of bleeding.
5. Prostaglandins are formed in response to tissue injury and include vasodilators (e.g., prostacyclin) and vasoconstrictors (e.g., thromboxane A_2).

SECTION II: APPLYING YOUR KNOWLEDGE
Activity D CASE STUDIES

Case Study 1
1. Hypertension is persistently high blood pressure that results from abnormalities in regulatory mechanisms. Hypertension is usually defined as a systolic pressure greater than 140 mm Hg or a diastolic pressure greater than 90 mm Hg on multiple blood pressure measurements.
2. Secondary hypertension may result from renal, endocrine, or central nervous system disorders or from drugs that stimulate the SNS or cause retention of sodium and water.

Case Study 2

1. A systolic pressure of 140 mm Hg or greater, with a diastolic pressure lower than 90 mm Hg, is called *isolated systolic hypertension* and is more common in the elderly.
2. Hypertension profoundly alters cardiovascular function by increasing the workload of the heart and causing thickening and sclerosis of arterial walls.

SECTION III: PRACTICING FOR NCLEX

Activity E

1. **Answer: a**
   RATIONALE: The FDA has issued a black box warning for minoxidil, because the drug can exacerbate angina and precipitate effusion (which can progress to cardiac tamponade).

2. **Answer: a**
   RATIONALE: The FDA has issued a black box warning for ACE inhibitors and ARBs during pregnancy, because their use can cause injury and even death to a developing fetus.

3. **Answer: c**
   RATIONALE: The FDA has issued a black box warning for patients with CAD who are withdrawing from oral forms of atenolol, metoprolol, nadolol, propranolol, and timolol; abrupt withdrawal has resulted in exacerbation of angina, increased incidence of ventricular dysrhythmias, and the occurrence of MIs.

4. **Answer: a, b, and c**
   RATIONALE: African Americans are more likely to have severe hypertension and to require multiple drugs as a result of having low circulating renin, increased salt sensitivity, and a higher incidence of obesity. There is no evidence that African Americans have an increased level of anxiety.

5. **Answer: d**
   RATIONALE: In general, people of Asian descent with hypertension require much smaller doses of beta-blockers, because they metabolize and excrete the drugs slowly.

6. **Answer: b**
   RATIONALE: Beta-adrenergic blockers are the drugs of first choice for patients younger than 50 years of age who have high-renin hypertension, tachycardia, angina pectoris, myocardial infarction, or left ventricular hypertrophy.

7. **Answer: c**
   RATIONALE: Captopril is an ACE inhibitor, and it is used to treat hypertension in patients with type 1 diabetes mellitus because it reduces proteinuria and slows progression of renal impairment.

8. **Answer: b**
   RATIONALE: Alpha$_1$-adrenergic receptor blocking agents should be administered at bedtime to minimize the first-dose phenomenon.

9. **Answer: b**
   RATIONALE: Key behavioral determinants of blood pressure are related to dietary consumption of calories and salt; the prevalence of hypertension rises proportionally to average body mass index.

10. **Answer: b**
    RATIONALE: Yohimbe, used to treat erectile dysfunction, is a central nervous system stimulant and can affect blood pressure.

11. **Answer: b, c, and d**
    RATIONALE: Whether the patient or another member of the household is taking antihypertensive medications, the home care nurse may be helpful in teaching about the drugs, monitoring for drug effects, and promoting compliance with the prescribed regimen (pharmacologic and lifestyle modifications). The nurse would not provide financial assistant with daily expenses though the nurse would help the patient and family discover resources that might provide what is needed.

12. **Answer: d**
    RATIONALE: There are risks with severe hypertension, there are also risks associated with lowering blood pressure excessively or too rapidly, including stroke, myocardial infarction, and acute renal failure. Therefore, the goal of management is usually to lower blood pressure over several minutes to several hours, with careful titration of drug dosage to avoid precipitous drops.

13. **Answer: c**
    RATIONALE: Nitroglycerin is especially beneficial in patients with both severe hypertension and myocardial ischemia. The dose is titrated according to blood pressure response and may range from 5 to 100 mcg/min. Tolerance develops to IV nitroglycerin over 24 to 48 hours.

14. **Answer: a**
    RATIONALE: Emergencies can be treated with oral antihypertensive agents such as captopril 25 to 50 mg every 1 to 2 hours or clonidine 0.2 mg initially and then 0.1 mg hourly until the diastolic blood pressure falls to less than 110 mm Hg or 0.7 mg has been given.

15. **Answer: c**
    RATIONALE: Patients who have jaundice or marked elevations of hepatic enzymes while taking an ACE inhibitor should have the drug discontinued, because these drugs have been associated with cholestatic jaundice, which can progress to hepatic necrosis and possibly death.

16. **Answer: d**
    RATIONALE: Approximately 25% of patients taking an ACE inhibitor for heart failure experience an increase in BUN and serum creatinine levels. These patients usually do not require drug discontinuation unless they have severe, preexisting renal impairment.

17. Answer: c, d, and e

RATIONALE: Other factors that may contribute to hypertension include the use of nasal decongestants, herbal supplements, and OTC appetite suppressants. Meditation and a walking program may help to decrease or control hypertension.

18. Answer: a, b, and c

RATIONALE: Nonpharmacologic management of hypertension should be tried alone or with drug therapy. For example, weight reduction, limited alcohol intake, moderate sodium restriction, and smoking cessation may be the initial treatment of choice if the patient is hypertensive and overweight. The hot water in a hot tub may actually increase blood pressure.

19. Answer: b

RATIONALE: The National High Blood Pressure Education Program Working Group on High Blood Pressure in Children and Adolescents produced the fourth report on the diagnosis, evaluation, and treatment of high blood pressure in children and adolescents in 2004. These guidelines established parameters for blood pressure in children and adolescents of comparable age, body size (height and weight), and sex. Normal blood pressure is defined as systolic and diastolic values less than the 90th percentile; prehypertension is defined as an average of systolic or diastolic pressures within the 90th to 95th percentiles; hypertension is defined as pressures beyond the 95th percentile.

20. Answer: b

RATIONALE: It is recommended that patient with early or prehypertension should follow the Dietary Approaches to Stop Hypertension (DASH) diet, which encourages the patient to eat a diet abundant in fresh fruits and vegetables and low-fat dairy products. Most patients with hypertension are encouraged to eat food low in sodium. A restricted-calorie diet is only recommended if the patient is overweight. A high-protein diet is not recommended because of the effect on the kidneys.

CHAPTER 29

SECTION I: ASSESSING YOUR UNDERSTANDING

Activity A FILL IN THE BLANKS

1. common cold
2. rhinoviruses
3. Sinusitis
4. Rhinitis
5. Nasal congestion

Activity B MATCHING

1. e **2.** d **3.** a **4.** c **5.** b

Activity C SHORT ANSWERS

1. Colds can be caused by many types of viruses, most often the rhinoviruses. Shedding of these viruses by infected people, mainly from nasal mucosa, can result in rapid spread to other people. The viruses can enter the body through mucous membranes. Cold viruses can survive for several hours on the skin and on hard surfaces such as wood or plastic. There may also be airborne spread from sneezing and coughing, but this source is considered secondary. After the viruses gain entry, the incubation period is usually 5 days, the most contagious period is about 3 days after symptoms begin, and the cold usually lasts about 7 days.

2. Sinusitis is inflammation of the paranasal sinuses, air cells that connect with the nasal cavity and are lined by similar mucosa. As in other parts of the respiratory tract, ciliated mucous membranes help move fluid and microorganisms out of the sinuses and into the nasal cavity. This movement becomes impaired when sinus openings are blocked by nasal swelling, and the impairment is considered a major cause of sinus infections. Another contributing factor is a lower oxygen content in the sinuses, which aids the growth of microorganisms and impairs local defense mechanisms.

3. Rhinorrhea is defined as the secretions discharged from the nose.

4. Rhinitis is defined as inflammation of nasal mucosa and is usually accompanied by nasal congestion, rhinorrhea, and sneezing.

5. Cough is a forceful expulsion of air from the lungs. It is normally a protective reflex for removing foreign bodies, environmental irritants, or accumulated secretions from the respiratory tract.

SECTION II: APPLYING YOUR KNOWLEDGE

Activity D CASE STUDY

1. Many combination products are available for treating symptoms of the common cold. Many of the products contain an antihistamine, a nasal decongestant, and an analgesic. Some contain antitussives, expectorants, and other agents as well. Many cold remedies are over-the-counter (OTC) formulations. Commonly used ingredients include chlorpheniramine (antihistamine), pseudoephedrine (adrenergic nasal decongestant), acetaminophen (analgesic and antipyretic), dextromethorphan (antitussive), and guaifenesin (expectorant).

2. Although antihistamines are popular OTC drugs because they dry nasal secretions, they are not recommended because they can also dry lower respiratory secretions and worsen secretion retention and cough. Allergy remedies contain an antihistamine; "nondrowsy" or "daytime" formulas contain a nasal decongestant but do not contain an antihistamine; "PM" or "night" formulas contain a sedating

antihistamine to promote sleep. Pain, fever, and multisymptom formulas usually contain acetaminophen; the term "maximum strength" usually refers only to the amount of acetaminophen per dose, usually 1000 mg for adults.

3. The use of OTC products containing pseudoephedrine to manufacture methamphetamine has increased at an alarming rate. Most states have passed laws placing these products behind pharmacy counters to restrict sales. Mrs. Hoyer would have to ask the pharmacist for the drug.

4. Many products come in several formulations, with different ingredients, and are advertised for different purposes (e.g., allergy, sinus disorders, multisymptom cold and flu remedies). In addition, labels on OTC combination products list ingredients by generic name, without identifying the type of drug. As a result of these bewildering products, consumers, including nurses and other health care providers, may not know what medications they are taking or whether some drugs increase or block the effects of other drugs.

5. The use of antiviral agents for cold treatment has increased in popularity. Oseltamivir (Tamiflu) limits spread of virus within the respiratory tract and may also prevent virus penetration of respiratory secretions to initiate replication. Oseltamivir has activity against influenza A and B. Although the drug was effective in treating community-acquired colds caused by rhinoviruses in two placebo-controlled trials, there is not sufficient evidence to support its use in viral upper respiratory tract infections.

SECTION III: PRACTICING FOR NCLEX
Activity E

1. **Answer: b**
   RATIONALE: Several OTC cough and cold medicines for use in infants have been recalled voluntarily due to concerns about possible misuse that could result in overdoses.

2. **Answer: d**
   RATIONALE: There is limited or no support for the use of dietary or herbal supplements to prevent or treat symptoms of the common cold.

3. **Answer: a, b, and c**
   RATIONALE: First-generation antihistamines (e.g., chlorpheniramine, diphenhydramine) have anticholinergic effects that may reduce sneezing, rhinorrhea, and cough. They do not have antipyretic effects.

4. **Answer: c**
   RATIONALE: Rebound nasal swelling can occur with excessive or extended use of nasal sprays.

5. **Answer: b, c, and d**
   RATIONALE: An adequate fluid intake, humidification of the environment, and sucking on hard candy or throat lozenges can help relieve mouth dryness and cough. The use of astringent mouthwash will only increase mouth dryness.

6. **Answer: d**
   RATIONALE: Nonrespiratory conditions that predispose to secretion retention include immobility, debilitation, cigarette smoking, and postoperative status.

7. **Answer: c**
   RATIONALE: Retention of secretions commonly occurs with influenza, pneumonia, upper respiratory infections, acute and chronic bronchitis, emphysema, and acute attacks of asthma.

8. **Answer: a**
   RATIONALE: Most upper respiratory infections are viral in origin, and antibiotics are not generally recommended.

9. **Answer: b**
   RATIONALE: Before recommending a particular product, the nurse needs to assess the intended recipient for conditions or other medications that contraindicate the product's use.

10. **Answer: b and c**
    RATIONALE: A major consideration is that older adults are at high risk of adverse effects from oral nasal decongestants (e.g., hypertension, cardiac dysrhythmias, nervousness, insomnia).

11. **Answer: b**
    RATIONALE: Parents often administer a medication (e.g., acetaminophen, ibuprofen) for pain and fever when a child has cold symptoms, whether the child has pain and fever or not. Some pediatricians suggest treating fevers higher than 101 degrees if the child seems uncomfortable but not to treat them otherwise. Parents may need to be counseled that fever is part of the body's defense mechanism and may help the child recover from an infection.

12. **Answer: c**
    RATIONALE: Nasal congestion may interfere with an infant's ability to nurse. Phenylephrine nasal solution, applied just before feeding time, is usually effective.

13. **Answer: a**
    RATIONALE: Excessive amounts or too-frequent administration of topical agents (i.e., phenylephrine) may result in rebound nasal congestion and systemic effects of cardiac and central nervous system stimulation. Therefore, the drug should be given to infants only when recommended by a pediatric specialist.

14. **Answer: d**
    RATIONALE: For sore throat, a throat culture for streptococcal organisms should be performed and the results obtained before an antibiotic is prescribed.

15. **Answer: b**
    RATIONALE: Single-drug formulations allow flexibility and individualization of dosage, whereas combination products may contain unneeded ingredients and are more expensive. However, many people find combination products more convenient to use.

16. **Answer: c**
    RATIONALE: With nasal decongestants, topical preparations (i.e., nasal solutions or sprays) are often preferred for short-term use. They are rapidly effective because they come into direct contact with nasal mucosa.

17. **Answer: a**
    RATIONALE: Antihistamines are clearly useful in allergic conditions, but their use to relieve cold symptoms is controversial. First-generation antihistamines (e.g., chlorpheniramine, diphenhydramine) have anticholinergic effects that may reduce sneezing, rhinorrhea, and cough. Also, their sedative effects may aid sleep. Many multi-ingredient cold remedies contain an antihistamine.

18. **Answer: b, c, and e**
    RATIONALE: Older adults may experience hypertension, heart rhythm abnormalities, nervousness, and insomnia when they use oral nasal decongestants.

19. **Answer: c**
    RATIONALE: Cough syrups serve as vehicles for antitussive drugs and may exert antitussive effects of their own by soothing irritated pharyngeal mucosa.

20. **Answer: a, b, and d**
    RATIONALE: People with diabetes, cardiovascular disorders, and glaucoma should be advised to avoid medications that contain pseudoephedrine.

CHAPTER 30

SECTION I: ASSESSING YOUR UNDERSTANDING

Activity A FILL IN THE BLANKS

1. Antihistamines
2. Histamine
3. mast cells
4. Hypersensitivity
5. H_1

Activity B MATCHING

1. c   2. e   3. a   4. b   5. d

Activity C SHORT ANSWERS

1. Histamine is the first chemical mediator to be released in immune and inflammatory responses. It is synthesized and stored in most body tissues, with high concentrations in tissues exposed to environmental substances (such as the skin and mucosal surfaces of the eyes, nose, lungs, and gastrointestinal tract). It is also found in the central nervous system (CNS). In these tissues, histamine is located mainly in secretory granules of mast cells (tissue cells surrounding capillaries) and basophils (circulating blood cells).

2. When H_2 receptors are stimulated, the main effects are increased secretion of gastric acid and pepsin, increased rate and force of myocardial contraction, and decreased immunologic and proinflammatory reactions (e.g., decreased release of histamine from basophils, decreased movement of neutrophils and basophils into areas of injury, inhibited T- and B-lymphocyte function). Stimulation of both H_1 and H_2 receptors causes peripheral vasodilation (with hypotension, headache, and skin flushing) and increased bronchial, intestinal, and salivary secretion of mucus.

3. Hypersensitivity or allergic reactions are exaggerated responses by the immune system that produce tissue injury and may cause serious disease. The mechanisms that eliminate pathogens in adaptive immune responses are essentially identical to those of natural immunity. Allergic reactions may result from specific antibodies, sensitized T lymphocytes, or both, formed during exposure to an antigen.

4. Type I immune response (also called immediate hypersensitivity because it occurs within minutes after exposure to the antigen) is an immunoglobulin E (IgE)-induced response triggered by the interaction of antigen with antigen-specific IgE bound on mast cells, causing mast cell activation. Histamine and other mediators are released immediately, and cytokines, chemokines, and leukotrienes are synthesized after activation.

5. Type II responses are mediated by IgG or IgM generating direct damage to the cell surface. These cytotoxic reactions include blood transfusion reactions, hemolytic disease of newborns, autoimmune hemolytic anemia, and some drug reactions. Hemolytic anemia (caused by destruction of erythrocytes) and thrombocytopenia (caused by destruction of platelets), both type II hypersensitivity responses, are adverse effects of certain drugs (e.g., penicillin, methyldopa, heparin).

SECTION II: APPLYING YOUR KNOWLEDGE

Activity D CASE STUDY

1. Allergic rhinitis is inflammation of nasal mucosa caused by a type I hypersensitivity reaction to inhaled allergens.

2. There are two types of allergic rhinitis. Seasonal disease (often called hay fever) produces acute symptoms in response to the protein components of airborne pollens from trees, grasses, and weeds, mainly in the spring or fall. Perennial disease produces chronic symptoms in response to nonseasonal allergens such as dust mites, animal dander, and molds.

3. Allergic rhinitis is an immune response in which normal nasal breathing and filtering of air brings inhaled antigens into contact with mast cells and basophils in nasal mucosa, blood vessels, and submucosal tissues. With initial exposure, the inhaled antigens are processed by lymphocytes that produce IgE, an antigen-specific antibody that binds to mast cells. With later exposures, the IgE interacts with inhaled antigens and triggers the breakdown of the mast cell.

4. In people with allergies, mast cells and basophils are increased in both number and reactivity. Therefore, these cells may be capable of releasing large amounts of histamine and other mediators.

5. Allergic rhinitis that is not effectively treated may lead to chronic fatigue, impaired ability to perform usual activities of daily living, difficulty sleeping, sinus infections, postnasal drip, cough, and headache. In addition, this condition is a strong risk factor for asthma.

SECTION III: PRACTICING FOR NCLEX

Activity E

1. **Answer: b**
   RATIONALE: For children with allergies, provide all family members, day care, and school personnel with an emergency plan.

2. **Answer: c**
   RATIONALE: Systemic lupus erythematosus has been induced by hydralazine.

3. **Answer: a**
   RATIONALE: Azelastine (Astelin) is the only antihistamine formulated as a nasal spray for topical use.

4. **Answer: d**
   RATIONALE: Second-generation H_1 antagonists cause less CNS depression because they are selective for peripheral H_1 receptors and do not cross the blood–brain barrier.

5. **Answer: c**
   RATIONALE: First-generation antihistamines have substantial anticholinergic effects; therefore, they may cause dry mouth, urinary retention, constipation, and blurred vision.

6. **Answer: c**
   RATIONALE: First-generation antihistamines (e.g., diphenhydramine) may cause drowsiness and decreased mental alertness in children as in adults.

7. **Answer: a, b, c, and e**
   RATIONALE: Some food allergens such as shellfish, egg, milk, peanut, and tree nuts have a higher inherent risk for triggering anaphylaxis than others.

8. **Answer: d**
   RATIONALE: Allergic rhinitis is inflammation of nasal mucosa caused by a type I hypersensitivity reaction to inhaled allergens.

9. **Answer: c**
   RATIONALE: Macrolides increase the plasma concentration of fexofenadine.

10. **Answer: a**
    RATIONALE: A first-generation antihistamine may cause drowsiness and safety hazards in the environment (e.g., operating a car or other potentially hazardous machinery). In most people, tolerance develops to the sedative effects within a few days if they are not taking other sedative-type drugs or alcoholic beverages.

11. **Answer: d**
    RATIONALE: Diphenhydramine may be given by injection, usually as a single dose, to a patient who is having a blood transfusion or a diagnostic test, to prevent allergic reactions. Hydroxyzine or promethazine may be given by injection for nausea and vomiting or to provide sedation, but they are not usually the first drugs of choice for these indications.

12. **Answer: c**
    RATIONALE: Patients with hepatic impairment who take promethazine should be aware that cholestatic jaundice has been reported and the drug should be used with caution.

13. **Answer: a**
    RATIONALE: The dosing interval of diphenhydramine should be extended to 12 to 18 hours in patients with severe kidney failure.

14. **Answer: a**
    RATIONALE: Second-generation antihistamines should be used for older adults. They are much safer because they do not impair consciousness, thinking, or ability to perform activities of daily living (e.g., driving a car or operating various machines).

15. **Answer: a and c**
    RATIONALE: First-generation antihistamines (e.g., diphenhydramine) may cause confusion (with impaired thinking, judgment, and memory), dizziness, hypotension, sedation, syncope, unsteady gait, and paradoxical CNS stimulation in older adults. Pulmonary edema is not a side effect of first-generation antihistamines.

16. **Answer: a and d**
    RATIONALE: First-generation antihistamines (e.g., diphenhydramine) may cause drowsiness and decreased mental alertness in children as in adults. Young children may experience paradoxical excitement. These reactions may occur with therapeutic dosages. In overdosage, hallucinations, convulsions, and death may occur. Close supervision and appropriate dosages are required for safe drug usage in children. Headache is not usually experienced after administration of diphenhydramine in either children or adults.

17. **Answer: b**
    RATIONALE: For treatment of the common cold, studies have demonstrated that antihistamines do not relieve symptoms and are not recommended. However, an antihistamine is often included in prescription and OTC combination products for the common cold.

18. **Answer: c**
    RATIONALE: For chronic allergic symptoms (e.g., allergic rhinitis), long-acting preparations provide more consistent relief. A patient may respond better to one antihistamine than to another. Therefore, if one antihistamine does not relieve symptoms or produces excessive sedation, another may be effective.

19. **Answer: b**
    RATIONALE: Fexofenadine and related drugs should not be taken with fruit juice.

20. **Answer: c**
    RATIONALE: Promethazine is most commonly used in the treatment of nausea and vomiting.

CHAPTER 31

SECTION I: ASSESSING YOUR UNDERSTANDING

Activity A FILL IN THE BLANKS

1. Occupational asthma
2. hyperreactivity
3. Wheezing
4. bronchoconstriction
5. sulfites

Activity B MATCHING

1. c   2. e   3. a   4. b   5. d

Activity C SHORT ANSWERS

1. Asthma is an airway disorder that is characterized by bronchoconstriction, inflammation, and hyperreactivity to various stimuli. Resultant symptoms include dyspnea, wheezing, chest tightness, cough, and sputum production. Wheezing is a high-pitched, whistling sound caused by turbulent airflow through an obstructed airway.
2. Symptoms of asthma vary in incidence and severity, from occasional episodes of mild respiratory distress with normal functioning between "attacks" to persistent, daily, or continual respiratory distress if not adequately controlled. Inflammation and damaged airway mucosa are chronically present, even when patients appear symptom free.
3. Viral infections of the respiratory tract are often the causative agents of asthma, especially in infants and young children, whose airways are small and easily obstructed. Asthma symptoms may persist for days or weeks after the viral infection resolves.
4. Patients with severe asthma should be cautioned against ingesting food and drug products containing sulfites or metabisulfites.
5. Gastroesophageal reflux disease (GERD), a common disorder characterized by heartburn and esophagitis, is also associated with asthma. Asthma that worsens at night may be associated with nighttime acid reflux.

SECTION II: APPLYING YOUR KNOWLEDGE

Activity D CASE STUDY

1. The main xanthine used clinically is theophylline. Despite many years of use, the drug's mechanism of action is unknown. Various mechanisms have been proposed, such as inhibiting phosphodiesterase enzymes that metabolize cyclic AMP, increasing endogenous catecholamines, inhibiting calcium ion movement into smooth muscle, inhibiting prostaglandin synthesis and release, or inhibiting the release of bronchoconstrictive substances from mast cells and leukocytes.
2. Theophylline should be used cautiously in those with cardiovascular disorders that could be aggravated by drug-induced cardiac stimulation.

3. Theophylline increases the ability of the body to clear mucus from the airways. In addition to bronchodilation, other effects that may be beneficial in asthma and COPD include inhibiting pulmonary edema by decreasing vascular permeability, increasing the ability of cilia to clear mucus from the airways, strengthening contractions of the diaphragm, and decreasing inflammation.
4. Mrs. Livingston should be taught that it is important to keep all her appointments, because her serum drug levels need to be monitored. Theophylline increases cardiac output, causes peripheral vasodilation, exerts a mild diuretic effect, and stimulates the CNS. The cardiovascular and CNS effects are adverse effects. Serum drug levels should be monitored to help regulate dosage and avoid adverse effects.
5. Theophylline is metabolized in the liver; metabolites and some unchanged drug are excreted through the kidneys. In a patient with impaired liver function, metabolism of the drug can be compromised. Theophylline preparations are contraindicated in patients with acute gastritis or peptic ulcer disease.

SECTION III: PRACTICING FOR NCLEX

Activity E

1. **Answer: c**
   RATIONALE: The FDA has issued a black box warning that initiating salmeterol in people with significantly worsening or acutely deteriorating asthma may be life threatening.
2. **Answer: a**
   RATIONALE: The FDA has issued a black box warning for the drug omalizumab because of its propensity to cause anaphylaxis.
3. **Answer: a**
   RATIONALE: Cigarette smoking and drugs that stimulate drug-metabolizing enzymes in the liver (e.g., phenobarbital, phenytoin) increase the rate of metabolism and therefore the dosage requirements of aminophylline.
4. **Answer: d**
   RATIONALE: Almost all over-the-counter aerosol products promoted for use in asthma contain epinephrine, which may produce hazardous cardiac stimulation and other adverse effects.
5. **Answer: c**
   RATIONALE: Asthma may aggravate GERD, because antiasthma medications that dilate the airways also relax muscle tone in the gastroesophageal sphincter and may increase acid reflux.
6. **Answer: a, b, c, and e**
   RATIONALE: Because aerosol products act directly on the airways, drugs given by inhalation can usually be given in smaller doses and produce fewer adverse effects than oral or parenteral drugs. Aerosol products also produce a relief of asthma symptoms in a quick fashion.

7. Answer: a
RATIONALE: A selective, short-acting, inhaled beta$_2$-adrenergic agonist (e.g., albuterol) is the initial rescue drug of choice for acute broncho-spasm; subcutaneous epinephrine may also be considered.

8. Answer: c
RATIONALE: Theophylline is a xanthine, which has properties that are close to caffeine; there-fore, the nurse will ensure that the patient doesn't have anything on the tray that has caffeine in it.

9. Answer: d
RATIONALE: Albuterol is the initial drug of choice for acute broncospasm.

10. Answer: c
RATIONALE: A specific monitoring plan for patients with asthma should be in place, whether through peak-flow or symptom monitoring.

11. Answer: a, b, and d
RATIONALE: With theophylline, the home care nurse needs to assess the patient and the environ-ment for substances that may affect metabolism of theophylline and decrease therapeutic effects or increase adverse effects. Issues with excretion of theophylline are rarely an issue.

12. Answer: a
RATIONALE: The nurse needs to reinforce the importance of not exceeding the prescribed dose, not crushing long-acting formulations, reporting adverse effects, and keeping appointments for follow-up care.

13. Answer: b, c, and d
RATIONALE: In children, high doses of nebulized albuterol have been associated with tachycardia, hypokalemia, and hyperglyce-mia. Lowered or elevated blood pressure is not a usual issue with high doses of nebulized albuterol in children.

14. Answer: d
RATIONALE: Montelukast and zafirlukast produce higher blood levels and are eliminated more slowly in patients with hepatic impairment. However, no dosage adjustment is recommended for patients with mild to moderate hepatic impairment.

15. Answer: a
RATIONALE: Cromolyn is eliminated by renal and biliary excretion; the drug should be given in reduced doses, if at all, in patients with renal impairment.

16. Answer: a and d
RATIONALE: Older adults often have chronic pulmonary disorders for which bronchodilators and antiasthmatic medications are used. The main risks with adrenergic bronchodilators are excessive cardiac and CNS stimulation. Ana-phylaxis is not usually a risk with adrenergic bronchodilators.

17. Answer: b
RATIONALE: If the patient is obese, the dosage of theophylline should be based on lean or ideal body weight, because theophylline is not highly distributed in fatty tissue.

18. Answer: b
RATIONALE: Combination therapy for asthma is used to allow for smaller doses of each agent to be given. This way the patient can receive a larger dose if an exacerbation of the asthma occurs.

19. Answer: c
RATIONALE: Adrenal insufficiency is most likely to occur with systemic or high doses of inhaled corticosteroids.

20. Answer: b
RATIONALE: For theophylline overdose in patients without seizures, induce vomiting unless the level of consciousness is impaired. Precautions to pre-vent aspiration are needed, especially in children. If overdose is identified within 1 hour after drug ingestion, gastric lavage may be helpful if vomiting cannot be induced or is contraindicated. Adminis-tration of activated charcoal and a cathartic is also recommended, especially for overdoses of sus-tained-release formulations, if benefit exceeds risk.

CHAPTER 32

SECTION I: ASSESSING YOUR UNDERSTANDING

Activity A FILL IN THE BLANKS

1. output
2. composition
3. glomerulus
4. capillaries
5. Bowman's capsule

Activity B MATCHING

1. c   2. e   3. a   4. b   5. d

Activity C SHORT ANSWERS

1. The tubules are often called *convoluted tubules* be-cause of their many twists and turns. The convolu-tions provide a large surface area that brings the blood flowing through the peritubular capillaries and the glomerular filtrate flowing through the tubular lumen into close proximity. Consequently, substances can be readily exchanged through the walls of the tubules.

2. The nephron functions by three processes: glo-merular filtration, tubular reabsorption, and tubular secretion. These processes normally maintain the fluid volume, electrolyte concentration, and pH of body fluids within a relatively narrow range. They also remove waste products of cellular metabolism. A minimum daily urine output of approximately 400 mL is required to remove normal amounts of metabolic end products.

3. Arterial blood enters the glomerulus via the afferent arteriole at the relatively high pressure of approximately 70 mm Hg. This pressure pushes water, electrolytes, and other solutes out of the capillaries into Bowman's capsule and then to the proximal tubule. This fluid, called glomerular filtrate, contains the same components as blood except for blood cells, fats, and proteins that are too large to be filtered.

4. The glomerular filtration rate (GFR) is about 180 L/d, or 125 mL/min. Most of this fluid is reabsorbed as the glomerular filtrate travels through the tubules. The end product is about 2 L of urine daily. Because filtration is a nonselective process, the reabsorption and secretion processes determine the composition of the urine. After it is formed, urine flows into collecting tubules, which carry it to the renal pelvis, then through the ureters, bladder, and urethra for elimination from the body.

5. Blood that does not become part of the glomerular filtrate leaves the glomerulus through the efferent arteriole. The efferent arteriole branches into the peritubular capillaries that eventually empty into veins, which return the blood to systemic circulation.

SECTION II: APPLYING YOUR KNOWLEDGE
Activity D CASE STUDY

1. About 20% of the glomerular filtrate enters the loop of Henle. In the descending limb of the loop of Henle, water is reabsorbed; in the ascending limb, sodium is reabsorbed. A large fraction of the total amount of sodium (up to 30%) filtered by the glomeruli is reabsorbed in the loop of Henle.

2. Furosemide and other loop diuretics inhibit sodium and chloride reabsorption in the ascending limb of the loop of Henle, where reabsorption of most filtered sodium occurs. Thus, these potent drugs produce significant diuresis, their sodium-losing effect being up to 10 times greater than that of thiazide diuretics. Uses include the management of acute pulmonary edema, heart failure, as well as hepatic and renal disease.

3. Adverse effects of furosemide include fluid and electrolyte imbalances (e.g., hyponatremia, hypokalemia, fluid volume deficit) and ototoxicity.

4. In most instances, it is necessary to initiate measures to limit sodium intake. Key considerations should include not adding salt to food during preparation or at the dinner table, reading food labels carefully to be aware of hidden sources of sodium, and avoiding processed or high-sodium foods. The nurse instructs the patient in the use of equipment needed to take routine blood pressure readings. Too little potassium (hypokalemia) may result from the use of potassium-losing diuretics such as hydrochlorothiazide, furosemide (Lasix), and several others. To prevent or treat hypokalemia, your physician may prescribe a potassium chloride supplement or a combination of a potassium-losing and a potassium-saving diuretic (either separately or as a combined product such as Dyazide, Maxzide, or Aldactazide). He or she may also recommend increased dietary intake of potassium-containing foods (e.g., bananas, orange juice). If you are taking a diuretic to lower your blood pressure, especially with other antihypertensive drugs, you may feel dizzy or faint when you stand up suddenly. This can be prevented or decreased by changing positions slowly. If dizziness is severe, notify your health care provider. Do not drive or operate dangerous machinery until the effects of the drug are known.

SECTION III: PRACTICING FOR NCLEX
Activity E

1. **Answer: c**
   RATIONALE: When digoxin and diuretics are given concomitantly, the risk of digoxin toxicity is increased due to diuretic-induced hypokalemia.

2. **Answer: a**
   RATIONALE: High-dose furosemide continuous IV infusions should be given at a rate of 4 mg/min or less to decrease or avoid risks of adverse effects, including ototoxicity.

3. **Answer: c**
   RATIONALE: Thiazides and related diuretics are the drugs of choice for most patients who require diuretic therapy, especially for long-term management of heart failure and hypertension.

4. **Answer: a**
   RATIONALE: There is a known cross-sensitivity of some sulfonamide-allergic patients to sulfonamide nonantibiotics, such as thiazides.

5. **Answer: b**
   RATIONALE: Potassium-sparing diuretics are contraindicated in patients with renal impairment because of the high risk of hyperkalemia.

6. **Answer: d**
   RATIONALE: Loop diuretics have a sodium-losing effect up to 10 times greater than that of thiazide diuretics.

7. **Answer: b**
   RATIONALE: Excessive table salt and salty foods (e.g., ham, packaged sandwich meats, potato chips, dill pickles, most canned soups) may aggravate edema or hypertension.

8. **Answer: a, c, and d**
   RATIONALE: Mannitol is an osmotic diuretic that is used to treat oliguria and anuria in an effort to prevent renal failure. It is also used to reduce intracranial pressure, reduce intraocular pressure, and assist in the urinary excretion of toxic substances. It is not used to reduce mild to moderate swelling or to reduce venous jugular pressure.

9. **Answer: b**
   RATIONALE: When hydrochlorothiazide is taken with a beta-blocker such as propranolol, there is an increase in the effectiveness of the hydrochlorothiazide.

10. **Answer: a and b**

    RATIONALE: Diuretics are often taken in the home setting. The home care nurse may need to assist patients and caregivers in using the drugs safely and effectively; monitor patient responses (e.g., with each home visit, assess nutritional status, blood pressure, weight, use of over-the-counter medications that may aggravate edema or hypertension); and provide information as indicated. The nurse would teach the patient and family to administer the medication in the morning to prevent nighttime trips to the bathroom.

11. **Answer: a and d**

    RATIONALE: Fast-acting, potent diuretics such as furosemide and bumetanide are the most likely diuretics to be used in critically ill patients (e.g., those with pulmonary edema).

12. **Answer: b**

    RATIONALE: Although IV bolus doses of the drugs are often given to critically ill patients, continuous IV infusions may be more effective and less likely to produce adverse effects in critically ill patients.

13. **Answer: c**

    RATIONALE: Diuretics are often used to manage edema and ascites in patients with hepatic impairment. These drugs must be used with caution, because diuretic-induced fluid and electrolyte imbalances may precipitate or worsen hepatic encephalopathy and coma.

14. **Answer: a**

    RATIONALE: For patients with cirrhosis, diuretic therapy should be initiated in a hospital setting, with small doses and careful monitoring. To prevent hypokalemia and metabolic alkalosis, supplemental potassium or spironolactone may be needed.

15. **Answer: b**

    RATIONALE: Potassium-sparing diuretics are contraindicated in patients with renal impairment because of the high risk of hyperkalemia. If they are used at all, frequent monitoring of serum electrolytes, creatinine, and BUN is needed.

16. **Answer: c**

    RATIONALE: For continuous infusion, furosemide should be mixed with normal saline or lactated Ringer's solution, because D5W may accelerate degradation of furosemide.

17. **Answer: c**

    RATIONALE: With loop diuretics, older adults are at greater risk of excessive diuresis, hypotension, fluid volume deficit, and possibly thrombosis or embolism.

18. **Answer: d**

    RATIONALE: The smallest effective dose to treat elder adults in need of diuresis is recommended, usually a daily dose of 12.5 to 25 mg of hydrochlorothiazide or equivalent doses of other thiazides and related drugs.

19. **Answer: a**

    RATIONALE: Thiazides may be useful in managing edema caused by renal disorders such as nephrotic syndrome and acute glomerulonephritis. However, their effectiveness decreases as the GFR decreases, and the drugs become ineffective when the GFR is less than 30 mL/min.

20. **Answer: b**

    RATIONALE: Furosemide is the loop diuretic used most often in children. Oral therapy is preferred when feasible, and doses greater than 6 mg/kg of body weight per day are not recommended.

CHAPTER 33

SECTION I: ASSESSING YOUR UNDERSTANDING

Activity A FILL IN THE BLANKS

1. Proteins
2. Carbohydrates
3. kilocalories
4. proteins
5. Vitamins

Activity B MATCHING

1. d   **2.** e   **3.** a   **4.** b   **5.** c

Activity C SHORT ANSWERS

1. Nurses encounter many patients who are unable to ingest, digest, absorb, or use sufficient nutrients to improve or maintain health. Debilitating illnesses such as cancer; AIDS; and chronic lung, kidney, or cardiovascular disorders often interfere with appetite and gastrointestinal (GI) function. Therapeutic drugs often cause anorexia, nausea, vomiting, diarrhea, or constipation. Nutritional deficiencies may impair the function of essentially every body organ. Signs and symptoms include unintended weight loss, increased susceptibility to infection, weakness and fatigability, impaired wound healing, impaired growth and development in children, edema, and decreased hemoglobin.

2. Numerous liquid enteral formulas are available over-the-counter or in health care settings for oral or tube feedings. Many are nutritionally complete, except for water, when given in sufficient amounts (e.g., Ensure, Isocal, Sustacal, Resource). Additional water must be given to meet fluid needs. Most oral products are available in a variety of flavors and contain 1 kcal/mL. Additional products are formulated for patients with special conditions (e.g., renal or hepatic failure, malabsorption syndromes) or special needs (e.g., high protein, increased calories).

3. Intravenous fluids are used when oral or tube feedings are contraindicated. Most are nutritionally incomplete and are used in the short term to supply fluids, electrolytes, and a few calories. Dextrose or dextrose and sodium chloride solutions are often used. When nutrients must be provided intravenously for more than a few days, a special

parenteral nutritional formula can be designed to meet all nutritional needs or to supplement other feeding methods.

4. Pancreatic enzymes (amylase, protease, lipase) are required for absorption of carbohydrates, proteins, and fats. Pancrelipase and others are commercial preparations used as replacement therapy in deficiency states, including cystic fibrosis, chronic pancreatitis, pancreatectomy, and pancreatic obstruction. Dosage is one to three capsules or tablets with each meal or snack.

5. Vitamins are obtained from foods or supplements. Although foods are considered the best source, studies indicate that most adults and children do not consume enough fruits, vegetables, cereal grains, dairy products, and other foods to consistently meet their vitamin requirements. In addition, some conditions increase requirements above the usual recommended amounts (e.g., pregnancy, lactation, various illnesses).

SECTION II: APPLYING YOUR KNOWLEDGE

Activity D   CASE STUDY

1. Iron preparations are used to prevent or treat iron deficiency anemia. For prevention, they are often given during periods of increased need, such as childhood or pregnancy.

2. The drug is well absorbed. Oral ferrous salts (sulfate, gluconate, fumarate) are preferred because of their absorption. Action starts in about 4 days, peaks in 7 to 10 days, and lasts 2 to 4 months. The drugs are not metabolized; a portion of a dose is lost daily in feces. Otherwise, the iron content is recycled and its half-life is unknown. Sustained-release or enteric-coated formulations are not as well absorbed as other preparations. Available ferrous salts differ in the amount of elemental iron they contain.

3. Adverse effects include nausea and other symptoms of GI irritation. Oral preparations also discolor feces, producing a black-green color that may be mistaken for blood in the stool. A guaiac test can tell whether the discoloration is from blood or from the iron preparation. Iron preparations are contraindicated in patients with peptic ulcer disease, inflammatory intestinal disorders, anemias other than iron deficiency anemia, multiple blood transfusions, hemochromatosis, or hemosiderosis. Ferrous gluconate (Fergon) may be less irritating to GI mucosa and therefore better tolerated than ferrous sulfate. It contains 12% elemental iron (i.e., 36 mg per 325 mg tablet).

SECTION III: PRACTICING FOR NCLEX

Activity E

1. **Answer: b**
   RATIONALE: Although most adults and children probably benefit from a daily multivitamin, large doses of single vitamins do not prevent cancer or cardiovascular disease and should be avoided.

2. **Answer: d**
   RATIONALE: Nutrients are best obtained from foods; when they cannot be obtained from foods, they can be provided by oral, enteral (via GI tubes), or parenteral (IV) feedings to meet a patient's nutritional needs.

3. **Answer: a**
   RATIONALE: The symptoms of vitamin A toxicity are double vision, headache, vomiting, hair loss, and dry, itching skin.

4. **Answer: c**
   RATIONALE: Large amounts of vitamin E are relatively nontoxic but can interfere with vitamin K action (blood clotting) by decreasing platelet aggregation and producing a risk of bleeding. Excessive doses can also cause fatigue, headache, blurred vision, nausea, and diarrhea.

5. **Answer: c**
   RATIONALE: Health promotion may involve assessing the nutritional status of all members of the household, especially children, older adults, and those with obvious deficiencies, and providing assistance to improve nutritional status.

6. **Answer: b, c, and e**
   RATIONALE: The nurse must teach the patient and family that the patient must be in a sitting position for administration of the tube feeding, it should not be over 500 mL, and it should be administered over 30 to 60 minutes. The container should be changed every 24 hours, and the family/patient should keep a record of the amount given each day.

7. **Answer: b**
   RATIONALE: Electrolyte and acid–base imbalances often occur in critically ill patients and are usually treated, as in other patients, with very close monitoring of serum electrolyte levels and avoidance of excessive amounts of replacement products.

8. **Answer: d**
   RATIONALE: With parenteral nutrition, adequate types and amounts of nutrients are needed. When IV fat emulsions are given, they should be infused slowly, over 24 hours.

9. **Answer: a**
   RATIONALE: The Nutrition Advisory Group of the American Medical Association (NAG-AMA) has established guidelines for daily intake of vitamins, and parenteral multivitamin formulations are available for adults and children. Those for adults do not contain vitamin K, which is usually injected weekly. The usual dose is 2 to 4 mg. Vitamin K is included in pediatric parenteral nutrition solutions.

10. **Answer: b**
    RATIONALE: Patients with respiratory impairment may need an enteral formula that contains less carbohydrate and more fat than other products and produces less carbon dioxide (e.g., Pulmocare).

11. Answer: b
RATIONALE: Taking an iron preparations with orange juice assists in the absorption of iron.

12. Answer: d
RATIONALE: Protein restriction is usually needed in patients with cirrhosis to prevent or treat hepatic encephalopathy, which is caused by excessive protein or excessive production of ammonia (from protein breakdown in the GI tract).

13. Answer: d
RATIONALE: The nurse would anticipate administering both insulin, which moves the potassium back into the cell, and glucose to prevent hypoglycemia. This is an extremely high, dangerous level of potassium, so it must be attended to immediately.

14. Answer: b
RATIONALE: IV fat emulsions should not be given to patients with ARF if serum triglyceride levels exceed 300 mg/dL.

15. Answer: a
RATIONALE: With the high incidence of atherosclerosis, cardiovascular disease, and diabetes mellitus in older adults, it is especially important that intake of animal fats and high-calorie sweets be reduced.

16. Answer: b
RATIONALE: Accidental ingestion of iron-containing medications and dietary supplements is a common cause of poisoning death in children younger than 6 years of age. To help prevent poisoning, products containing iron must be labeled with a warning, and products with 30 mg or more of iron (e.g., prenatal products) must be packaged as individual doses. All iron-containing preparations should be stored in places that are inaccessible to young children.

17. Answer: b
RATIONALE: Niacin may cause vasodilation, so it is important for the patient to lie down for approximately 30 minutes after niacin has been administered to prevent falling or fainting. The patient should use care when arising. It can cause facial flushing, and the patient can take 325 mg of aspirin to help with this.

18. Answer: b
RATIONALE: Preterm infants need proportionately more vitamins than term infants, because their growth rate is faster and their absorption of vitamins from the intestine is less complete. A multivitamin product containing the equivalent of DRIs for term infants is recommended.

19. Answer: b
RATIONALE: Folic acid decreases effects of phenytoin and may decrease absorption and effects of zinc.

20. Answer: c
RATIONALE: Deferoxamine is used for acute overdoses of iron. Deferasirox is used for chronic iron overload.

CHAPTER 34

SECTION I: ASSESSING YOUR UNDERSTANDING

Activity A FILL IN THE BLANKS
1. Overweight
2. Obese
3. BMI
4. BMI
5. obesity

Activity B MATCHING
1. b   **2.** a   **3.** c   **4.** e   **5.** d

Activity C SHORT ANSWERS
1. Obesity may occur in anyone but is more likely to occur in women, members of minority groups, and poor people. It results from consistent ingestion of more calories than are used for energy, and it substantially increases risks for development of numerous health problems.
2. Most obesity-related disorders are attributed mainly to the multiple metabolic abnormalities associated with obesity. Abdominal fat out of proportion to total body fat (also called central or visceral obesity), which often occurs in men and postmenopausal women, is considered a greater risk factor for disease and death than lower body obesity. In addition to the many health problems associated with obesity, obesity is increasingly being considered a chronic disease in its own right.
3. The prevalence of overweight people and obesity has dramatically increased during the past 25 years. Some authorities estimate that 60% of American adults are overweight or obese. There are differences in prevalence by gender, ethnicity, and socioeconomic status. In general, more women than men are obese, whereas more men than women are overweight; African American women and Mexican Americans of both sexes have the highest rates of overweight and obesity in the United States; and women in lower socioeconomic classes are more likely to be obese than those in higher socioeconomic classes.
4. The etiology of excessive weight is thought to involve complex and often overlapping interactions among physiologic, genetic, environmental, psychosocial, and other factors.
5. In general, increased weight is related to an energy imbalance in which energy intake (food/calorie consumption) exceeds energy expenditure. Total energy expenditure represents the energy expended at rest (i.e., the basal or resting metabolic rate), during physical activity, and during food consumption.

SECTION II: APPLYING YOUR KNOWLEDGE
Activity D CASE STUDY

1. "The drug decreases absorption of dietary fat from the intestine." Orlistat (Xenical, Alli) differs from phentermine and sibutramine because it decreases absorption of dietary fat from the intestine by binding to gastric and pancreatic lipases in the gastrointestinal tract lumen and making them unavailable to break down dietary fats into absorbable free fatty acids and monoglycerides.

2. The drug blocks absorption of approximately 30% of the fat ingested in a meal; increasing the dosage does not increase this percentage. Decreased fat absorption leads to decreased caloric intake, resulting in weight loss and improved serum cholesterol values (e.g., decreased total and low-density lipoprotein cholesterol levels). The improvement in cholesterol levels is thought to be independent of weight-loss effects.

3. Orlistat is not absorbed systemically, and its action occurs in the GI tract. Consequently, it does not cause systemic adverse effects or drug interactions as phentermine and sibutramine do. Orlistat's main disadvantages are the requirement for frequent administration (three times daily) and gastrointestinal symptoms (abdominal pain, oily spotting, fecal urgency, flatulence with discharge, fatty stools, fecal incontinence, and increased defecation). Adverse gastrointestinal effects occur in almost all orlistat users but usually subside after a few weeks of continued drug usage.

4. The patient should consult with her physician about other supplements to take with orlistat. The drug prevents absorption of the fat-soluble vitamins, A, D, E, and K, so people taking orlistat should also take a multivitamin containing these vitamins daily. The multivitamin should be taken 2 hours before or after the orlistat dose. If it is taken at the same time, the orlistat will prevent absorption of the fat-soluble vitamins. High-fat foods need to be decreased, because total caloric intake is a major determinant of weight, and adverse effects (e.g., diarrhea, fatty and malodorous stools) worsen with high fat consumption.

SECTION III: PRACTICING FOR NCLEX
Activity E

1. **Answer: a, b, d, and e**
   RATIONALE: Many people lose weight but regain it within a few months if they do not change their lifestyle habits toward eating more healthfully and exercising more. It is also important to review the patient's drinking history because alcohol is high in calories and may contribute to weight gain.

2. **Answer: b**
   RATIONALE: Weight-loss drugs are generally recommended only for people who are seriously overweight or have health problems associated with or aggravated by obesity.

3. **Answer: d**
   RATIONALE: The main ingredient in "energy drinks" is caffeine. Drinking too much caffeine can cause palpitations, tachycardia, and insomnia.

4. **Answer: d**
   RATIONALE: Ingesting 500 calories more per day than those used in exercise and physical activity leads to a weight gain of 1 pound in 1 week; decreasing caloric intake or increasing caloric output of 500 calories per day for 1 week leads to a weight loss of 1 pound.

5. **Answer: a, b, and e**
   RATIONALE: Overweight and obesity are major concerns because of their association with numerous health problems, including diabetes, hypertension, other cardiovascular disorders, and muscle and joint disorders. It has also been associated with the development of gallstones.

6. **Answer: d**
   RATIONALE: Fluoxetine promotes weight loss only with short-term use. Phenelzine and amitriptyline are associated with weight gain. Bupropion is associated with weight gain when used with patients who are using the medication for smoking cessation, but in patients who have taken it for depression, more patients have experienced weight loss than weight gain.

7. **Answer: b**
   RATIONALE: Sibutramine is no longer available because of cardiovascular problems associated with the drug.

8. **Answer: a, b, and c**
   RATIONALE: With orlistat, the manufacturer recommends conservative use and dosage because older adults often have decreased renal, cardiac, and pancreatic function. There is no evidence that older adults have decreased cognitive function.

9. **Answer: c**
   RATIONALE: Treatment of childhood obesity should focus on healthy eating and increasing physical activity. In general, children should not be put on "diets." For a child who is overweight, the recommended goal is to maintain weight or slow the rate of weight gain so that weight-for-height and BMI gradually decline as the child grows in height.

10. **Answer: a**
    RATIONALE: If the child already exceeds the optimal adult weight, the goal of treatment should be a slow weight loss of 10 to 12 pounds per year until the optimal adult weight is reached.

11. **Answer: b**
    RATIONALE: Although drug therapy has not been generally recommended for treatment of childhood obesity, orlistat is approved for use in children aged 12 to 16 years and is considered safe and effective for weight reduction in overweight

adolescents. As with adults, common adverse effects in clinical trials were gastrointestinal effects (e.g., diarrhea, flatulence) and reduced concentrations of fat-soluble vitamins.

12. Answer: b
RATIONALE: A weight-loss strategy that helps patients keep to a weight loss program is to keep a food and physical activity diary.

13. Answer: d
RATIONALE: The National Institutes of Health do not recommend combining weight-loss medications except in the context of clinical trials. Thus far, studies indicate that combining phentermine and orlistat has no additional benefit over using one of the drugs alone.

14. Answer: b
RATIONALE: For people who already have type 2 diabetes, weight loss reduces blood levels of glucose and glycosylated (A_{1c}) hemoglobin. These effects make the diabetes easier to manage, reduce complications of diabetes, and may allow smaller doses of antidiabetic medications.

15. Answer: a, c, and d
RATIONALE: Emphasize health benefits of weight reduction. There is strong evidence that weight loss reduces risk factors for cardiovascular disease, including blood pressure, serum triglycerides, and total and LDL cholesterol. It also increases HDL cholesterol. Weight loss will not cause a patient's hemoglobin to increase.

16. Answer: b
RATIONALE: Drug therapy and bariatric surgery are recommended only for seriously overweight people with major medical problems that can be improved by weight loss. In addition, neither of these treatments is a substitute for the necessary changes in eating and physical activity patterns.

17. Answer: a
RATIONALE: Laxative and diuretic herbs (e.g., aloe, rhubarb root, buckthorn, cascara, senna, parsley, juniper, dandelion leaves) are found in several products such as Super Dieter's Tea, Trim-Maxx Tea, and Water Pill. These products cause a significant loss of body fluids and electrolytes, not fat. Adverse effects may include low serum potassium levels, with subsequent cardiac dysrhythmias and other heart problems.

18. Answer: c
RATIONALE: Guar gum is a dietary fiber that is included in weight-loss products because it is bulk-forming and produces feelings of fullness. Several small studies indicated it is no more effective than placebo for weight loss. It may cause esophageal or intestinal obstruction if not taken with an adequate amount of water and may interfere with the absorption of other drugs if taken at the same time. Adverse effects include nausea, diarrhea, flatulence, and abdominal discomfort.

19. Answer: b, d, and e
RATIONALE: Metabolic syndrome includes three or more of the following abnormalities:
- Central obesity (waist circumference over 40 inches for men and over 35 inches for women)
- Serum triglycerides of 150 mg/dL or more
- HDL cholesterol below 40 mg/dL in men and below 50 mg/dL in women
- Blood pressure of 135/85 mm Hg or higher
- Serum glucose of 110 mg/dL or higher

CHAPTER 35

SECTION I: ASSESSING YOUR UNDERSTANDING
Activity A FILL IN THE BLANKS
1. Peptic ulcer disease
2. duodenal
3. protective
4. pepsin
5. Gastric acid

Activity B MATCHING
1. e **2.** c **3.** d **4.** a **5.** b

Activity C SHORT ANSWERS
1. Antacids are alkaline substances that neutralize acids. They react with hydrochloric acid in the stomach to produce neutral, less acidic, or poorly absorbed salts and to raise the pH (alkalinity) of gastric secretions. Raising the pH to approximately 3.5 neutralizes more than 90% of gastric acid and inhibits conversion of pepsinogen to pepsin. Commonly used antacids are aluminum, magnesium, and calcium compounds.

2. Histamine is a substance that is found in almost every body tissue and is released in response to certain stimuli (e.g., allergic reactions, tissue injury). After it is released, histamine causes contraction of smooth muscle in the bronchi, GI tract, and uterus; dilation and increased permeability of capillaries; dilation of cerebral blood vessels; and stimulation of sensory nerve endings to produce pain and itching. Histamine also causes strong stimulation of gastric acid secretion. Vagal stimulation causes release of histamine from cells in the gastric mucosa. The histamine then acts on receptors located on the parietal cells to increase production of hydrochloric acid. These receptors are called the histamine$_2$ (H_2) receptors.

3. PPIs are strong inhibitors of gastric acid secretion. These drugs bind irreversibly to the gastric proton pump (e.g., the enzyme H^+,K^+-ATPase) to prevent the "pumping" or release of gastric acid from parietal cells into the stomach lumen, thereby blocking the final step of acid production.

Inhibition of the proton pump suppresses gastric acid secretion in response to all primary stimuli including histamine, gastrin, and acetylcholine. Therefore, the drugs inhibit both daytime (including meal-stimulated) and nocturnal (unstimulated) acid secretion.

4. Naturally occurring prostaglandin E, which is produced in mucosal cells of the stomach and duodenum, inhibits gastric acid secretion and increases mucus and bicarbonate secretion, mucosal blood flow, and perhaps mucosal repair. It also inhibits the mucosal damage produced by gastric acid, aspirin, and NSAIDs.

5. Sucralfate is a preparation of sulfated sucrose and aluminum hydroxide that binds to normal and ulcerated mucosa. It is used to prevent and treat peptic ulcer disease. It is effective even though it does not inhibit secretion of gastric acid or pepsin and has little neutralizing effect on gastric acid. Its mechanism of action is unclear, but it is thought to act locally on the gastric and duodenal mucosa. Possible mechanisms include binding to the ulcer and forming a protective barrier between the mucosa and gastric acid, pepsin, and bile salts; neutralizing pepsin; stimulating prostaglandin synthesis in the mucosa; and exerting healing effects through the aluminum component. Sucralfate is effective in healing duodenal ulcers and in maintenance therapy to prevent ulcer recurrence. In general, the rates of ulcer healing with sucralfate are similar to the rates with H₂RAs.

SECTION II: APPLYING YOUR KNOWLEDGE
Activity D CASE STUDY

1. Misoprostol is a synthetic form of prostaglandin E that is approved for concurrent use with NSAIDs to protect gastric mucosa from NSAID-induced erosion and ulceration. Prostaglandin E, which is produced in mucosal cells of the stomach and duodenum, inhibits gastric acid secretion and increases mucus and bicarbonate secretion, mucosal blood flow, and perhaps mucosal repair. It also inhibits the mucosal damage produced by gastric acid, aspirin, and NSAIDs. When synthesis of prostaglandin E is inhibited, erosion and ulceration of gastric mucosa may occur.

2. You should know more about Mrs. Dinwiddie before advising her husband. The FDA has issued a black box warning to alert health care professionals that misoprostol is contraindicated in women of childbearing potential (unless effective contraceptive methods are being used) and during pregnancy, because it may induce abortion, premature birth, or birth defects.

3. The most common adverse effects of misoprostol use are diarrhea (in 10%–40% of recipients) and abdominal cramping. It is indicated for patients who are at high risk of GI ulceration and bleeding, such as those taking high doses of NSAIDs.

SECTION III: PRACTICING FOR NCLEX
Activity E

1. **Answer: a**
   RATIONALE: Sucralfate forms a protective barrier over mucosal ulcerations, protecting them from exposure to gastric juices. It requires an acid pH to be effective.

2. **Answer: a, b, and d**
   RATIONALE: The risk factors for the development of a peptic ulcer include smoking, psychological stress, physiological stress, and the use of NSAIDs such as aspirin or ibuprofen. The use of acetaminophen or sucralfate is not a risk factor.

3. **Answer: a, c, and d**
   RATIONALE: PPIs are considered drugs of choice for treatment of heartburn, gastric and duodenal ulcers, GERD, esophagitis, and hypersecretory syndromes such as Zollinger-Ellison syndrome. It is not used in the treatment of anaphylaxis.

4. **Answer: b**
   RATIONALE: The combination of an opioid analgesic and cimetidine will cause an increase in respiratory depression.

5. **Answer: a**
   RATIONALE: The treatment of choice for *Helicobacter pylori* infection is a PPI and clarithromycin plus either amoxicillin or metronidazole.

6. **Answer: b**
   RATIONALE: Calcium antacids have high neutralizing capacity and rapid onset. They may cause rebound acidity and hypercalcemia.

7. **Answer: c**
   RATIONALE: Magnesium antacids have high neutralizing capacity and may cause diarrhea and hypermagnesemia.

8. **Answer: d**
   RATIONALE: The PPI that is suggested for use with NG tubes is esomeprazole because the contents of this capsule can be opened and used successfully in NG tube.

9. **Answer: d**
   RATIONALE: Gastroesophageal reflux disease (GERD) is characterized by regurgitation of acidic gastric contents into the esophagus resulting in esophagitis or esophageal ulceration.

10. **Answer: c**
    RATIONALE: Misoprostol can cause uterine contractions and emptying of any uterine contents, so it is important to know if there is a possibility that the patient is pregnant before administering the medication.

11. **Answer: b**
    RATIONALE: Sucralfate must be taken for 4 to 8 weeks to ensure healing of the ulcer has occurred.

12. **Answer: c**
    RATIONALE: It is important for the patient to take the ciprofloxacin 2 hours prior to taking sucralfate to ensure full absorption of the ciprofloxacin.

13. **Answer: b**
RATIONALE: The home care nurse can assist patients by providing information about taking the drugs correctly and monitoring responses. If cimetidine is being taken, the home care nurse needs to assess for potential drug–drug interactions.

14. **Answer: b**
RATIONALE: PPIs are metabolized in the liver and may cause transient elevations in liver function tests.

15. **Answer: b**
RATIONALE: Antacids containing magnesium are contraindicated in patients with impaired renal function.

16. **Answer: c**
RATIONALE: Sucralfate is well tolerated by older adults. PPIs are also well tolerated, but long-term use (greater than 1 year) is associated with increased risk of hip fractures in adults older than 50 years of age. The risk of fractures increases the longer the medications are taken. The risk of hip fractures is also greater in those taking higher dosages of PPIs.

17. **Answer: a**
RATIONALE: With H_2RAs, older adults are more likely to experience adverse effects, especially confusion, agitation, and disorientation, with cimetidine. In addition, older adults often have decreased renal function, and doses need to be reduced.

18. **Answer: a**
RATIONALE: Smaller doses of antacids may be effective in older adults, because they usually secrete less gastric acid than younger adults do.

19. **Answer: b**
RATIONALE: When a patient has a nasogastric tube in place, antacid dosage may be titrated by aspirating stomach contents, determining pH, and then basing the dose on the pH. (Most gastric acid is neutralized and most pepsin activity is eliminated at a pH greater than 3.5.)

20. **Answer: c**
RATIONALE: Recommended doses of PPIs heal most gastric and duodenal ulcers in about 4 weeks. Large gastric ulcers may require 8 weeks.

CHAPTER 36

SECTION I: ASSESSING YOUR UNDERSTANDING

Activity A FILL IN THE BLANKS

1. Antiemetic
2. Nausea
3. Vomiting
4. adverse effects
5. vomiting center

Activity B MATCHING

1. b   2. d   3. c   4. a   5. e

Activity C SHORT ANSWERS

1. Nausea and vomiting are the most common adverse effects of drug therapy. Although the symptoms may occur with most drugs, they are especially associated with alcohol, aspirin, digoxin, anticancer drugs, antimicrobials, estrogen preparations, and opioid analgesics.

2. Nausea and vomiting may be caused by pain and other noxious stimuli, such as unpleasant sights and odors; emotional disturbances; physical or mental stress; radiation therapy; motion sickness; postoperative status, which may include pain; impaired GI motility; and pregnancy.

3. The vomiting center, CTZ, and GI tract contain benzodiazepine, cholinergic, dopamine, histamine, opiate, substance P/neurokinin, and serotonin receptors, which are stimulated by emetogenic drugs and toxins.

4. When stimulated, the vomiting center initiates efferent impulses that stimulate the salivary center, causing closure of the glottis; contraction of abdominal muscles and the diaphragm; relaxation of the gastroesophageal sphincter; and reverse peristalsis, which moves stomach contents toward the mouth for ejection.

5. Anticipatory nausea is triggered by memories, and fear of nausea and vomiting is mediated by afferent signals from the higher centers of the cerebral cortex to the vomiting center.

SECTION II: APPLYING YOUR KNOWLEDGE

Activity D CASE STUDY

1. Aprepitant exerts its antiemetic effect by blocking the activity of substance P at NK_1 receptors in the brain, inhibiting the signal to the brain that causes nausea. Prescribers often order aprepitant as part of combination therapy along with a $5-HT_3$ receptor antagonist and corticosteroids to treat both acute and delayed nausea and vomiting associated with chemotherapy.

2. Patients should take aprepitant by mouth as directed with a full glass of water, with or without food. Typically, the first dose is taken 1 hour before chemotherapy and then daily in the morning for the next 2 days after the chemotherapy treatment.

3. Aprepitant may cause fatigue, weakness, dizziness, headache, or hiccups, so it may make it difficult for the patient to return to work.

SECTION III: PRACTICING FOR NCLEX

Activity E

1. **Answer: a**
RATIONALE: Scopolamine is an anticholinergic drug that is effective in relieving nausea and vomiting associated with motion sickness and radiation therapy for cancer.

2. **Answer: d**
RATIONALE: Dronabinol is a cannabinoid used in the management of nausea and vomiting associated with chemotherapy unrelieved by other antiemetic drugs. It is a Schedule III drug under federal narcotic laws.

3. **Answer: c**
RATIONALE: Promethazine may cause urinary retention, which may be problematic in a patient who already has benign prostatic hypertrophy.

4. **Answer: c**
RATIONALE: Chlorpromazine, which is a phenothiazine, is used in the treatment of intractable hiccups.

5. **Answer: a**
RATIONALE: Aprepitant is often used in combination therapy with a 5-HT$_3$ serotonin receptor antagonist (ondansetron) and a corticosteroid (dexamethasone).

6. **Answer: a, b, and c**
RATIONALE: Benzodiazepines such as lorazepam produce relaxation, relieve anxiety, and inhibit cerebral cortex input to the vomiting center. They are prescribed for anticipatory nausea associated with cancer chemotherapy. Lorazepam is not associated with amnesia.

7. **Answer: b**
RATIONALE: A nonpharmacologic therapy that is helpful to women who are experiencing morning sickness is the use of acupressure wristbands. Other measures include eating dry crackers before getting out of bed. Phosphorated carbohydrate solution is a medication called Emetrol that may be purchased OTC.

8. **Answer: b**
RATIONALE: The nurse should immediately help the patient rinse out his mouth which helps take away the taste and sensation of vomit.

9. **Answer: a, d, and e**
RATIONALE: The home care nurse would reinforce medication teaching which would include how much medication and when to take the medication. It is usually taken 30 to 60 minutes before the event that causes nausea. The patient should sit or lie quietly after taking the medication because it may cause sedation. This is also a reason that the patient should not drive. The patient should be encouraged to drink clear liquids to prevent dehydration.

10. **Answer: a**
RATIONALE: Phenothiazines are metabolized in the liver and eliminated in urine. In the presence of liver disease (e.g., cirrhosis, hepatitis), metabolism may be slowed and drug elimination half-lives prolonged, with resultant accumulation and increased risk of adverse effects. Therefore, the drugs should be used cautiously in patients with hepatic impairment. Cholestatic jaundice has been reported with promethazine.

11. **Answer: a**
RATIONALE: Most antiemetic drugs are metabolized in the liver and should be used cautiously in patients with impaired hepatic function. With oral ondansetron, do not exceed an 8-mg dose; with IV use, a single, maximal daily dose of 8 mg is recommended.

12. **Answer: b**
RATIONALE: The use of acupuncture is the nonpharmacologic technique that is the most accepted and widely studied in the treatment of nausea.

13. **Answer: b**
RATIONALE: Most antiemetic drugs cause drowsiness, especially in older adults, and therefore should be used cautiously. Efforts should be made to prevent nausea and vomiting when possible. Older adults are at risk of fluid volume depletion and electrolyte imbalances with vomiting.

14. **Answer: a, c, and d**
RATIONALE: Patients who have been taking dronabinol may go through withdrawal symptoms if it is discontinued suddenly. The patient will experience insomnia, sleep disturbances, irritability, and restlessness.

15. **Answer: c**
RATIONALE: A black box warning alerts nurses that promethazine is contraindicated in children younger than 2 years of age because of the risk of potentially fatal respiratory depression. When using promethazine, the lowest effective dosage should be used, and other drugs with respiratory depressant effects should not be given concurrently. Excessive doses may cause hallucinations, convulsions, and sudden death.

16. **Answer: b**
RATIONALE: A patient taking both aprepitant and oral contraceptives must use an alternative form of birth control for at least 1 month after taking aprepitant.

17. **Answer: a, b, c, and e**
RATIONALE: If nausea and vomiting are likely to occur because of travel, administration of emetogenic anticancer drugs, diagnostic tests, or therapeutic procedures, an antiemetic drug should be given before the emetogenic event. Pretreatment usually increases patient comfort and allows use of lower drug doses. It also may prevent aspiration and other potentially serious complications of vomiting. It is also used to decrease the patient's anxiety concerning the upcoming treatment.

18. **Answer: c**
RATIONALE: It takes dimenhydrinate up to 4 hours to be fully effective, so it should be given approximately 4 hours before getting in the car.

19. **Answer: d**
RATIONALE: Antihistamines such as meclizine and dimenhydrinate are useful for vomiting caused by labyrinthitis, uremia, or postoperative status.

20. **Answer: c**
RATIONALE: The patient who has liver disease and receives promethazine may develop cholestatic jaundice.

CHAPTER 37

SECTION I: ASSESSING YOUR UNDERSTANDING

Activity A FILL IN THE BLANKS

1. Constipation
2. impaction
3. laxative
4. cathartic
5. gastrocolic, duodenocolic

Activity B MATCHING

1. c   **2.** e   **3.** d   **4.** b   **5.** a

Activity C SHORT ANSWERS

1. Risk factors associated with the development of constipation include diet and lifestyle, particularly decreased levels of physical activity. Female sex, nonwhite status, advanced age, and low levels of education and income are related risk factors. In addition, certain drugs and disease process are associated with constipation.
2. Voluntary control inhibits the external anal sphincter to allow defecation or contracts the sphincter to prevent defecation. When the external sphincter remains contracted, the defecation reflex dissipates, and the urge to defecate usually does not recur until additional feces enter the rectum or several hours later. In people who often inhibit the defecation reflex or fail to respond to the urge to defecate, constipation develops as the reflex weakens.
3. Symptoms of constipation include fewer than three stools per week, straining at the stool, a sensation of incomplete evacuation, a sensation of anorectal blockage, hard stools, and the use of manual evacuation.
4. Advancing age may lead to abdominal muscles that have become weak or atrophied, making it harder to defecate. Older adults also may have issues with limited mobility and a lessened sense of thirst, which decreases fluid intake.
5. Lifestyle changes that will promote regular bowel elimination include increased activity and exercise, increase intake of dietary fiber, a fluid intake of at least 2 L/d, and a regular routine for bowel elimination.

SECTION II: APPLYING YOUR KNOWLEDGE

Activity D CASE STUDY

1. The nurse explains that bisacodyl works by irritating the GI mucosa and pulling water into the bowel, which causes stool to move rapidly through the bowel, which decreases absorption of fecal water. The pain medication she has been taking for her broken leg slows the movement of feces through the bowel, which leads to constipation.

2. Mrs. Fuller may experience abdominal pain and cramping. She also may have some nausea, diarrhea, and weakness.
3. The nurse instructs the patient that milk will cause the enteric coating of the tablet to dissolve earlier than it is supposed to, which can result in earlier release of the drug. The nurse will advise Mrs. Fuller to wait a full hour after drinking milk before taking bisacodyl.
4. The nurse will advise Mrs. Fuller to make sure she gets an adequate amount of fluids each day (at least 2000 mL) and to increase the amount of fiber-rich foods she is eating. The nurse will also encourage the patient to establish a time to use the bathroom for bowel elimination. The best time is right after breakfast.

SECTION III: PRACTICING FOR NCLEX

Activity E

1. **Answer: c**
   RATIONALE: Docusate sodium is a stool softener that decreases the surface tension of the fecal mass to allow water to penetrate into the stool. Stools are softer and easier to pass. Its main value is to prevent straining at the stool. This makes the drug most appropriate for the patient who has had a heart attack who should avoid straining at the stool.
2. **Answer: d**
   RATIONALE: Psyllium should be taken with a full glass of liquid; therefore, it should be mixed in 240 mL (8 ounces) of liquid.
3. **Answer: a**
   RATIONALE: Bisacodyl is contraindicated in patients under the age of 12.
4. **Answer: a, d, and e**
   RATIONALE: Critically ill patients are more at risk for constipation because of decreased activity, decreased access to a high-fiber diet, the use of opioid medications, and changes in usual bowel routines.
5. **Answer: b**
   RATIONALE: Laxatives and cathartics are contraindicated in patients with abdominal pain. The presence of fever would also be a possible indication of infection.
6. **Answer: a, c, and d**
   RATIONALE: Nonpharmacologic treatments for constipation include an increase in the use of high-fiber foods, an adequate fluid intake of at least 2 L, the use of both prebiotics and probiotics, and regular daily exercise.
7. **Answer: c**
   RATIONALE: Patients with hepatic encephalopathy are prescribed lactulose which helps to decrease the amount of ammonia in the intestine.
8. **Answer: d**
   RATIONALE: Patients with chronic idiopathic constipation are prescribed lubiprostone.

9. Answer: b
RATIONALE: Patients taking lactulose should have two to three soft stools per day.

10. Answer: a
RATIONALE: The patient should refrigerate the solution to increase the palatability and also to ensure its potency.

11. Answer: b, c, and e
RATIONALE: Chronic idiopathic constipation is characterized by hard, lumpy stools that the patient strains to pass, abnormal GI motility, and abdominal cramping and bloating.

12. Answer: b
RATIONALE: Sodium polystyrene sulfonate is prescribed for the treatment of increased potassium levels.

13. Answer: a
RATIONALE: Constipation is associated with fluid intake less than 2000 mL/d.

14. Answer: a and c
RATIONALE: Drugs that reduce intestinal function and motility include opioid analgesics, antacids containing aluminum or calcium, anticholinergics, calcium channel blockers, clozapine, diuretics, iron, phenothiazines, cholestyramine, colestipol, sucralfate, tricyclic antidepressants, and vincristine.

15. Answer: b
RATIONALE: Patients with hypothyroidism are at high risk for constipation because of the decreased intestinal motility associated with this condition.

16. Answer: b
RATIONALE: Patients should attempt to have a bowel movement immediately after breakfast for best results.

17. Answer: d
RATIONALE: Psyllium is the best medication for long-term use in the treatment of constipation.

18. Answer: b
RATIONALE: Polyethylene glycol–electrolyte solution is contraindicated in patients who have colitis.

19. Answer: b
RATIONALE: Patients with decreased renal function may develop hypermagnesemia if mail of magnesia is used frequently.

20. Answer: c
RATIONALE: Patients who believe that a daily bowel movement is necessary need further instruction.

CHAPTER 38

SECTION I: ASSESSING YOUR UNDERSTANDING

Activity A FILL IN THE BLANKS
1. Diarrhea
2. ground beef
3. hemolytic uremic
4. enterotoxigenic
5. *Campylobacter jejuni*

Activity B MATCHING
1. c   2. d   3. e   4. b   5. a

Activity C SHORT ANSWERS
1. *Salmonella* infections may occur when contaminated poultry and other meats, eggs, and dairy products are ingested. Elderly patients are especially susceptible to *Salmonella*-associated colitis.
2. Several strains of *Shigella* may produce diarrhea. Infection most often results from direct person-to-person contact, but it may also occur via food or water contamination. Hand washing is especially important in preventing the spread of *Shigella* from person to person.
3. Deficiency of pancreatic enzymes inhibits digestion and absorption of carbohydrates, proteins, and fats. Deficiency of lactase, which breaks down lactose to simple sugars (i.e., glucose and galactose) that can be absorbed by GI mucosa, inhibits digestion of milk and milk products. Lactase deficiency commonly occurs among people of African or Asian descent.
4. In inflammatory bowel disorders, such as gastroenteritis, diverticulitis, ulcerative colitis, and Crohn's disease, the inflamed mucous membrane secretes large amounts of fluids into the intestinal lumen, along with mucus, proteins, and blood, and absorption of water and electrolytes is impaired. In addition, when the ileum is diseased or a portion is surgically excised, large amounts of bile salts reach the colon, where they act as cathartics and cause diarrhea. Bile salts are normally reabsorbed from the ileum.
5. IBS is a functional disorder of intestinal motility with no evidence of inflammation or tissue changes. A change in bowel pattern (constipation, diarrhea, or a combination of both) accompanied by abdominal pain, bloating, and distention is the presenting symptom. The cause is unknown; however, activation of 5-HT$_3$ (serotonin) receptors, which affect the regulation of visceral pain, colonic motility, and GI secretions, is thought to be involved in the pathophysiology of IBS.

SECTION II: APPLYING YOUR KNOWLEDGE
Activity D CASE STUDY
1. Alosetron (Lotronex) is a selective 5-HT$_3$ receptor antagonist that is indicated for treating women with chronic severe diarrhea-predominant irritable bowel syndrome (IBS) that has not responded to conventional therapy. This drug has recently become available for treatment of your condition.
2. The patient is likely to show signs of alosetron toxicity. Alosetron is extensively metabolized by the cytochrome P450 enzyme system (CYP2C9, CYP3A4, and CYP1A2) with multiple metabolites produced that are excreted primarily in the urine. Caution must be used with concurrent administration of CYP1A2 and CYP3A4 inhibitors. Concurrent administration with fluvoxamine is

contraindicated. The physician will consult the psychiatrist and reduce the dose of the fluvoxamine. Alosetron should not be given to patients with a history of GI disorders, including chronic or severe constipation or sequelae of constipation, intestinal obstruction, stricture, toxic megacolon, GI perforation and/or adhesions, ischemic colitis, impaired intestinal circulation, thrombophlebitis or hypercoagulable state, Crohn's disease, ulcerative colitis, or diverticulitis.

3. Reduced dosages may be needed in some women older than 65 years of age to prevent drug accumulation and toxicity. Each patient must sign a patient–physician agreement indicating that she understands the risks of taking alosetron and agrees to take the medication, will discontinue taking alosetron and immediately notify the physician if constipation or signs of ischemic colitis occur, and will stop taking alosetron and contact the physician after 4 weeks of therapy with alosetron if the symptoms of IBS are not controlled. The medication guide and patient–physician agreement are available at http://www.lotronex.com.

SECTION III: PRACTICING FOR NCLEX

Activity E

1. **Answer: b**
   RATIONALE: In bacterial gastroenteritis or diarrhea, the choice of antibacterial drug depends on the causative organism and susceptibility tests.

2. **Answer: a, b, and e**
   RATIONALE: Diarrhea may occur in patients who have intestinal infections, hyperthyroidism, lack of digestive enzymes, highly spiced foods, and laxative abuse.

3. **Answer: c**
   RATIONALE: Adverse effect of diphenoxylate include tachycardia, urinary retention, flushing, headache, and dizziness as well as nausea and vomiting.

4. **Answer: d**
   RATIONALE: Bismuth subsalicylate has antisecretory, antimicrobial, and possibly anti-inflammatory effects. It is used in the control of travelers' diarrhea and relief of abdominal cramping.

5. **Answer: b**
   RATIONALE: Octreotide, a synthetic form of somatostatin, decreases GI secretion and motility. It is used for diarrhea associated with carcinoid syndrome, intestinal tumors, or HIV/AIDS and diarrhea that does not respond to other antidiarrheal drugs.

6. **Answer: a**
   RATIONALE: Diphenoxylate is contraindicated in patients who have pathogenic *Escherichia coli* intestinal infection.

7. **Answer: b and d**
   RATIONALE: Patients with HIV often develop diarrhea related to drug therapy and also as a part of an opportunistic intestinal infection.

8. **Answer: d**
   RATIONALE: With loperamide, monitor patients with hepatic impairment for signs of CNS toxicity. Loperamide normally undergoes extensive first-pass metabolism, which may be lessened by liver disease. As a result, a larger portion of the dose reaches the systemic circulation and may cause adverse effects.

9. **Answer: a**
   RATIONALE: Diphenoxylate should be used with extreme caution in patients with severe hepatorenal disease because hepatic coma may be precipitated.

10. **Answer: a**
    RATIONALE: Diphenoxylate contains atropine, and signs of atropine overdose may occur with usual doses. Diphenoxylate is contraindicated in children younger than 2 years of age.

11. **Answer: b**
    RATIONALE: Patients with anorexia nervosa and bulimia suffer diarrhea due to chronic laxative abuse as a way to lose weight or prevent gaining any additional weight related to binging.

12. **Answer: b**
    RATIONALE: The following oral drugs and dosages are approximately equivalent in antidiarrheal effectiveness: 4 mg morphine, 30 mg codeine, 10 mL paregoric, 5 mg diphenoxylate, and 2 mg loperamide.

13. **Answer: b**
    RATIONALE: In antibiotic-associated colitis, stopping the causative drug is the initial treatment.

14. **Answer: c**
    RATIONALE: In antibiotic-associated colitis, stopping the causative drug is the initial treatment. If symptoms do not improve within 3 or 4 days, oral metronidazole or vancomycin is given for 7 to 10 days.

15. **Answer: d**
    RATIONALE: In ulcerative colitis, sulfonamides, adrenal corticosteroids, and other anti-inflammatory agents such as balsalazide (Colazal), mesalamine (Pentasa), and olsalazine (Dipentum) are the drugs of choice.

16. **Answer: a and d**
    RATIONALE: For symptomatic treatment of diarrhea, diphenoxylate with atropine (Lomotil) or loperamide (Imodium) is probably the drug of choice for most people.

17. **Answer: c**
    RATIONALE: Patients who are allergic to aspirin should not use bismuth salts.

18. **Answer: a**
    RATIONALE: In most cases of acute, nonspecific diarrhea in adults, fluid losses are not severe and patients need only simple replacement of fluids and electrolytes lost in the stool. Acceptable replacement fluids during the first 24 hours include 2 to 3 L of clear liquids (e.g., flat ginger ale, decaffeinated cola drinks or tea, broth, gelatin).

19. Answer: a, b, and d

RATIONALE: Contraindications to the use of antidiarrheal drugs include diarrhea caused by toxic materials, microorganisms that penetrate intestinal mucosa (e.g., pathogenic *E. coli, Salmonella, Shigella*), and antibiotic-associated colitis.

20. Answer: c

RATIONALE: Nitazoxanide (Alinia) is an antiprotozoal agent used specifically for treating diarrhea resulting from infection with *Giardia lamblia* or *Cryptosporidium parvum*.

CHAPTER 39

SECTION I: ASSESSING YOUR UNDERSTANDING

Activity A FILL IN THE BLANKS

1. Insulin
2. Amylin
3. liver
4. fat
5. glomeruli

Activity B MATCHING

1. d   **2.** b   **3.** a   **4.** e   **5.** c

Activity C SHORT ANSWERS

1. Metformin increases the use of glucose by muscle and fat cells, decreases hepatic glucose production, and decreases intestinal absorption of glucose. It is preferably called an antihyperglycemic rather than a hypoglycemic agent, because it does not cause hypoglycemia, even in large doses, when used alone. Metformin is absorbed from the small intestine, circulates without binding to plasma proteins, and has a serum half-life of 1.3 to 4.5 hours. It is not metabolized in the liver and is excreted unchanged in the urine.

2. Thiazolidinediones include pioglitazone and rosiglitazone. They are sometimes called "glitazones" and are also referred to as insulin sensitizers. Thiazolidinediones decrease insulin resistance, a major factor in the pathophysiology of type 2 diabetes. The drugs stimulate receptors on muscle, fat, and liver cells. This stimulation increases or restores the effectiveness of circulating insulin and results in increased uptake of glucose by peripheral tissues and decreased production of glucose by the liver. Thiazolidinediones may be used as monotherapy with diet and exercise or in combination with insulin, metformin, a sulfonylurea, an amylin analogue (pramlintide), or an incretin mimetic (exenatide).

3. Pramlintide (Symlin) is a synthetic analogue of amylin, a peptide hormone secreted with insulin by the beta cells of the pancreas that is important in the regulation of glucose control during the postprandial period. Pramlintide is used as an adjunctive treatment with mealtime insulin for adult patients with type 1 or type 2 diabetes who have not achieved optimal glucose control with insulin therapy alone. Pramlintide slows gastric emptying, helping to regulate the postprandial rise in blood glucose. The drug also suppresses postprandial glucagon secretion, thus helping maintain better blood glucose control. Pramlintide increases the sense of satiety, possibly reducing food intake and promoting weight loss. Pramlintide and insulin therapy may be combined with metformin or sulfonylureas for patients with type 2 diabetes.

4. Exenatide acts as a natural helper hormone by stimulating the pancreas to secrete the right amount of insulin based on the food that was just eaten. This helps to reduce the problem of high blood glucose after meals. Exenatide also halts gluconeogenesis by the liver, keeping it from making too much glucose after a meal. Exenatide slows gastric emptying, which serves to reduce the sudden rise of blood glucose after a meal and also quickly stimulates a feeling of satiety when eating. This fosters a sense of fullness, which causes the patient to eat less and potentially lose weight. Exenatide may reduce the absorption of concurrently administered oral medications.

5. Certain supplements may increase blood glucose levels. Bee pollen may cause hyperglycemia and decrease the effects of antidiabetic medications; it should not be used by people with diabetes. *Ginkgo biloba* extract is thought to increase blood sugar in patients with diabetes by increasing hepatic metabolism of insulin and oral hypoglycemic drugs, thereby making the drugs less effective. It is not recommended for use. Glucosamine, as indicated by animal studies, may cause impaired beta-cell function and insulin secretion similar to that observed in humans with type 2 diabetes. Long-term effects in humans are unknown, but the product is considered potentially harmful to people with diabetes or prediabetes. Adverse effects on blood sugar and drug interactions with antidiabetic medications have not been reported. However, blood sugar should be monitored carefully. With chondroitin, which is often taken with glucosamine for osteoarthritis, there is no information about effects on blood sugar, use by patients with diabetes, or interactions with antidiabetic drugs.

SECTION II: APPLYING YOUR KNOWLEDGE

Activity D CASE STUDY

1. Type 2 is a heterogenous disease, and its etiology probably involves multiple factors such as a genetic predisposition and environmental factors. Obesity is a major cause. With obesity and chronic ingestion of excess calories, along with a sedentary lifestyle, more insulin is required. The increased need leads to prolonged stimulation and eventual "fatigue" of pancreatic beta cells. As a result, the cells become less responsive to elevated blood glucose levels and less able to produce enough insulin to

meet metabolic needs. Therefore, insulin is secreted but is inadequate or ineffective, especially when insulin demand is increased by obesity, pregnancy, aging, or other factors.

2. Most signs and symptoms stem from a lack of effective insulin and the subsequent metabolic abnormalities. Their incidence and severity depend on the amount of effective insulin, and they may be precipitated by infection, rapid growth, pregnancy, or other factors that increase demand for insulin. Most early symptoms result from disordered carbohydrate metabolism, which causes excess glucose to accumulate in the blood (hyperglycemia). Hyperglycemia produces glucosuria, which, in turn, produces polydipsia, polyuria, dehydration, and polyphagia.

3. When large amounts of glucose are present, as in the hyperglycemic state of diabetes, water is pulled into the renal tubule. This results in a greatly increased urine output (polyuria). The excessive loss of fluid in urine leads to increased thirst (polydipsia) and, if fluid intake is inadequate, to dehydration. Dehydration also occurs because high blood glucose levels increase osmotic pressure in the bloodstream, and fluid is pulled out of the cells in the body's attempt to regain homeostasis.

4. Exenatide is administered subcutaneously twice a day and has been approved to be administered with oral medications such as sulfonylureas, metformin, and/or thiazolidinediones. Major advantages of exenatide over insulin are increased satiety and weight loss. Exenatide is available via a prefilled injection pen in two doses (5 or 10 mcg) and does not need to be adjusted based on blood glucose levels or the amount of food a patient was able to consume. The drug should be taken twice a day within 60 minutes of the morning and evening meal (at least 6 hours apart). Exenatide can be injected into the subcutaneous tissue of the upper arm or leg or the abdominal area. It should be stored at all times in the original packaging in a refrigerator at 36°F to 46°F, protected from light, kept dry, and discarded once opened after 30 days.

SECTION III: PRACTICING FOR NCLEX
Activity E

1. **Answer: b, c, and d**
   RATIONALE: People with impaired glucose tolerance can significantly reduce the risk of developing type 2 diabetes through intervention with diet and exercise.

2. **Answer: d**
   RATIONALE: A FPG result (126 mg/dL) on two separate occasions is diagnostic of diabetes, values of 100 to 125 mg/dL are termed impaired fasting glucose, and values less than 100 mg/dL are considered normal.

3. **Answer: a**
   RATIONALE: Fasting plasma glucose test (FPG) is the simplest and least expensive screening test.

4. **Answer: b**
   RATIONALE: The American Diabetes Association (ADA) suggests a target A1C of less than 7%. A1C should be measured every 3 to 6 months. An A1C of 9 indicates that the patient's average blood glucose is consistently above normal.

5. **Answer: b, c, and d**
   RATIONALE: The home care nurse would assist the patient and family to know how to plan meals that meet the needs of the patient and the family. The nurse would also want to assure that the patient knows how to administer insulin correctly and would need to make sure that the patient understands how to deal with hypoglycemia.

6. **Answer: a and b**
   RATIONALE: Hyperglycemia may complicate the progress of the critically ill patient, resulting in increased complications such as postoperative infections, poor recovery, and increased mortality. Tight glycemic control is a key factor in preventing complications and improving mortality in patients with diabetes in the intensive care unit.

7. **Answer: a**
   RATIONALE: Sulfonylureas and their metabolites are excreted mainly by the kidneys; renal impairment may lead to accumulation and hypoglycemia. They should be used cautiously, with close monitoring of renal function, in patients with mild to moderate renal impairment and are contraindicated in severe renal impairment.

8. **Answer: d**
   RATIONALE: Renal insufficiency may increase risks of adverse effects with antidiabetic drugs, and treatment with thiazide diuretics, corticosteroids, estrogens, and other drugs may cause hyperglycemia, thereby increasing dosage requirements for antidiabetic drugs.

9. **Answer: c**
   RATIONALE: Type 2 diabetes is being increasingly identified in children. This trend is attributed mainly to obesity and inadequate exercise, because most children with type 2 are seriously overweight and have poor eating habits.

10. **Answer: a, c, and e**
    RATIONALE: In young children, hypoglycemia may be manifested by changes in behavior, including severe hunger, irritability, and lethargy. In addition, mental functioning may be impaired in all age groups, even with mild hypoglycemia. Anytime hypoglycemia is suspected, blood glucose should be tested.

11. **Answer: b**
    RATIONALE: Recognition of hypoglycemia may be delayed because signs and symptoms are vague and the children may be unable to communicate them to parents or caregivers. Because of these difficulties, most pediatric diabetologists recommend maintaining blood glucose levels between 100 and 200 mg/dL to prevent hypoglycemia. In addition, the bedtime snack and blood glucose measurement should never be skipped.

12. Answer: c
RATIONALE: When drawing up both regular and NPH insulin, the regular insulin is drawn up first and then the NPH. Remember: clear to cloudy.

13. Answer: d
RATIONALE: Administration of insulin for infants and toddlers who weigh less than 10 kg or require less than 5 units of insulin per day can be difficult because small doses are hard to measure in a U-100 syringe. Use of diluted insulin allows more accurate administration. The most common dilution strength is U-10 (10 units/mL), and a diluent is available from insulin manufacturers for this purpose. Vials of diluted insulin should be clearly labeled and should be discarded after 1 month.

14. Answer: a
RATIONALE: During illness, children are highly susceptible to dehydration, and an adequate fluid intake is very important. Many clinicians recommend sugar-containing liquids (e.g., regular sodas, clear juices, regular gelatin desserts) if blood glucose values are lower than 250 mg/dL. If blood glucose values are above 250 mg/dL, diet soda, unsweetened tea, and other fluids without sugar should be given.

15. Answer: b
RATIONALE: Corticosteroids increase insulin needs so the patient may develop hyperglycemia.

16. Answer: b
RATIONALE: Patients who take acarbose should take the medication with the first bite of each main meal to prevent bloating and diarrhea.

17. Answer: c
RATIONALE: Patients who take pramlintide should not be injected into the same site where insulin is administered.

18. Answer: c
RATIONALE: Studies indicate that insulin is absorbed fastest from the abdomen, followed by the deltoid, thigh, and hip.

19. Answer: b
RATIONALE: With regular insulin before meals, it is very important that the medication be injected 30 to 45 minutes before meals so that the insulin will be available when blood sugar increases after the meal.

20. Answer: c
RATIONALE: BIDS stands for bedtime insulin plus daytime sulfonylurea.

CHAPTER 40

SECTION I: ASSESSING YOUR UNDERSTANDING

Activity A   FILL IN THE BLANKS

1. thyroxine
2. iodine, tyrosine
3. cellular metabolism
4. Primary hypothyroidism

5. Congenital hypothyroidism

Activity B   MATCHING
1. a   2. d   3. e   4. b   5. c

Activity C   SHORT ANSWERS

1. Hyperthyroidism is characterized by excessive secretion of thyroid hormone and usually involves an enlarged thyroid gland that has an increased number of cells and an increased rate of secretion. It may be associated with Graves' disease, nodular goiter, thyroiditis, overtreatment with thyroid drugs, functioning thyroid carcinoma, or a pituitary adenoma that secretes excessive amounts of TSH. The hyperplastic thyroid gland may secrete 5 to 15 times the normal amount of thyroid hormone. As a result, body metabolism is greatly increased.

2. Thyroid storm or thyrotoxic crisis is a rare but severe complication characterized by extreme symptoms of hyperthyroidism, such as severe tachycardia, fever, dehydration, heart failure, and coma. It is most likely to occur in patients with hyperthyroidism that has been inadequately treated, especially when stressful situations occur (e.g., trauma, infection, surgery, emotional upset).

3. Thyroid drugs such as the synthetic drug levothyroxine provide an exogenous source of thyroid hormone. Antithyroid drugs act by decreasing production or release of thyroid hormones. The thioamide drugs inhibit synthesis of thyroid hormone. Iodine preparations inhibit the release of thyroid hormones and cause them to be stored within the thyroid gland. Radioactive iodine emits rays that destroy the thyroid gland tissue.

4. Thyroid drugs are indicated for primary or secondary hypothyroidism, cretinism, and myxedema. Antithyroid drugs may be necessary for hyperthyroidism associated with Graves' disease, nodular goiter, thyroiditis, overtreatment with thyroid drugs, functioning thyroid carcinoma, or a pituitary adenoma that secretes excessive amounts of TSH. Antithyroid drugs may also be indicated for thyroid storm.

5. Iodine preparations and thioamide antithyroid drugs are contraindicated in pregnancy, because they can lead to goiter and hypothyroidism in the fetus or newborn. Radioactive iodine is contraindicated during lactation as well. Because radioactive iodine may cause cancer and chromosome damage in children, it should be used only for hyperthyroidism that cannot be controlled by other drugs or surgery.

SECTION II: APPLYING YOUR KNOWLEDGE

Activity D   CASE STUDIES

Case Study 1

1. Subclinical hypothyroidism involves a mildly elevated serum TSH and normal serum thyroxine levels.
2. Thyroid replacement therapy in the patient with hypothyroidism is lifelong; no clear-cut guidelines

exist regarding duration of antithyroid drug therapy because of exacerbations and remissions. Replacement therapy usually continues until the patient has been euthyroid for 6 to 12 months.

Case Study 2

1. Subclinical hyperthyroidism is defined as a reduced TSH level (less than 0.1 microunit/L) and normal T_3 and T_4 levels.

2. The most common cause of hyperthyroidism is excess thyroid hormone therapy. Subclinical hyperthyroidism is a risk factor for osteoporosis in postmenopausal women who do not take estrogen replacement therapy, because it leads to reduced bone mineral density. Subclinical hyperthyroidism also greatly increases the risk for atrial fibrillation in patients older than 60 years of age.

SECTION III: PRACTICING FOR NCLEX

Activity E

1. **Answer: a**
   RATIONALE: The FDA has issued a black box warning regarding the use of thyroid hormones for the treatment of obesity or for weight loss, either alone or with other therapeutic agents. Significant and serious complications may develop in euthyroid people taking thyroid hormones.

2. **Answer: c**
   RATIONALE: People with hypothyroidism are especially likely to experience respiratory depression and myxedema coma with opioid analgesics and other sedating drugs.

3. **Answer: b**
   RATIONALE: For congenital hypothyroidism (cretinism), drug therapy should be started within 6 weeks after birth.

4. **Answer: d**
   RATIONALE: For congenital hypothyroidism (cretinism), drug therapy should be started within 6 weeks of birth and continued for life, or mental retardation may result.

5. **Answer: a**
   RATIONALE: Thyroid replacement therapy in the patient with hypothyroidism is lifelong; no clear-cut guidelines exist regarding duration of antithyroid drug therapy because of exacerbations and remissions. Replacement therapy usually continues until the patient has been euthyroid for 6 to 12 months.

6. **Answer: b, c, and d**
   RATIONALE: Symptoms that support a diagnosis of congenital hypothyroidism include subnormal temperature, low heart rate, feeding difficulties, lethargy, and constipation.

7. **Answer: a**
   RATIONALE: Patients who are taking antithyroid drugs should be monitored closely for hypothyroidism, which usually develops within 1 year after starting treatment for hyperthyroidism.

8. **Answer: a, c, and e**
   RATIONALE: Symptoms of myxedema coma include coma, hypothermia, cardiovascular collapse, hypoventilation, hypoglycemia, and lactic acidosis.

9. **Answer: a, b, and d**
   RATIONALE: The home care nurse may be involved in a wide range of activities, including assessing the patient's response to therapy, teaching about the disease process, managing of symptoms, and preventing and managing adverse drug effects. The nurse would not modify medications without a physician's order or provide information about weight loss especially if the patient has hyperthyroidism.

10. **Answer: b**
    RATIONALE: People in thyroid storm or thyrotoxic crisis are commonly managed in the critical care unit. Increased rates of cellular metabolism and oxygen consumption occur, with a resultant increase in heat production. The hypermetabolic state increases the metabolism of medications, so increased or more frequent dosing may be necessary.

11. **Answer: c**
    RATIONALE: Drug metabolism in the liver is delayed in patients with hypothyroidism and liver disease, so most drugs given to these patients have a prolonged effect.

12. **Answer: a**
    RATIONALE: Vital signs would be the most important assessment because cardiac difficulties may occur early in treatment for hypothyroidism.

13. **Answer: a**
    RATIONALE: For hypothyroidism, levothyroxine is given. Thyroid hormone replacement increases the workload of the heart and may cause serious adverse effects in older adults, especially those with cardiovascular disease.

14. **Answer: a, b, and e**
    RATIONALE: For hyperthyroidism, PTU or methimazole is used. Potential risks for adverse effects are similar to those in adults. Radioactive iodine may cause cancer and chromosome damage in children; therefore, this agent should be used only for hyperthyroidism that cannot be controlled by other antithyroid drugs or surgery. It also may lead to the development of hypothyroidism.

15. **Answer: d**
    RATIONALE: Treatment of hyperthyroidism changes the rate of body metabolism, including the rate of metabolism of many drugs. In the hyperthyroid state, drug metabolism may be very rapid, and higher doses of most drugs may be necessary to achieve therapeutic results. When the patient becomes euthyroid, the rate of drug metabolism is decreased. Consequently, doses of all medications should be evaluated and probably reduced to avoid severe adverse effects.

16. Answer: b
RATIONALE: Diagnostic tests to evaluate thyroid function or a trial withdrawal may be implemented to determine whether the patient is likely to remain euthyroid without further drug therapy. If a drug is to be discontinued, this is usually done gradually over weeks or months.

17. Answer: c
RATIONALE: When hypothyroidism and adrenal insufficiency coexist, the adrenal insufficiency should be treated with a corticosteroid drug before starting thyroid replacement. Thyroid hormones increase tissue metabolism and tissue demands for adrenocortical hormones. If adrenal insufficiency is not treated first, administration of thyroid hormone may cause acute adrenocortical insufficiency, a life-threatening condition.

18. Answer: c
RATIONALE: Levothyroxine should be held if the patient's heart rate is over 100 beats per minute.

19. Answer: b, d, and e
RATIONALE: Adverse effects of levothyroxine include irritability, fever, weight loss, insomnia, and intolerance to heat.

20. Answer: c
RATIONALE: Sodium iodide[131] I is used in the diagnosis of thyroid disease and also in the treatment of hyperthyroidism.

CHAPTER 41

SECTION I: ASSESSING YOUR UNDERSTANDING

Activity A FILL IN THE BLANKS

1. homeostasis
2. hypophyseal
3. hypothalamus
4. target tissues
5. nerve

Activity B MATCHING

1. e   **2.** c   **3.** a   **4.** b   **5.** c

Activity C SHORT ANSWERS

1. FSH, one of the gonadotropins, stimulates functions of sex glands. FSH is produced by the anterior pituitary gland of both sexes, beginning at puberty. It acts on the ovaries in a cyclical fashion during the reproductive years, stimulating growth of ovarian follicles. These follicles then produce estrogen, which prepares the endometrium for implantation of a fertilized ovum. FSH acts on the testes to stimulate the production and growth of sperm (spermatogenesis), but it does not stimulate secretion of male sex hormones.
2. LH (also called interstitial cell–stimulating hormone) is another gonadotropin that stimulates hormone production by the gonads of both sexes. In women, LH is important in the maturation and rupture of the ovarian follicle (ovulation). After ovulation, LH acts on the cells of the collapsed follicular sac to produce the corpus luteum, which then produces progesterone during the last half of the menstrual cycle. When blood progesterone levels rise, a negative feedback effect is exerted on hypothalamic and anterior pituitary secretion of gonadotropins. Decreased pituitary secretion of LH causes the corpus luteum to die and stop producing progesterone. Lack of progesterone causes slough and discharge of the endometrial lining as menstrual flow. (Of course, if the ovum has been fertilized and attached to the endometrium, menstruation does not occur.) In men, LH stimulates the Leydig's cells in the spaces between the seminiferous tubules to secrete androgens, mainly testosterone.
3. Prolactin plays a part in milk production by nursing mothers. It is not usually secreted in nonpregnant women because of the hypothalamic hormone PIF. During late pregnancy and lactation, various stimuli, including suckling, inhibit the production of PIF, allowing prolactin to be synthesized and released.
4. Melanocyte-stimulating hormone (MSH) plays a role in skin pigmentation and has recently been found to play important roles in feeding and energy metabolism as well as in inflammation. Recently, MSH, particularly gamma-MSH, has been linked to cardiovascular regulation and sodium metabolism.
5. Oxytocin functions in childbirth and lactation. It initiates uterine contractions at the end of gestation to induce childbirth, and it causes milk to move from breast glands to nipples so the infant can obtain the milk by suckling.

SECTION II: APPLYING YOUR KNOWLEDGE

Activity D CASE STUDY

1. The drugs goserelin (Zoladex), histrelin (Vantas), leuprolide (Lupron), nafarelin (Synarel), and triptorelin (Trelstar) are equivalent to GnRH. After initial stimulation of LH and FSH secretion, chronic administration of therapeutic doses inhibits gonadotropin secretion.
2. After initial stimulation of LH and FSH secretion, chronic administration of therapeutic doses inhibits gonadotropin secretion. This action results in decreased production of testosterone and estrogen, which is reversible when administration is stopped.
3. These GnRH equivalents cannot be given orally, because they would be destroyed by enzymes in the GI tract. Goserelin (Zoladex), histrelin (Vantas), leuprolide (Lupron), nafarelin (Synarel), and triptorelin (Trelstar) are given by injection and are available in depot preparations that can be given once monthly or less often.
4. Adverse effects of Lupron are basically those of testosterone or estrogen deficiency. When given for prostate cancer, the drug may cause increased bone pain and increased difficulty in urinating during the first few weeks of treatment.

SECTION III: PRACTICING FOR NCLEX

Activity E

1. Answer: b
RATIONALE: Somatropin is used in a child with chronic renal insufficiency prior to a renal transplant.

2. Answer: b
RATIONALE: The nurse needs to be alert for signs of hyponatremia, which include diminished mental status. Decrease in urine output, decrease in thirst, and increase in urine specific gravity are all therapeutic effects.

3. Answer: c and d
RATIONALE: Conditions resulting from excessive amounts of pituitary hormones (hyperpituitarism) are most often treated with surgery or radiation.

4. Answer: a
RATIONALE: Dosage of all pituitary hormones must be individualized, because the responsiveness of affected tissues varies.

5. Answer: c
RATIONALE: Middle-aged and older adults who use GH for treatment of a growth hormone deficiency are at high risk for the development of hyperglycemia.

6. Answer: a
RATIONALE: There is concern about a possible link between GH, which stimulates tumor growth, and cancer. GH stimulates the release of IGF-1 (also called somatomedin), a substance that circulates in the blood and stimulates cell division. Most tumor cells have receptors that recognize IGF-1, bind it, and allow it to enter the cell, where it could trigger uncontrolled cell division. This concern may be greater for middle-aged and older adults, because malignancies are more common in these groups than in adolescents and young adults.

7. Answer: a, b, and d
RATIONALE: Caution is used when administering somatropin to patients with Turner's syndrome, obesity, and a family history of diabetes mellitus because these patients have increased insulin sensitivity.

8. Answer: d
RATIONALE: Oxytocin (Pitocin) is a synthetic drug that exerts the same physiologic effects as the posterior pituitary hormone. It promotes uterine contractility and is used clinically to induce labor and in the postpartum period to control bleeding. Oxytocin must be used only when clearly indicated and when the recipient can be supervised by well-trained personnel, as in a hospital.

9. Answer: b
RATIONALE: Desmopressin is contraindicated in patients with a history of cardiovascular disorders because a *black box warning* stipulates that changes in fluid volume status may result in cardiac arrest in patients with known cardiovascular disease.

10. Answer: c
RATIONALE: Desmopressin (DDAVP, Stimate) and vasopressin (Pitressin) are synthetic equivalents of ADH. A major clinical use is the treatment of neurogenic diabetes insipidus, a disorder characterized by a deficiency of ADH and the excretion of large amounts of dilute urine.

11. Answer: a
RATIONALE: Pegvisomant (Somavert) is a GH receptor antagonist used in the treatment of acromegaly in adults who are unable to tolerate or are resistant to other management strategies. The drug selectively binds to GH receptors, blocking the binding of endogenous GH. In general, dosage should be individualized according to response. Dosage reduction of hypoglycemic agents may be required, because the drug may increase glucose tolerance.

12. Answer: b, c, and d
RATIONALE: The most common adverse effect associated with leuprolide acetate are pain at the injection site. Other adverse effects include vasodilation, labile emotions, acne, and rash. The drug is used to treat enlargement of the genitals.

13. Answer: b and d
RATIONALE: Octreotide (Sandostatin) has pharmacologic actions similar to those of somatostatin. Indications for use include acromegaly, in which the drug reduces blood levels of GH and insulin-like growth factor-1 (IGF-1); carcinoid tumors, in which it inhibits diarrhea and flushing; and vasoactive intestinal peptide tumors, in which it relieves diarrhea (by decreasing GI secretions and motility). It is also used to treat diarrhea in acquired immunodeficiency syndrome (AIDS) and other conditions.

14. Answer: c
RATIONALE: Growth hormone is only indicated for use in older adults who have had their pituitary gland removed.

15. Answer: a, c, and d
RATIONALE: Prior to beginning therapy for the treatment of diabetes insipidus, the nurse should obtain the patient's weight, urine specific gravity, and the ratio of the patient's intake to output. The patient's BMI and renal function tests are not necessary.

16. Answer: c
RATIONALE: Desmopressin is also used in the treatment of nocturnal enuresis in children.

17. Answer: a and c
RATIONALE: The patient taking octreotide will need ongoing blood glucose monitoring and follow-up ultrasounds of the gallbladder to monitor for gallstones.

18. Answer: a
RATIONALE: GH is often considered an insulin antagonist because it suppresses the abilities of insulin to stimulate uptake of glucose in peripheral tissues and enhance glucose synthesis in the liver. Paradoxically, administration of GH produces hyperinsulinemia by stimulating insulin secretion.

19. Answer: b

RATIONALE: Somatropin is not used in patients with growth impairment who have closure of the epiphyseal plates.

20. Answer: b

RATIONALE: Alcohol decreases the diuretic effect of desmopressin.

CHAPTER 42

SECTION I: ASSESSING YOUR UNDERSTANDING

Activity A FILL IN THE BLANKS

1. parathyroid hormone (PTH)
2. PTH
3. hypoparathyroidism
4. hyperparathyroidism
5. hypocalcemia

Activity B MATCHING

1. e   2. b   3. a   4. c   5. d

Activity C SHORT ANSWERS

1. PTH secretion is stimulated by low serum calcium levels and inhibited by normal or high levels (a negative feedback system). Because phosphate is closely related to calcium in body functions, PTH also regulates phosphate metabolism. In general, when serum calcium levels increase, serum phosphate levels decrease, and vice versa. Thus, an inverse relationship exists between calcium and phosphate.

2. When the serum calcium level falls below the normal range, PTH raises the level by acting on bone, intestines, and kidneys. In bone, breakdown is increased, so that calcium moves from bone into the serum. In the intestines, there is increased absorption of calcium ingested in food (PTH activates vitamin D, which increases intestinal absorption). In the kidneys, there is increased reabsorption of calcium in the renal tubules and less urinary excretion. The opposite effects occur with phosphate (e.g., PTH decreases serum phosphate and increases urinary phosphate excretion).

3. Hyperparathyroidism is most often caused by a tumor or hyperplasia of a parathyroid gland. It also may result from ectopic secretion of PTH by malignant tumors (e.g., carcinomas of the lung, pancreas, kidney, ovary, prostate gland, or bladder). Clinical manifestations and treatment of hypoparathyroidism are the same as those of hypocalcemia. Clinical manifestations and treatment of hyperparathyroidism are the same as those of hypercalcemia.

4. Calcitonin is a hormone from the thyroid gland whose secretion is controlled by the concentration of ionized calcium in the blood flowing through the thyroid gland. When the serum level of ionized calcium is increased, secretion of calcitonin is increased. The function of calcitonin is to lower serum calcium in the presence of hypercalcemia, which it does by decreasing movement of calcium from bone to serum and increasing urinary excretion of calcium. The action of calcitonin is rapid but of short duration. Therefore, this hormone has little effect on long-term calcium metabolism.

5. Vitamin D (*calciferol*) is a fat-soluble vitamin that includes both ergocalciferol (obtained from foods) and cholecalciferol (formed by exposure of skin to sunlight). It functions as a hormone and plays an important role in calcium and bone metabolism. The main action of vitamin D is to raise serum calcium levels by increasing intestinal absorption of calcium and mobilizing calcium from bone. It also promotes bone formation by providing adequate serum concentrations of minerals. Vitamin D is not physiologically active in the body. It must be converted to an intermediate metabolite in the liver and then to an active metabolite (1,25-dihydroxyvitamin D or calcitriol) in the kidneys. PTH and adequate hepatic and renal function are required to produce the active metabolite.

SECTION II: APPLYING YOUR KNOWLEDGE

Activity D CASE STUDY

1. Osteoporosis results when bone strength (bone density and bone quality) is impaired, leading to increased porousness and vulnerability to fracture.

2. Hormonal deficiencies, some diseases, and some medications (e.g., glucocorticoids) can also increase resorption, resulting in loss of bone mass and osteoporosis.

3. Bone tissue is constantly being formed and broken down in a process called *remodeling*. During childhood, adolescence, and early adulthood, formation usually exceeds breakdown (resorption) as the person attains adult height and peak bone mass. After approximately 35 years of age, resorption is greater than formation.

4. Alendronate (Fosamax), ibandronate (Boniva), pamidronate (Aredia), risedronate (Actonel), and zoledronate (Zometa) are drugs that bind to bone and inhibit calcium resorption from bone. Bisphosphonates are poorly absorbed from the intestinal tract. Bisphosphonates must be taken on an empty stomach, with water, at least 30 minutes before any other fluid, food, or medication. The drugs are not metabolized. The drug bound to bone is slowly released into the bloodstream. Most of the drug that is not bound to bone is excreted in the urine.

SECTION III: PRACTICING FOR NCLEX

Activity E

1. Answer: a

RATIONALE: For men, corticosteroids decrease testosterone levels by approximately one half, and replacement therapy may be needed.

2. **Answer: b**
RATIONALE: Both men and women who take corticosteroids are at risk for osteoporosis.

3. **Answer: d**
RATIONALE: Postmenopausal women are at high risk for osteoporosis.

4. **Answer: a, c, and d**
RATIONALE: Calcium deficiency commonly occurs in the elderly because of long-term dietary deficiencies of calcium and vitamin D, impaired absorption of calcium from the intestine, lack of exposure to sunlight, and impaired liver or kidney metabolism of vitamin D to its active form. It is not connected to sodium intake.

5. **Answer: b**
RATIONALE: Hypomagnesemia must be corrected before the hypocalcemia can be corrected.

6. **Answer: a, d, and e**
RATIONALE: Excess amounts of vitamin D may cause headache, somnolence, weakness, irritability, hypertension, cardiac dysrhythmias, kidney stones, polydipsia, polyuria, and bone and muscle pain.

7. **Answer: d**
RATIONALE: Deficiency of vitamin D causes inadequate absorption of calcium and phosphorus.

8. **Answer: a, c, and e**
RATIONALE: Hyperparathyroidism is most often caused by a tumor or hyperplasia of a parathyroid gland. It may also be caused by ectopic secretion of PTH caused by metastatic cancer in other glands or organs.

9. **Answer: a**
RATIONALE: Patients with renal impairment or failure often have disturbances in calcium and bone metabolism. If hypercalcemia develops in patients with severely impaired renal function, hemodialysis or peritoneal dialysis with calcium-free solution is effective and safe. Calcium acetate may be used to prevent or treat hyperphosphatemia. The calcium reduces blood levels of phosphate by reducing its absorption from foods.

10. **Answer: a, b, and c**
RATIONALE: Calcium deficiency commonly occurs because of long-term dietary deficiencies of calcium and vitamin D, impaired absorption of calcium from the intestine, lack of exposure to sunlight, and impaired liver or kidney metabolism of vitamin D to its active form. It is not associated with chronic use of ampicillin.

11. **Answer: d**
RATIONALE: Patients diagnosed with osteoporosis require adequate calcium and vitamin D (at least the recommended dietary allowance), whether obtained from the diet or from supplements. Calcium 600 mg and vitamin D 200 international units once or twice daily are often recommended for postmenopausal women with osteoporosis, and pharmacologic doses of vitamin D are sometimes used to treat patients with serious osteoporosis.

If such doses are used, caution should be exercised, because excessive amounts of vitamin D can cause hypercalcemia and hypercalciuria.

12. **Answer: c**
RATIONALE: Preventive measures are necessary for patients taking phenytoin (Dilantin) and phenobarbital, because these drugs may contribute to osteoporosis through their effects on calcium metabolism. These anticonvulsant medications increase hepatic metabolism of vitamin D, which leads to a decrease in calcium absorption in the intestine. Supplemental calcium and vitamin D as well as specific drugs for osteoporosis should be considered if bone density is low.

13. **Answer: a, c, and d**
RATIONALE: Preventive measures are necessary for patients on chronic corticosteroid therapy (e.g., prednisone 7.5 mg daily; equivalent amounts of other systemic drugs; high doses of inhaled drugs). For both men and women, most of the guidelines for prevention of osteoporosis apply (e.g., calcium supplements, regular exercise, a bisphosphonate drug). In addition, low doses and nonsystemic routes help prevent osteoporosis and other adverse effects. For men, corticosteroids decrease testosterone levels by approximately one half, and replacement therapy may be needed.

14. **Answer: b**
RATIONALE: Dairy products are high in phosphorus.

15. **Answer: d**
RATIONALE: Calcium levels at 12 mg/dL or above are considered medical emergencies, and rehydration must be started immediately.

16. **Answer: a and c**
RATIONALE: Calcium preparations and digoxin have similar effects on the myocardium. Therefore, if calcium is given to a patient taking digoxin, the risks of digitalis toxicity and cardiac dysrhythmias are increased. This combination must be used very cautiously. Oral calcium preparations decrease effects of oral tetracycline drugs by combining with the antibiotic and preventing its absorption. They should not be given at the same time or within 2 to 3 hours of each other. Pulmonary edema is not caused by the combination of calcium and digoxin.

17. **Answer: b, c, and e**
RATIONALE: Contraindications to calcium preparations include cancer with bone metastases, as well as ventricular fibrillation, hypercalcemia, hypophosphatemia, and renal calculi.

18. **Answer: a**
RATIONALE: Sodium chloride (0.9%) injection (normal saline) is an IV solution that contains water, sodium, and chloride. It is included here because it is the treatment of choice for hypercalcemia and is usually effective. The sodium contained in the solution inhibits the reabsorption of calcium in renal tubules and thereby increases urinary excretion of calcium.

19. Answer: d
RATIONALE: Phosphates should be given only when hypercalcemia is accompanied by hypophosphatemia (serum phosphorus less than 3 mg/dL) and renal function is normal, to minimize the risk of soft tissue calcification.

20. Answer: b, c, and e
RATIONALE: Calcium is used to decrease stomach acid and reduce heartburn. It also is used in the treatment of chronic nonemergent hypocalcemia. It decreases bone loss and assists in reducing fractures in women.

CHAPTER 43

SECTION I: ASSESSING YOUR UNDERSTANDING

Activity A FILL IN THE BLANKS
1. Corticosteroids
2. Exogenous
3. slows, stops
4. negative feedback mechanism
5. Corticosteroids

Activity B MATCHING
1. c   2. d   3. a   4. b   5. e

Activity C SHORT ANSWERS
1. Corticosteroid secretion is controlled by the hypothalamus, the anterior pituitary, and adrenal cortex (the hypothalamic–pituitary–adrenal, or HPA, axis). Various stimuli (e.g., low plasma levels of corticosteroids, pain, anxiety, trauma, illness, anesthesia) activate the system. These stimuli cause the hypothalamus of the brain to secrete corticotropin-releasing hormone or factor (CRH or CRF), which stimulates the anterior pituitary gland to secrete corticotropin, and corticotropin then stimulates the adrenal cortex to secrete corticosteroids.
2. The stress response activates the sympathetic nervous system (SNS) to produce more epinephrine and norepinephrine and the adrenal cortex to produce as much as 10 times the normal amount of cortisol. The synergistic interaction of these hormones increases the person's ability to respond to stress. However, the increased SNS activity continues to stimulate cortisol production (the main glucocorticoids secreted as part of the body's response to stress) and overrules the negative feedback mechanism. Excessive and prolonged corticosteroid secretion damages body tissues.
3. Glucocorticoids are important in metabolic, inflammatory, and immune processes. Glucocorticoids include cortisol, corticosterone, and cortisone. Cortisol accounts for at least 95% of glucocorticoid activity; corticosterone and cortisone account for a small amount of activity. Glucocorticoids are secreted cyclically, with the largest amount being produced in the early morning and the smallest

amount during the evening hours (in people with a normal day–night schedule). At the cellular level, glucocorticoids account for most of the characteristics and physiologic effects of the corticosteroids.
4. Mineralocorticoids are a class of steroids that play a vital role in the maintenance of fluid and electrolyte balance through their influence on salt and water metabolism. Aldosterone is the main mineralocorticoid and is responsible for approximately 90% of mineralocorticoid activity.
5. The adrenal cortex secretes male (androgens) and female (estrogens and progesterone) sex hormones. Compared with the effect of hormones produced by the testes and ovaries, the adrenal sex hormones have an insignificant effect on normal body function. Adrenal androgens, secreted continuously in small quantities by both sexes, are responsible for most of the physiologic effects exerted by the adrenal sex hormones. They increase protein synthesis (anabolism), which increases the mass and strength of muscle and bone tissue; they affect development of male secondary sex characteristics; and they increase hair growth and libido in women.

SECTION II: APPLYING YOUR KNOWLEDGE

Activity D CASE STUDY
1. Systemic lupus erythematosus is a collagen disorder, as are scleroderma and periarteritis nodosa. Collagen is the basic structural protein of connective tissue, tendons, cartilage, and bone, and it is therefore present in almost all body tissues and organ systems. The collagen disorders are characterized by inflammation of various body tissues, particularly tendons, cartilage, and connective tissues. Signs and symptoms depend on which body tissues or organs are affected and the severity of the inflammatory process.
2. Dermatologic disorders that may be treated with systemic corticosteroids include acute contact dermatitis, erythema multiforme, herpes zoster (prophylaxis of postherpetic neuralgia), lichen planus, pemphigus, skin rashes caused by drugs, and toxic epidermal necrolysis.
3. The effectiveness of corticosteroids in neoplastic diseases, such as acute and chronic leukemias, Hodgkin's disease, other lymphomas, and multiple myelomas, probably stems from their ability to suppress lymphocytes and other lymphoid tissue.
4. Corticosteroids suppress cellular and humoral immune responses and help prevent rejection of transplanted tissue. Drug therapy is usually continued as long as the transplanted tissue is in place.
5. In patients with asthma, corticosteroids increase the number of beta-adrenergic receptors and increase or restore the responsiveness of beta receptors to beta-adrenergic bronchodilating drugs. In cases of asthma, COPD, and rhinitis, the drugs decrease mucus secretion and inflammation. In anaphylactic shock resulting from an

allergic reaction, corticosteroids may increase or restore cardiovascular responsiveness to adrenergic drugs.

SECTION III: PRACTICING FOR NCLEX

Activity E

1. Answer: d
RATIONALE: A black box warning has been issued by the FDA for people who are transferred from systemically active corticosteroids to flunisolide inhaler; deaths from adrenal insufficiency have been reported.

2. Answer: b and c
RATIONALE: Adverse effects of systemic corticosteroids may include infections, hypertension, glucose intolerance, obesity, cosmetic changes, bone loss, growth retardation in children, cataracts, pancreatitis, peptic ulcerations, and psychiatric disturbances.

3. Answer: b
RATIONALE: Strategies to minimize HPA suppression and risks of acute adrenal insufficiency include administering a systemic corticosteroid during high-stress situations in patients who are on long-term systemic therapy (i.e., are steroid dependent).

4. Answer: a
RATIONALE: Strategies to minimize HPA suppression and risks of acute adrenal insufficiency include giving short courses of systemic therapy for acute disorders.

5. Answer: c
RATIONALE: Strategies to minimize HPA suppression and risks of acute adrenal insufficiency include gradually tapering the dose of any systemic corticosteroid.

6. Answer: d
RATIONALE: Strategies to minimize HPA suppression and risks of acute adrenal insufficiency include using local rather than systemic therapy when possible, alone or in combination with low doses of systemic drugs.

7. Answer: d
RATIONALE: Mitotane is prescribed for patients who are diagnosed with inoperable adrenocortical carcinoma.

8. Answer: d
RATIONALE: Daily administration of corticosteroids and mineralocorticoids is required in cases of chronic adrenocortical insufficiency (Addison's disease).

9. Answer: c
RATIONALE: A patient who presents with the sudden development of unexplained severe hypoglycemia may have adrenal insufficiency.

10. Answer: a, b, and d
RATIONALE: The most frequently desired pharmacologic effects of exogenous corticosteroids are anti-inflammatory, immunosuppressive, antiallergic, and antistress effects.

11. Answer: a
RATIONALE: Because of potentially serious adverse effects, especially with oral drugs, it is extremely important that corticosteroids be used as prescribed. A major responsibility of home care nurses is to teach, demonstrate, supervise, monitor, or do whatever is needed to facilitate correct use.

12. Answer: b
RATIONALE: Corticosteroids improve survival and decrease the risk of respiratory failure with pneumocystosis, a common cause of death in patients with AIDS.

13. Answer: b
RATIONALE: Sepsis may be complicated by impaired corticosteroid production. There is sufficient evidence to support the idea that giving a long course of low-dose corticosteroids in patients with septic shock can improve survival without causing harm. However, overall, corticosteroids do not affect mortality.

14. Answer: d
RATIONALE: Although corticosteroids have been widely used, several well-controlled studies demonstrated that the drugs are not beneficial in early treatment or in prevention of adult respiratory distress syndrome (ARDS).

15. Answer: a
RATIONALE: Some studies support the use of IV methylprednisolone. So, if other medications do not produce adequate bronchodilation, it seems reasonable to try an IV corticosteroid during the first 72 hours of the illness. However, corticosteroid therapy increases the risks of pulmonary infection.

16. Answer: b
RATIONALE: In adrenal insufficiency, hypotension is a common symptom in critically ill patients, and hypotension caused by adrenal insufficiency may mimic either hypovolemic or septic shock. If adrenal insufficiency is the cause of the hypotension, administration of corticosteroids can eliminate the need for vasopressor drugs to maintain adequate tissue perfusion.

17. Answer: a
RATIONALE: A patient in addisonian crisis will display hypotension, nausea, vomiting, muscle weakness, and vascular collapse. The patient will also crave salt.

18. Answer: c
RATIONALE: A diagnosis of Addison's disease is confirmed by an ACTH stimulation test.

19. Answer: a, c, and d
RATIONALE: Corticosteroids are used for the same conditions in older adults as in younger ones. Older adults are especially likely to have conditions that are aggravated by the drugs (e.g., congestive heart failure, hypertension, diabetes mellitus, arthritis, osteoporosis, increased susceptibility to infection, concomitant drug therapy

that increases risks of gastrointestinal ulceration and bleeding). Consequently, risk–benefit ratios of systemic corticosteroid therapy should be carefully considered, especially for long-term therapy. Corticosteroids do not aggravate macular degeneration.

20. Answer: a, b, and c

RATIONALE: The nurse assesses the patient's blood pressure, blood glucose, and symptoms of sexual dysfunction as well as muscle strength and skin irritation, pruritus, GI symptoms, and headache.

CHAPTER 44

SECTION I: ASSESSING YOUR UNDERSTANDING

Activity A FILL IN THE BLANKS

1. Estrogen, progesterone
2. adipose tissue
3. reproductive, sexual
4. endogenous
5. Estradiol

Activity B MATCHING

1. d   **2.** a   **3.** e   **4.** c   **5.** b

Activity C SHORT ANSWERS

1. Estrogens are secreted in a monthly cycle called the menstrual cycle. During the first half of the cycle, before ovulation, estrogens are secreted in progressively larger amounts. During the second half of the cycle, estrogens and progesterone are secreted in increasing amounts until 2 to 3 days before the onset of menstruation. At that time, secretion of both hormones decreases abruptly. When the endometrial lining of the uterus loses its hormonal stimulation, it is discharged vaginally as menstrual flow.

2. In nonpregnant women, progesterone is secreted by the corpus luteum during the last half of the menstrual cycle, which occurs after ovulation. This hormone continues the changes in the endometrial lining of the uterus begun by estrogens during the first half of the menstrual cycle. These changes provide for implantation and nourishment of a fertilized ovum.

3. Progesterones decrease high-density lipoprotein (HDL) cholesterol and increase low-density lipoprotein (LDL) cholesterol, both of which increase the risk of cardiovascular disease.

4. The use of exogenous estrogen is contraindicated in conditions such as undiagnosed vaginal or uterine bleeding; fibroid tumors of the uterus; active liver disease, including liver cancer, impaired liver function; history of cerebrovascular disease, coronary artery disease, thrombophlebitis, hypertension, or conditions predisposing to these disease processes; and tobacco use. Women who smoke cigarettes have a greater risk of thromboembolic disorders if they take estrogen supplements, possibly because of increased platelet aggregation with estrogen ingestion and cigarette smoking. In addition, estrogen increases hepatic production of blood clotting factors and a family history of breast or reproductive system cancer.

5. Initially, the hypothalamus releases gonadotropin-releasing hormone (GnRH), which causes the anterior pituitary gland to produce FSH in the follicular phase of the cycle. FSH results in the maturing of ovarian follicles, which in turn produce estrogens. Increasing estrogen levels result in the continued maturation of the ovarian follicle and increasing growth of the endometrium. A negative feedback system responds to the increasing amounts of estrogen by decreasing the amount of FSH. At mid-cycle (typically day 14 of a 28-day menstrual cycle), the anterior pituitary gland releases LH, resulting in the rupture of the ovarian follicle and the development of the corpus luteum. This process is ovulation. The corpus luteum releases progesterone and estrogen, which causes the endometrial lining to continue to increase in thickness and vascularity. If fertilization of the ovum does not occur, the corpus luteum atrophies, resulting in the reduced production of estrogen and progesterone. As estrogen and progesterone levels continue to decrease, the endometrium begins to regress, causing menstruation, and the beginning of another menstrual cycle.

SECTION II: APPLYING YOUR KNOWLEDGE

Activity D CASE STUDY

1. This patient is experiencing symptoms of menopause that occurs as a result of a decrease in ovarian function, which is related to aging. There is a significant decrease in the production of estrogen, which leads to decreasing menstrual periods and symptoms such as hot flashes and vaginal dryness.

2. If the woman still has an intact uterus, hormone replacement therapy consists of an estrogen–progestin combination. If the woman is experiencing menopausal symptoms but has had a hysterectomy, then estrogen alone may be used.

3. Hormone replacement therapy is contraindicated in patients who have any history of cardiovascular disease, such as hypertension, or any history of breast, uterine, or ovarian cancers. It is used cautiously in patients who smoke.

4. The most common adverse effect is nausea and vomiting. The patient should also understand the signs and symptoms of cardiovascular complications since these must be treated promptly. Other adverse effects include weight gain and fluid retention, migraines or mental depression, ophthalmic disorders, skin conditions such as acne and hirsutism, and osteoporosis.

5. The latest research indicates that hormone replacement does not adequately prevent the occurrence of cardiovascular disease and may increase its incidence. HRT is recommended only

if the symptoms of menopause greatly impact the patient's standard of living and should be used for the shortest possible period of time.

SECTION III: PRACTICING FOR NCLEX
Activity E

1. **Answer: b**
   RATIONALE: Progestin use often results in inaccurate liver function and endocrine function tests.
2. **Answer: d**
   RATIONALE: To reduce the GI effects of medroxyprogesterone, this medication should be taken with food or at bedtime.
3. **Answer: a**
   RATIONALE: Patients who use transdermal estradiol should avoid prolonged sun exposure because the total amount of drug absorbed and the resulting plasma drug concentrations from transdermal estrogen can increase during exposure to heat.
4. **Answer: b**
   RATIONALE: Birth control pills are used for the treatment of menstrual orders such as dysfunctional uterine bleeding. It is contraindicated in patients with thrombophlebitis, breast lumps, and heart rhythm irregularities.
5. **Answer: c**
   RATIONALE: Estrogen is used cautiously in patients with renal disorder because of the adverse effect of fluid retention. Estrogen has also been associated with dilated kidneys especially in higher doses.
6. **Answer: a, c, and e**
   RATIONALE: Central nervous system adverse reactions such as migraine headache, dizziness, and mental depression may be caused or aggravated in some women who take estrogen.
7. **Answer: c and d**
   RATIONALE: Estrogen use has been associated with the development of breast and endometrial cancer.
8. **Answer: a and c**
   RATIONALE: Women who smoke cigarettes have a greater risk of thromboembolic disorders if they take estrogen supplements, possibly because of increased platelet aggregation with estrogen ingestion and cigarette smoking. In addition, estrogen increases hepatic production of blood clotting factors.
9. **Answer: b, c, and e**
   RATIONALE: Prior to the use of estrogen therapy, the nurse must know if the patient has any symptoms of cardiovascular disease such as heart attack or thrombophlebitis because estrogen use is contraindicated in these conditions. It is also contraindicated in pregnancy and is used with caution in a patient who has a family history of stroke.
10. **Answer: c**
    RATIONALE: Amenorrhea is the lack of menstruation so an indication that the estrogen has been effective is the occurrence of menstruation.

11. **Answer: a**
    RATIONALE: Patients who use progestins are at an increased risk for cardiovascular complications. This adverse effect is similar for both estrogens and progestins.
12. **Answer: b**
    RATIONALE: Medroxyprogesterone is associated with loss of bone density, which can lead to an increased incidence of bone breakage.
13. **Answer: b**
    RATIONALE: Combination estrogen–progestin use in patients with diabetes mellitus may cause an increase in blood glucose.
14. **Answer: a**
    RATIONALE: Triphasic oral contraceptives are used because they mimic normal variations of hormone secretions.
15. **Answer: d**
    RATIONALE: Antibiotics lessen the effectiveness of oral contraceptives so the patient should use alternative methods of birth control until the antibiotics are completed, and the patient begins a new cycle of oral contraceptives.
16. **Answer: b**
    RATIONALE: Depo-Provera is often used in teenagers because it is given by injection and provides effective birth control for 3 months from the first injection.
17. **Answer: b**
    RATIONALE: Vaginal estrogen is prescribed because it treats vaginal tissue with little systemic effects.
18. **Answer: a, d, and e**
    RATIONALE: The FDA has issued a black box warning that estrogens increase the risk of developing cancer of the uterus. The warning instructs women who take estrogens with or without progestins that there is an increased risk of dementia, myocardial infarctions, strokes, breast cancer, and blood clots.
19. **Answer: a**
    RATIONALE: The patient should be instructed to take medroxyprogesterone acetate for 5 days beginning on the 16th day of her cycle.
20. **Answer: c**
    RATIONALE: Decreasing estrogen causes a decrease in subcutaneous fat in the arms and the thighs.

CHAPTER 45

SECTION I: ASSESSING YOUR UNDERSTANDING
Activity A FILL IN THE BLANKS

1. Testosterone
2. Leydig cells
3. sexual, reproduction, metabolism
4. sperm
5. proteins

Activity B MATCHING

1. e   **2.** b   **3.** a   **4.** c   **5.** d

Activity C SHORT ANSWERS

1. Primary hypogonadism results from a testicular disorder. Common diseases that can cause primary hypogonadism are mumps, testicular inflammation, and trauma.

Secondary hypogonadism results from a problem in the hypothalamus or the pituitary gland, areas of the brain that signal the testicles to produce testosterone. A lack of production of gonadotropin-releasing hormone from the hypothalamus or a deficiency of follicle-stimulating hormone (FSH) and LH from the anterior pituitary may result from thyroid disorders, Cushing's syndrome, or estrogen-secreting tumors. Chronic diseases (e.g., metabolic syndrome, diabetes) can lead to secondary hypogonadism.

2. Causes may include drugs (antidepressants, antihypertensive agents, histamine receptor antagonists), lifestyle factors (alcohol, tobacco, or cocaine use), diseases (diabetes, thyroid conditions, prostate cancer, cardiovascular conditions, obesity), and spinal cord injuries.

3. ED and cardiovascular disease share many risk factors; the pathophysiology of both conditions is mediated through endothelial dysfunction. Cardiovascular disease enhances the risk of developing ED; conversely, ED is thought to be a powerful predictor of coronary artery disease, especially in men older than 60 years of age.

4. It is thought that BPH is a normal element of the male aging process. Causes include changes in hormone balance and cell growth. Testosterone undergoes reduction to form the more potent androgen DHT, which has greater affinity for androgen receptors than testosterone. During the formation and growth of an embryo, DHT plays a critical role in the formation of the male external genitalia, whereas in the adult, DHT acts as the primary androgen in the prostate and in hair follicles.

5. Pregnant caregivers, nurses, or pharmacists should not handle the crushed drug, which can be absorbed and harmful to a male fetus.

SECTION II: APPLYING YOUR KNOWLEDGE

Activity D CASE STUDY

1. The prostate undergoes two main growth periods, first in puberty, when the prostate doubles in size, and second in early adulthood, at about 25 years of age, when the gland begins another growth phase that often results years later in BPH. A surrounding layer of tissue limits overgrowth of the epithelial or glandular tissue of the prostate, causing the gland to put pressure against the urethra. In addition, the bladder wall becomes thicker and more easily irritated; it contracts even when it contains small amounts of urine, leading to more frequent urination. At some point, the bladder weakens and loses the capacity to empty, and urine is retained in the bladder. The narrowing of the urethra and partial emptying of the bladder cause many of the problems associated with BPH.

2. The 5-alpha reductase inhibitors and the alpha$_1$-adrenergic blockers are the two major drug classes used to treat BPH. Use of drugs from both classes in combination has demonstrated to be more effective than either drug class alone and is the gold standard for treatment of the symptoms associated with BPH. It may take 3 to 6 months before the patient notices the full therapeutic effect of the drugs.

3. The nurse assesses for improved urinary function with patient voiding insufficient amounts with no palpable bladder distention. Patients should report less urinary frequency, hesitancy, urgency, dribbling, nocturia, and an improved force of the urinary stream.

SECTION III: PRACTICING FOR NCLEX

Activity E

1. Answer: b, c, and e
   RATIONALE: The adverse effects of anabolic steroids include hypertension, jaundice, and liver disorders; aggression and other central nervous system disorders; testicular atrophy; and fluid retention.

2. Answer: c
   RATIONALE: The patient should take sildenafil approximately 20 to 60 minutes prior to an erection.

3. Answer: c
   RATIONALE: The patient should contact the doctor if priapism occurs or if the patient has an erection for longer than 4 hours. Lack of erection indicates the medication has not been effective, and flushing of the face and nasal congestion are adverse effects of the medication but would not require contacting the physician.

4. Answer: a
   RATIONALE: The physician will most likely order doxazosin, which works quickly, and the patient has therapeutic effects in 1 to 2 weeks.

5. Answer: b
   RATIONALE: Sildenafil is less effective if given with a high-fat meal. The meal of fried catfish and a baked potato with butter and sour cream has the highest concentration of fat.

6. Answer: a
   RATIONALE: Patients taking DHEA may display symptoms such as hirsutism, insomnia, irritability, and nervousness.

7. Answer: c
   RATIONALE: Testolactone is a derivative of progesterone and is used in the treatment of advanced breast cancer.

8. Answer: b
   RATIONALE: Testosterone therapy would be discontinued if the child demonstrated signs of precocious sexual puberty such as enlargement

of the penis. It would also be discontinued if the epiphyseal plate showed signs of early closure.

9. Answer: a, b, and d
RATIONALE: Signs of androgen deficiency include hypogonadism, cryptorchidism, impotence, and oligospermia.

10. Answer: a
RATIONALE: Older adults who receive testosterone should be evaluated for the development of benign prostatic hypertrophy.

11. Answer: b
RATIONALE: Approximately 50% of all men between the ages of 40 and 70 years complain of erectile dysfunction.

12. Answer: b
RATIONALE: Teenage patients who use testosterone often complain of acne. The best practice is for patients to practice frequent and thorough skin cleansing.

13. Answer: c
RATIONALE: Patients who take sildenafil should not take this medication with any beverage that includes alcohol. It increases the risk of orthostatic hypotension, tachycardia, dizziness, and headache.

14. Answer: b
RATIONALE: The physician should be notified if the patient is taking warfarin because warfarin increases the effect of tamsulosin and can increase the chances of orthostatic hypotension.

15. Answer: c
RATIONALE: Alprostadil is administered by self-injection into the penis or as a small pellet into the patient's urethra.

16. Answer: c
RATIONALE: Vardenafil is the only PDE5 inhibitor that prolongs the QT interval and should not be used with other drugs with similar effect, particularly class I and II antidysrhythmics.

17. Answer: c
RATIONALE: Tamsulosin is the prototype of the anti-BPH drugs and one of the drugs of choice in the treatment of BPH. Other drugs in the class are used to treat hypertension.

18. Answer: a, b, and d
RATIONALE: Patients taking finasteride may develop impotence, infertility, gynecomastia, reduced libido, and ejaculatory disorders, such as decreased volume of ejaculate.

19. Answer: c
RATIONALE: Finasteride in smaller doses is used to treat male pattern baldness under the name of Propecia.

20. Answer: b
RATIONALE: Testosterone replacement is available as an IM, transdermal, and topical gel. It is not available as an oral medication because it is metabolized too rapidly by the liver.

CHAPTER 46

SECTION I: ASSESSING YOUR UNDERSTANDING

Activity A FILL IN THE BLANKS

1. Cholinergic
2. acetylcholine
3. Myasthenia gravis
4. glutamatergic
5. cholinergic

Activity B MATCHING

1. b   **2.** e   **3.** c   **4.** d   **5.** a

Activity C SHORT ANSWERS

1. Cholinergic drugs stimulate the parasympathetic nervous system in the same manner as acetylcholine. Some drugs act directly to stimulate cholinergic receptors; others act indirectly by inhibiting the enzyme acetylcholinesterase, thereby slowing acetylcholine metabolism at autonomic nerve synapses.
2. In normal brain function, acetylcholine is an essential neurotransmitter and plays an important role in cognitive functions, including memory storage and retrieval.
3. Acetylcholine stimulates cholinergic receptors in the gut to promote normal secretory and motor activity. Cholinergic stimulation results in increased peristalsis and relaxation of the smooth muscle in sphincters to facilitate movement of flatus and feces. The secretory functions of the salivary and gastric glands are also stimulated.
4. Acetylcholine stimulates cholinergic receptors in the urinary system to promote normal urination. Cholinergic stimulation results in contraction of the detrusor muscle and relaxation of the urinary sphincter to facilitate emptying the urinary bladder.
5. Direct-acting cholinergic drugs are synthetic derivatives of choline. Most direct-acting cholinergic drugs are quaternary amines, carry a positive charge, and are lipid insoluble. Because they do not readily enter the central nervous system, their effects occur primarily in the periphery. Direct-acting cholinergic drugs are highly resistant to metabolism by acetylcholinesterase, the enzyme that normally metabolizes acetylcholine.

SECTION II: APPLYING YOUR KNOWLEDGE

Activity D CASE STUDY

1. Myasthenia gravis is an autoimmune disorder in which autoantibodies are thought to destroy nicotinic receptors for acetylcholine on skeletal muscle. As a result, acetylcholine is less able to stimulate muscle contraction, and muscle weakness occurs.
2. The anticholinesterase agents are used in the diagnosis and treatment of myasthenia gravis. Neostigmine (Prostigmin) is an anticholinesterase agent. Neostigmine, like bethanechol, is a quaternary

amine and carries a positive charge. This reduces its lipid solubility and results in poor absorption from the GI tract.

3. Oral doses of neostigmine are much larger than parenteral doses. When neostigmine is used for long-term treatment of myasthenia gravis, resistance to its action may occur and larger doses may be required.

SECTION III: PRACTICING FOR NCLEX

Activity E

1. **Answer: c and d**
   RATIONALE: Pralidoxime, a cholinesterase reactivator, is the specific treatment for neuromuscular blockade due to overdose with irreversible indirect cholinergic drugs.

2. **Answer: b**
   RATIONALE: Atropine will reverse muscarinic effects due to overdose of cholinergic drugs but will not reverse the nicotinic effects of skeletal-muscle weakness or paralysis due to overdose of indirect cholinergic drugs.

3. **Answer: a, c, and e**
   RATIONALE: Symptoms of myasthenia gravis, which vary in type and severity, may include a drooping of one or both eyelids (ptosis), blurred or double vision (diplopia) due to weakness of the muscles that control eye movements, unstable or waddling gait, a change in facial expression, difficulty in swallowing, shortness of breath, impaired speech (dysarthria), and weakness in the arms, hands, fingers, legs, and neck.

4. **Answer: c**
   RATIONALE: Indirect-acting cholinergic or anticholinesterase drugs are indicated to treat myasthenia gravis and Alzheimer's disease.

5. **Answer: b**
   RATIONALE: The direct-acting cholinergic drug, bethanechol, is used to treat urinary retention due to urinary bladder atony and postoperative abdominal distention due to paralytic ileus.

6. **Answer: c**
   RATIONALE: Indirect-acting cholinergic drugs also stimulate nicotinic receptors in skeletal muscles, resulting in improved skeletal muscle tone and strength.

7. **Answer: c**
   RATIONALE: A patient who is taking neostigmine and develops symptoms of respiratory depression is experiencing a cholinergic crisis.

8. **Answer: a**
   RATIONALE: The patient with myasthenia gravis may have diplopia or diminished muscle strength that makes it difficult to self-administer medications. Prepouring medications in an easy-to-open device facilitates medication administration.

9. **Answer: b**
   RATIONALE: The hepatic metabolism of neostigmine and pyridostigmine may be impaired by liver disease, resulting in increased adverse effects.

10. **Answer: d**
    RATIONALE: Cholinergic drugs are contraindicated in urinary or GI tract obstruction because they increase the contractility of smooth muscle in the urinary and GI systems and may result in injury to structures proximal to the obstruction.

11. **Answer: b**
    RATIONALE: A patient with benign prostatic hypertrophy may develop urinary retention, which is an adverse effect of neostigmine.

12. **Answer: d**
    RATIONALE: People with coronary artery disease should not take cholinergics because they can result in bradycardia, vasodilation, and hypotension.

13. **Answer: d**
    RATIONALE: Patients with hyperthyroidism should avoid cholinergic drugs. In the person with hyperthyroidism, the initial response to cholinergic medications (bradycardia and hypotension) triggers the baroreceptor reflex. As this reflex attempts to resolve the hypotension, norepinephrine is secreted from sympathetic nerves regulating the heart. Norepinephrine may trigger reflex tachycardia and other cardiac dysrhythmias.

14. **Answer: d**
    RATIONALE: Cholinergic drugs are contraindicated in people with asthma because they may cause bronchoconstriction and increased respiratory secretions.

15. **Answer: b**
    RATIONALE: Edrophonium is the drug that is used to help determine if a patient is experiencing a myasthenic or a cholinergic crisis.

16. **Answer: a, b, and e**
    RATIONALE: Direct-acting cholinergic drugs cause increased tone and contractility of smooth muscle (detrusor) in the urinary bladder and relaxation of the sphincter. This allows for increased emptying of the bladder.

17. **Answer: a**
    RATIONALE: In the case of a nerve gas attack, atropine is the antidote.

18. **Answer: d**
    RATIONALE: Patients who take memantine hydrochloride should not take sodium bicarbonate, which increases the serum level of memantine hydrochloride.

19. **Answer: a**
    RATIONALE: Indirect-acting cholinergic medications for Alzheimer's disease are widely distributed, including to the central nervous system. Thus, indirect-acting cholinergic drugs are able to improve cholinergic neurotransmission in the brain.

20. **Answer: b**
    RATIONALE: Neostigmine is used to treat myasthenia gravis, but it is also used to reverse the effects of tubocurarine that is used during surgery.

CHAPTER 47

SECTION I: ASSESSING YOUR UNDERSTANDING

Activity A FILL IN THE BLANKS

1. Parkinson's disease (also called parkinsonism)
2. increasing
3. increase
4. nicotinic
5. muscarinic

Activity B MATCHING

1. b   2. a   3. c   4. e   5. d

Activity C SHORT ANSWERS

1. The basal ganglia in the brain normally contain substantial amounts of the neurotransmitters dopamine and acetylcholine. The correct balance of dopamine and acetylcholine is important in regulating posture, muscle tone, and voluntary movement. People with Parkinson's disease have an imbalance in these neurotransmitters, resulting in a decrease in inhibitory brain dopamine and a relative increase in excitatory acetylcholine.
2. The first symptom of Parkinson's disease is often a resting tremor that begins in the fingers and thumb of one hand (pill-rolling movements); eventually it spreads over one side of the body and progresses to the contralateral limbs. Other common symptoms include slow movement (bradykinesia), inability to move (akinesia), rigid limbs, shuffling gait, stooped posture, mask-like facial expression, and a soft speaking voice. Less common symptoms may include depression, personality changes, loss of appetite, sleep disturbances, speech impairment, or sexual difficulty.
3. The U.S. Food and Drug Administration has issued a black box warning regarding an increased risk of suicidality in children and adolescents when treated with antidepressants including selegiline-transdermal.
4. Most anticholinergic medications are either tertiary amines or quaternary amines. Tertiary amines are uncharged, lipid-soluble molecules. Atropine and scopolamine are tertiary amines and therefore are able to cross cell membranes readily. They are well absorbed from the gastrointestinal (GI) tract and conjunctiva, and they cross the blood–brain barrier. Tertiary amines are excreted in the urine.
5. Some belladonna derivatives and synthetic anticholinergics are quaternary amines. These drugs carry a positive charge and are lipid insoluble. Consequently, they do not readily cross cell membranes. They are poorly absorbed from the GI tract and do not cross the blood–brain barrier. Quaternary amines are excreted largely in the feces.
6. Anticholinergic drugs cause decreased cardiovascular response to the parasympathetic (vagal) stimulation that slows heart rate. Atropine is the anticholinergic drug most often used for its cardiovascular effects. According to Advanced Cardiac Life Support (ACLS) protocol, atropine is the drug of choice to treat symptomatic sinus bradycardia. Low doses (less than 0.5 mg) may produce a slight and temporary decrease in heart rate; however, moderate to large doses (0.5–1 mg) increase heart rate by blocking parasympathetic vagal stimulation. Although the increase in heart rate may be therapeutic in bradycardia, it can be an adverse effect in patients with other types of heart disease, because atropine increases the myocardial oxygen demand. Atropine usually has little or no effect on blood pressure. Large doses cause facial flushing because of dilation of blood vessels in the neck.

SECTION II: APPLYING YOUR KNOWLEDGE

Activity D CASE STUDIES

Case Study 1

1. Rasagiline is the newest irreversible MAO inhibitor. It is indicated for initial treatment of idiopathic parkinsonism and, as an adjunct therapy with levodopa, to reduce "off time" when movements are poorly controlled.
2. Because rasagiline has not been determined to be selective for MAO-B in humans, care must be taken to avoid tyramine-containing foods.
3. Rasagiline has the potential to increase serotonin neurotransmission. When it is given with other drugs that enhance stimulation of serotonergic receptors (e.g., antidepressants, St. John's wort, dextromethorphan, and meperidine), serotonin syndrome, a potential fatal CNS toxicity reaction characterized by hyperpyrexia and death, can occur. Rasagiline should be discontinued at least 14 days before beginning treatment with most antidepressants or other MAO inhibitors. Fluoxetine should be discontinued at least 5 weeks before initiating rasagiline, because of its long half-life. Rasagiline is well absorbed orally, metabolized in the liver, and excreted primarily by the kidneys.

Case Study 2

1. An appropriate response is "Your medication will dilate your bronchi, which will help you to breathe better." Tiotropium bromide (Spiriva HandiHaler) is a long-acting, antimuscarinic and anticholinergic, quaternary ammonium compound that inhibits M3 receptors in smooth muscle, resulting in bronchodilation.
2. This statement indicates the need for more patient teaching. Tiotropium bromide (Spiriva HandiHaler) is a dry powder in capsule form intended for oral inhalation with the HandiHaler inhalation device. The capsule is to be used with the inhalation device only. Tiotropium bromide is not used in place of a rescue inhaler. It is indicated for daily maintenance treatment of bronchospasm associated with COPD.

It is not indicated for acute episodes of bronchospasm (i.e., rescue therapy).

3. The proper response should be "Your medication dose should not be modified; it is ordered once a day." Tiotropium bromide (Spiriva HandiHaler) is indicated for daily maintenance treatment of bronchospasm associated with COPD. The patient should be taught to follow the prescription.
4. The nurse would expect the physician to monitor the patient routinely for drug toxicity. Tiotropium is eliminated via the renal system, and patients with moderate to severe renal dysfunction should be carefully monitored for drug toxicity. No dosage adjustments are required for older patients or patients with hepatic impairment or mild renal impairment.

SECTION III: PRACTICING FOR NCLEX
Activity E

1. **Answer: a, c, d, and e**
   RATIONALE: Classic symptoms of Parkinson's disease include resting tremor, bradykinesia, rigidity, and postural instability.
2. **Answer: a**
   RATIONALE: The home care nurse can help patients and caregivers understand that the purpose of drug therapy for Parkinson's disease is to control symptoms and that noticeable improvement may not occur for several weeks.
3. **Answer: b**
   RATIONALE: Tolcapone therapy should not be initiated for any person with liver disease or elevated liver enzymes. Liver transaminase enzymes should be monitored frequently on the schedule described in the text.
4. **Answer: d**
   RATIONALE: With amantadine, excretion is primarily via the kidneys, and the drug should be used with caution in patients with renal failure.
5. **Answer: b**
   RATIONALE: Dosage of levodopa/carbidopa may need to be reduced because of an age-related decrease in peripheral AADC, the enzyme that carbidopa inhibits.
6. **Answer: a**
   RATIONALE: When centrally active anticholinergics are given for Parkinson's disease, agitation, mental confusion, hallucinations, and psychosis may occur.
7. **Answer: c**
   RATIONALE: The optimal dose is the lowest one that allows the patient to function adequately. Optimal dosage may not be established for 6 to 8 weeks with levodopa.
8. **Answer: b**
   RATIONALE: The levodopa/carbidopa combination is probably the most effective drug when bradykinesia and rigidity become prominent. However, because levodopa becomes less effective

after approximately 5 to 7 years, many clinicians use other drugs first and reserve levodopa for use when symptoms become more severe.

9. **Answer: d**
   RATIONALE: Pramipexole (Mirapex), ropinirole (Requip), and rotigotine-transdermal (Neupro) stimulate dopamine receptors in the brain. They are approved for both beginning and advanced stages of Parkinson's disease. In early stages, one of these drugs can be used alone to improve motor performance, improve ability to participate in usual activities of daily living, and delay levodopa therapy.
10. **Answer: a**
    RATIONALE: Levodopa is the most effective drug available for the treatment of Parkinson's disease. It relieves all major symptoms, especially bradykinesia and rigidity. Levodopa does not alter the underlying disease process, but it may improve a patient's quality of life.
11. **Answer: a, c, and d**
    RATIONALE: Anticholinergic overdose is characterized by hyperthermia, hot dry flushed skin, dry mouth, mydriasis, delirium, tachycardia, paralytic ileus, urinary retention, myoclonic movements, seizures, coma, and respiratory arrest.
12. **Answer: d**
    RATIONALE: Anticholinergic drugs are contraindicated for patients with BPH, myasthenia gravis, hyperthyroidism, narrow-angle glaucoma, tachydysrhythmias, myocardial infarction, heart failure, or conditions associated with esophageal reflux.
13. **Answer: b**
    RATIONALE: Anticholinergic drugs are given preoperatively to prevent anesthesia-associated complications such as bradycardia, excessive respiratory secretions, and hypotension.
14. **Answer: b**
    RATIONALE: Anticholinergic medications are indicated in the relief of central nervous system symptoms of Parkinson's disease or extrapyramidal symptoms associated with some antipsychotic drugs.
15. **Answer: a**
    RATIONALE: Ipratropium and tiotropium are anticholinergic medications given by inhalation for bronchodilation effects in the treatment of asthma and chronic bronchitis.
16. **Answer: c**
    RATIONALE: Anticholinergic drugs (e.g., dicyclomine, glycopyrrolate) are indicated for antispasmodic effects in GI disorders. Historically, they have also been used to treat peptic ulcer disease; however, they are weak inhibitors of gastric acid secretion and have been largely replaced other, more effective medications (e.g., proton pump inhibitors).
17. **Answer: d**
    RATIONALE: Anticholinergic drugs are commonly used in home care with children and adults. The home care nurse may need to teach older patients or caregivers that the drugs prevent sweating and

heat loss and increase risks of heat stroke if precautions to avoid overheating are not taken.

18. Answer: a
RATIONALE: Older adults are especially likely to have significant adverse reactions because of slowed drug metabolism and the frequent presence of several disease processes. A patient who complains of blurred vision may need help with ambulation, especially with stairs or in other potentially hazardous environments. Obstacles and hazards should be removed if possible.

19. Answer: d
RATIONALE: Normally, anticholinergics do not change intraocular pressure, but with narrow-angle glaucoma, they may increase intraocular pressure and precipitate an episode of acute glaucoma.

20. Answer: a
RATIONALE: In infections such as cystitis, urethritis, and prostatitis, anticholinergic drugs decrease the frequency and pain of urination. The drugs are also given to increase bladder capacity in enuresis, paraplegia, or neurogenic bladder.

CHAPTER 48

SECTION I: ASSESSING YOUR UNDERSTANDING

Activity A   FILL IN THE BLANKS

1. Pain
2. Opioid
3. Nociceptors
4. Nonopioid; nonopioids
5. black box warnings

Activity B   MATCHING

1. b   **2.** e   **3.** a   **4.** c   **5.** d

Activity C   SHORT ANSWERS

1. For a person to feel pain, the signal from the nociceptors in peripheral tissues must be transmitted to the spinal cord and then to the hypothalamus and cerebral cortex in the brain. The signal is carried to the spinal cord by two types of nerve cells, A-delta fibers and C fibers. A-delta fibers, which are myelinated and are found mainly in skin and muscle, transmit fast, sharp, well-localized pain signals. These fibers release glutamate and aspartate (excitatory amino acid neurotransmitters) at synapses in the spinal cord. C fibers, which are unmyelinated and are found in muscle, abdominal viscera, and periosteum, conduct the pain signal slowly and produce a poorly localized, dull, or burning type of pain. Tissue damage resulting from an acute injury often produces an initial sharp pain transmitted by A-delta fibers, followed by a dull ache or burning sensation transmitted by C fibers. C fibers release somatostatin and substance P at synapses in the spinal cord.

Glutamate, aspartate, substance P, and perhaps other chemical mediators enhance transmission of the pain signal.

2. Causes of tissue damage may be physical (e.g., heat, cold, pressure, stretch, spasm, ischemia) or chemical (e.g., pain-producing substances are released into the extracellular fluid surrounding the nerve fibers that carry the pain signal). These pain-producing substances activate pain receptors, increase the sensitivity of pain receptors, or stimulate the release of inflammatory substances.

3. Oral drugs undergo significant first-pass metabolism in the liver, which means that oral doses must be larger than injected doses to have equivalent therapeutic effects. The drugs are extensively metabolized in the liver, and metabolites are excreted in urine. Morphine and meperidine form pharmacologically active metabolites. Therefore, liver impairment can interfere with metabolism, and kidney impairment can interfere with excretion. Drug accumulation and increased adverse effects may occur if dosage is not reduced.

4. In the GI tract, opioids slow motility and may cause constipation and smooth muscle spasms in the bowel and biliary tract.

5. When opioids are used postoperatively, the goal is to relieve pain without excessive sedation, so that patients can do deep breathing exercises, cough, ambulate, and participate in other activities to promote recovery. Strong opioids are usually given parenterally for a few days. Then, oral opioids or nonopioid analgesics are given.

SECTION II: APPLYING YOUR KNOWLEDGE

Activity D   CASE STUDY

1. In severely burned patients, opioids should be used cautiously. A common cause of respiratory arrest in burned patients is excessive administration of analgesics. When opioids are necessary, they are usually given IV in small doses. Drugs given by other routes are absorbed erratically in the presence of shock and hypovolemia and may not relieve pain. In addition, unabsorbed drugs may be rapidly absorbed when circulation improves, with the potential for excessive dosage and toxic effects.

2. Agitation in a burned person may indicate hypoxia or hypovolemia rather than pain.

SECTION III: PRACTICING FOR NCLEX

Activity E

1. Answer: c
RATIONALE: Pain is a subjective experience. Stressors such as anxiety, depression, fatigue, anger, and fear tend to increase pain; rest, mood elevation, and diversionary activities tend to decrease pain. Pain is a complex physiologic, psychological, and sociocultural phenomenon that must be thoroughly assessed if it is to be managed effectively.

2. Answer: a
RATIONALE: With patients who are taking opioid analgesics for more than a few days, the nurse should assess periodically for drug tolerance and the need for higher doses or more frequent administration. Do not assume that increased requests for pain medication indicate inappropriate drug-seeking behavior associated with drug dependence.

3. Answer: b
RATIONALE: Because pain is a subjective experience and cannot be objectively measured, assessment of intensity or severity is based on the patient's description and the nurse's observations. Various scales have been developed to measure and quantify pain. These include verbal descriptor scales, in which the patient is asked to rate pain as mild, moderate, or severe; numeric scales, with 0 representing no pain and 10 representing severe pain; and visual analogue scales, in which the patient chooses the location indicating the level of pain on a continuum.

4. Answer: b
RATIONALE: The term referred pain is used when pain arising from tissue damage in one area of the body is felt in another area. Patterns of referred pain may be helpful in diagnosis. For example, pain of cardiac origin may radiate to the neck, shoulders, chest muscles, and down the arms, often on the left side. This type of pain usually results from myocardial ischemia due to atherosclerotic plaque in coronary arteries.

5. Answer: d
RATIONALE: The nurse must assess every patient in relation to pain, initially to determine appropriate interventions and later to determine whether the interventions were effective in preventing or relieving pain.

6. Answer: c
RATIONALE: When giving morphine to a child, it is most important for at least two licensed persons to perform independent calculations before administering the medication to the child.

7. Answer: a
RATIONALE: Breakthrough pain are periods of intense pain that occur while being treated for acute pain.

8. Answer: b, c, and d
RATIONALE: Morphine is not an appropriate treatment for chronic low back pain. Treatments for this condition include physical therapy and nonopioid medications.

9. Answer: c
RATIONALE: The most important assessment that the nurse can make prior to administration of an opioid is the respiratory rate because the most serious adverse complication of opioid use is respiratory depression.

10. Answer: b
RATIONALE: Nausea is a common side effect of morphine. Giving it with food helps to reduce the occurrence of the problem.

11. Answer: b, c, and e
RATIONALE: Constipation is a common problem that occurs with the use of opioids. The patient should be encouraged to eat a high-fiber diet, drink 2 to 3 quarts of water, take daily stool softener and laxative (if OK'd by physician), and establish a bowel routine.

12. Answer: c and d
RATIONALE: Signs of opioid withdrawal in a neonate include increased muscle tone, tachycardia, screaming, vomiting and diarrhea, and fever.

13. Answer: a, c, and d
RATIONALE: The nurse will notify the physician, administer naloxone, and prepare for endotracheal intubation. If the patient has an IV, the nurse would increase the rate. It is possible the nurse would insert a Foley catheter, but it is not a priority nursing intervention at this time. The priority interventions revolve around the patient's respiratory status.

14. Answer: c
RATIONALE: The patient should not receive morphine within 14 days of receiving an MOA inhibitor.

15. Answer: b, d, and e
RATIONALE: For patients who can't verbalize pain, the nurse assesses the patient's facial expression, limb movements, guarding, and grimacing.

16. Answer: a
RATIONALE: Naloxone is the drug of choice for opioid overdose.

17. Answer: d
RATIONALE: When opioids are needed, those with short half-lives (e.g., oxycodone, hydromorphone) are usedbecause they are less likely to accumulate.

18. Answer: a
RATIONALE: Expressions of pain may differ according to age and developmental level. Infants may cry and have muscular rigidity and thrashing behavior. Preschoolers may behave aggressively or complain verbally of discomfort. Young school-aged children may express pain verbally or behaviorally, often with regression to behaviors used at younger ages. Adolescents may be reluctant to admit they are uncomfortable or need help. With chronic pain, children of all ages tend to withdraw and regress to an earlier stage of development.

19. Answer: c
RATIONALE: Opioids administered during labor and delivery may depress fetal and neonatal respiration. The drugs cross the blood–brain barrier of the infant more readily than that of the mother. Therefore, doses that do not depress maternal respiration may profoundly depress the infant's respiration. Respiration should be monitored closely in neonates, and the opioid antagonist naloxone should be readily available.

20. **Answer: a**
    RATIONALE: Clonidine, an antihypertensive drug, is a nonopioid that may be used to treat opioid withdrawal. Clonidine reduces the release of norepinephrine in the brain and thus reduces symptoms associated with excessive stimulation of the sympathetic nervous system (e.g., anxiety, restlessness, insomnia). Blood pressure must be closely monitored during clonidine therapy.

CHAPTER 49

SECTION I: ASSESSING YOUR UNDERSTANDING

Activity A   FILL IN THE BLANKS

1. amide, ester
2. Spinal
3. epidural
4. Bier block
5. Topical

Activity B   MATCHING

1. c   2. e   3. b   4. a   5. d

Activity C   SHORT ANSWERS

1. The epidural route is also used to provide analgesia (often with a combination of a local anesthetic and an opioid) for patients with postoperative or other pain. When the combination is used, it is essential to reduce the dosage of the anesthetic and the opioid to avoid respiratory depression and other adverse effects.
2. The use of topical anesthetics is especially important in children, who are administered local anesthesia before suturing, insertion of an intravenous (IV) line, or vaccination administration.
3. Bier block anesthesia is regional limb anesthesia produced by a local anesthetic such as lidocaine and a pneumatic extremity tourniquet. The tourniquet prevents lidocaine and blood flow from the extremity from entering the general circulation.
4. Local anesthetic systemic toxicity (LAST) is the most severe and life-threatening effect associated with the use of lidocaine or any local anesthetic. LAST occurs when the local anesthetic is absorbed systemically, resulting in extreme central nervous system (CNS) excitation followed by cardiovascular excitation and cardiovascular collapse. Initial symptoms may include analgesia, circumoral numbness, metallic taste, tinnitus or auditory changes, and agitation. These may progress to seizure activity and then lead to symptoms of CNS depression, including coma, respiratory arrest, and cardiovascular depression.
5. Topical cocaine is an anesthetic administered to the ear, nose, or throat to produce adequate anesthesia and vasoconstriction of the mucous membranes. The drug has a rapid onset of action and reaches a peak in 5 minutes.

SECTION II: APPLYING YOUR KNOWLEDGE

Activity D   CASE STUDY

1. This cream-based mixture of lidocaine and prilocaine is applied to intact skin. The cream penetrates intact skin to provide local anesthesia and decrease pain of vaccinations and venipuncture.
2. With epidural anesthesia, the patient remains awake with no sensation to the point below the site of injection. It is used primarily for obstetrical procedures.
3. Symptoms of a hypersensitivity reaction include hives, redness, and a rash.

SECTION III: PRACTICING FOR NCLEX

Activity E

1. **Answer: b**
   RATIONALE: The nurse assesses for adverse effects, which include anxiety, tremors, and seizures.
2. **Answer: d**
   RATIONALE: Vital signs are monitored before, during, and after a procedure when local anesthetic is used.
3. **Answer: c**
   RATIONALE: The nurse keeps the patient NPO until the gag reflex returns to prevent aspiration.
4. **Answer: c**
   RATIONALE: Contraindications are sepsis or inflammation, meningitis, syphilis, increased abdominal pressure, and impaired cardiac function.
5. **Answer: a, c, and e**
   RATIONALE: Initial symptoms may include analgesia, circumoral numbness, metallic taste, tinnitus or auditory changes, and agitation.
6. **Answer: b**
   RATIONALE: Bronchospasm is more likely to occur when lidocaine is administered by the nebulizer route.
7. **Answer: a**
   RATIONALE: Epinephrine is used to prolong the effects of lidocaine.
8. **Answer: b**
   RATIONALE: Topical lidocaine is used to treat postherpetic neuralgia.
9. **Answer: d**
   RATIONALE: Sulfonamides and antihypertensive drugs may cause hypotension when procaine is administered.
10. **Answer: a, b, and d**
    RATIONALE: Benzocaine is used to treat minor burns, insect bites, hemorrhoid pain, and mouth pain.
11. **Answer: b**
    RATIONALE: The nurse must ensure that feeling and movement have returned to the patient's legs before allowing the patient to get out of the bed to prevent the patient from falling and becoming injured.

12. Answer: c
RATIONALE: The most appropriate nursing diagnosis is risk for impaired tissue perfusion related to the onset of LAST (local anesthetic systemic toxicity).

13. Answer: c
RATIONALE: Dibucaine is not absorbed systemically and is considered safe during pregnancy.

14. Answer: b
RATIONALE: The nurse will have IV lipid emulsion available to give a patient who develops severe symptoms of LAST such as cardiac collapse. This drug has been found to assist the patient.

15. Answer: d
RATIONALE: The patient understands the use of the Lido patch when he states that he will first remove the old patch, cleanse the skin, and then put on a new patch at the site that has the most pain.

16. Answer: c
RATIONALE: The patient should not eat or drink anything before feeling has returned to prevent injury to the oral tissues.

17. Answer: a
RATIONALE: EMLA cream must be applied 1 hour before the need for skin numbness, and it must be covered with an occlusive dressing.

18. Answer: b
RATIONALE: Compressed gas can be used to administer lidocaine. It is needle–free, and it provides a rapid loss of feeling to the skin.

19. Answer: a
RATIONALE: Prior to the application of a topical local anesthetic, the nurse must ensure that the area that the anesthetic will be applied to is intact to prevent systemic absorption of the medication.

20. Answer: b
RATIONALE: The nurse will notify the physician if the patient takes propranolol. Antidysrhythmic drugs, barbiturates, and darunavir will increase the effects of lidocaine.

CHAPTER 50

SECTION I: ASSESSING YOUR UNDERSTANDING

Activity A FILL IN THE BLANKS

1. General anesthesia
2. balanced anesthesia
3. induction
4. maintenance anesthesia
5. Emergence

Activity B MATCHING

1. c   2. a   3. d   4. e   5. b

Activity C SHORT ANSWERS

1. Balanced anesthesia refers to the following four elements of general anesthesia designed to work collectively to produce a superior outcome: amnesia, or memory loss (of limited duration in anesthesia); analgesia, or a reduction or absence of pain; hypnosis, or unconsciousness; and muscle relaxation, or immobility.

2. Adult patients usually receive a rapid-acting intravenous anesthetic medication. Pediatric patients more often breathe an inhalation anesthetic through a face mask. Called a mask induction, this allows an anesthesia provider or nurse to perform the venipuncture for intravenous solutions after the patient is under general anesthesia.

3. Isoflurane has a mild pungent or ethereal odor and can irritate the airways when concentration increases. Therefore, it does not lend itself to inhalation mask inductions.

4. Inhalation anesthetics such as isoflurane are associated with cardiovascular and respiratory depression. They can also cause airway irritation and progress to coughing, laryngospasm, or bronchospasm in susceptible patients such as smokers or asthmatics. In addition, inhalation anesthetics are known to cause vomiting, especially after two or more hours of exposure.

5. When an anesthesia provider administers propofol or similar medications for sedation, it is called *monitored anesthesia care*. During conscious or moderate sedation, the patient can be aroused with stimulation and maintains protective airway reflexes.

SECTION II: APPLYING YOUR KNOWLEDGE

Activity D CASE STUDY

1. A urine specimen is obtained in all women of childbearing age prior to surgery to check for pregnancy. If a woman is pregnant, surgery is canceled except for cesarean sections, because the medications used during surgery are teratogenic. Surgery is conducted only if the need for surgery outweighs the risk to the fetus.

2. The nurse anticipates that the patient will receive balanced anesthesia. Medications included are benzodiazepines, inhaled anesthetics, intravenous anesthetics, analgesics, and neuromuscular blocking agents.

3. Assess the patient's status in relation to the anesthesia administration and his or her surgical experience preoperatively.
   - Assess the patient's understanding of the perioperative process.
   - Assess the patient for comorbid conditions that increase the patient's risk related to anesthesia administration.
   - Assess the patient's health and surgical history, including allergies to medications, eggs or soy products, latex, or anesthesia-related products.
   - Interview the patient about the surgical experience and administration of anesthetics, including a family or patient history of malignant hyperthermia or atypical plasma cholinesterase.

- Assess medications, both prescription and over the counter, or complementary and alternative therapies taken in the last 2 weeks.
- Assess the time of the last fluid intake prior to surgery.
- Assess the time of the last meal and its contents.
- Assess medications taken the day of surgery.
- Implement preoperative assessments.
- Assess blood count, chemistry panel, coagulation profile, fasting blood sugar, glycated hemoglobin or HbA1c, electrocardiogram, chest x-ray, and pregnancy test (obtained depending on age, sex, and comorbidities).
- Assess baseline vital signs, level of consciousness, and orientation.
- Assess psychosocial status.
- Assess for pain using a pain scale.

SECTION III: PRACTICING FOR NCLEX

Activity E

1. **Answer: b, d, and e**
   RATIONALE: Medication categories that are a part of balanced anesthesia include benzodiazepines, inhaled and intravenous anesthetics, analgesics, and neuromuscular blocking agents.

2. **Answer: b**
   RATIONALE: Patients who smoke are at high risk for the development of bronchospasm after receiving isoflurane.

3. **Answer: a, c, and e**
   RATIONALE: The signs of malignant hyperthermia include tachycardia, elevated temperature, body rigidity, mixed metabolic and respiratory acidosis, mottling and sweating, masseter spasm (rigid jaw), hyperkalemia, elevated creatine kinase, myoglobinuria, and renal failure.

4. **Answer: c**
   RATIONALE: Patients who develop malignant hyperthermia will receive dantrolene sodium.

5. **Answer: b**
   RATIONALE: Patients who have had severe postoperative nausea and vomiting with previous surgeries may receive total intravenous anesthesia, which appears to cause less nausea than inhalation anesthetics.

6. **Answer: a**
   RATIONALE: Patients who receive both isoflurane and isoproterenol are more likely to develop cardiac dysrhythmias.

7. **Answer: b, c, d, and e**
   RATIONALE: Patients emerging from inhalation general anesthesia may develop hypotension and respiratory depression, shivering, and nausea and vomiting.

8. **Answer: c**
   RATIONALE: Children who receive sevoflurane by mask often emerge from anesthesia with agitation.

9. **Answer: d**
   RATIONALE: Propofol is the prototype drug for intravenous anesthesia.

10. **Answer: b**
    RATIONALE: Alcohol causes an increase in the effect of isoflurane so the patient will need to be monitored closely for delayed emergence from anesthesia.

11. **Answer: d**
    RATIONALE: Patients who receive propofol for a short surgery or diagnostic procedure usually recover from the anesthesia in approximately 10 minutes.

12. **Answer: a**
    RATIONALE: Propofol does not produce analgesia.

13. **Answer: a, b, and d**
    RATIONALE: Symptoms of propofol infusion syndrome are rhabdomyolysis, elevated CK and lactic acid levels, metabolic acidosis, and multiorgan failure.

14. **Answer: d**
    RATIONALE: Propofol is contraindicated in patients who are allergic to eggs.

15. **Answer: a**
    RATIONALE: Vecuronium is a neuromuscular blocking agent that causes paralysis of the muscles, so mechanical ventilation needs to be available for intubation.

16. **Answer: c**
    RATIONALE: Neostigmine reverses the effects of neuromuscular blocking agents so that the patient regains the muscles necessary for breathing on his own.

17. **Answer: d**
    RATIONALE: Patients at risk include those with liver and kidney disease, acid–base or electrolyte imbalance, hypothermia, critical illness, myopathic disorders, and neuromuscular diseases such as myasthenia gravis or myasthenic (Eaton-Lambert) syndrome. Also, elderly patients or those taking medications that may intensify or prolong the actions of neuromuscular blocking agents are at risk.

18. **Answer: a, b, and d**
    RATIONALE: Symptoms of recurarization include inability to sustain a head lift off the pillow for less than 5 seconds, difficulty taking a deep breath, a weak cough, difficulty swallowing, and double vision.

19. **Answer: a**
    RATIONALE: Midazolam is administered to reduce anxiety and to produce amnesia prior to surgery.

20. **Answer: b**
    RATIONALE: Fentanyl is an opioid analgesic, and the nurse will have naloxone on hand to reverse the effects of the opioid that is causing respiratory depression.

CHAPTER 51

SECTION I: ASSESSING YOUR UNDERSTANDING

Activity A FILL IN THE BLANKS

1. Cluster headaches
2. tension headaches
3. Migraine
4. aura
5. Menstrual

Activity B MATCHING

1. c   2. e   3. b   4. d   5. a

Activity C SHORT ANSWERS

1. Foods that precipitate migraine effects include aged cheeses, fermented foods, aspartame, monosodium glutamate, and chocolate.
2. Migraines demonstrate a familial pattern, and authorities believe that they are inherited as autosomal dominant traits with incomplete penetrance.
3. Cluster headaches are recurrent, severe, unilateral orbitotemporal headaches that are associated with histamine reactions. Migraine headaches are unilateral pain in the head that may or may not be accompanied by an aura.
4. An aura is a subjective sensation that immediately precedes the migraine headache consisting of a breeze, odor, or light.
5. Abortive therapy is the administration of medications to treat the symptoms of migraine headache. Preventive therapy is the administration of medications to prevent the development of a migraine headache.

SECTION II: APPLYING YOUR KNOWLEDGE

Activity D CASE STUDY

1. The current theory of chronic tension headache asserts that a person experiences a sensitization of the dorsal horn neurons related to increased nociceptive inputs from pericranial myofascial tissues. With a decreased pain threshold, the person misinterprets incoming signals as pain.
2. Pharmacological treatment of tension headaches includes acetaminophen, aspirin, and nonsteroidal anti-inflammatory agents.
3. Acute therapy for tension headaches entails the use of nonpharmacological methods such as rest, relaxation techniques, or stress-reduction strategies as well as medication.

SECTION III: PRACTICING FOR NCLEX

Activity E

1. **Answer: a**
   RATIONALE: The patient is in the prodrome phase of migraine headaches. The prodrome phase occurs hours or days before the onset of a migraine headache. Symptoms include depression, irritability, feeling cold, cravings, loss of appetite, alterations in activity, polyuria, diarrhea, and constipation.
2. **Answer: b**
   RATIONALE: Patients are diagnosed with chronic migraine headaches when they have symptoms of migraine headache at least eight times per month for at least 3 months.
3. **Answer: c**
   RATIONALE: When naproxen sodium and lithium carbonate are given together, there is an increased risk for lithium toxicity.
4. **Answer: b**
   RATIONALE: Ketorolac tromethamine is the only NSAID that may be given IV.
5. **Answer: b**
   RATIONALE: Caffeine causes vasoconstriction of blood vessels. This helps treat migraine headaches because migraine headaches are caused by vasodilation of cerebral vessels.
6. **Answer: a, b, and c**
   RATIONALE: Ergotamine may cause both cardiovascular and musculoskeletal adverse effects. The cardiovascular adverse effects of ergotamine include absence of pulse, bradycardia, cardiac valvular fibrosis, cyanosis, edema, heart rhythm changes, gangrene, hypertension, ischemia, precordial distress, chest pain, tachycardia, and vasospasm. Musculoskeletal adverse effects include muscle pain, numbness, paresthesia, and weakness.
7. **Answer: c**
   RATIONALE: Ergotamine is contraindicated in patients who are taking macrolide antibacterials.
8. **Answer: b**
   RATIONALE: Sumatriptan should be taken at the onset of migraine symptoms.
9. **Answer: c**
   RATIONALE: Almotriptan is a triptan that may be used with patients who are also taking MAOIs.
10. **Answer: a, d, and e**
    RATIONALE: Symptoms of serotonin syndrome include restlessness, hallucinations, fever, loss of consciousness, tachycardia, and a rapid change in blood pressure.
11. **Answer: a, c, and d**
    RATIONALE: The U.S. Food and Drug Administration has issued two *black box warnings*: (1) cardiovascular risk from sumatriptan, with an increased risk of adverse thrombotic events, including myocardial infarction and stroke, and (2) GI risk due to naproxen sodium, with an increased risk of GI irritation, inflammation, ulceration, bleeding, and perforation.
12. **Answer: b**
    RATIONALE: Estradiol is contraindicated in patients who have had a history of deep vein thrombosis because estradiol is a form of estrogen.
13. **Answer: c**
    RATIONALE: Valproic acid is a carboxylic acid derivative that is used as a preventative medication for migraines.

14. **Answer: b**
    RATIONALE: Propranolol is a beta-blocker and it may take up to 3 months to be effective as a migraine preventative.
15. **Answer: d**
    RATIONALE: It is important for the patient to use a barrier form of contraception while taking this medication to prevent birth defects.
16. **Answer: d**
    RATIONALE: Imipramine is a tricyclic antidepressant that is used as a migraine preventative and should be taken at bedtime because it may cause drowsiness.
17. **Answer: b**
    RATIONALE: The most appropriate nursing diagnosis for this patient is acute pain. There is no indication that the patient has fluid volume excess or activity intolerance related to muscle pain or that the patient is full of fear.
18. **Answer: b, c, and e**
    RATIONALE: Specific foods that may trigger a migraine headache are aged cheese, monosodium glutamate (found in Chinese foods), chocolate, aspartame (found in diet beverages), and fermented foods.
19. **Answer: c, d, and e**
    RATIONALE: The patient is instructed to report sore throat, fever, rash, itching, edema, visual changes, and black, tarry stools to the health care provider.
20. **Answer: c**
    RATIONALE: Acetaminophen, aspirin, and caffeine would be contraindicated in patients who are currently taking warfarin because of the risk of bleeding with the combination of aspirin and warfarin.

CHAPTER 52

SECTION I: ASSESSING YOUR UNDERSTANDING

Activity A FILL IN THE BLANKS

1. seizure
2. convulsion
3. epilepsy
4. Muscle spasms
5. clonic, tonic

Activity B MATCHING

1. b   2. e   3. a   4. d   5. c

Activity C SHORT ANSWERS

1. Seizures may occur as single events in response to hypoglycemia, fever, electrolyte imbalances, overdoses of numerous drugs (e.g., amphetamine, cocaine, isoniazid, lidocaine, lithium, methylphenidate, antipsychotics, theophylline), and withdrawal of alcohol or sedative–hypnotic drugs.
2. Epilepsy is characterized by sudden, abnormal, hypersynchronous firing of neurons; it is diagnosed by clinical signs and symptoms of seizure activity and by the presence of abnormal brain wave patterns on the electroencephalogram.
3. An absence seizure is characterized by abrupt alterations in consciousness that last only a few seconds. A tonic–clonic seizure is characterized by a loss of consciousness and consists of two parts: the tonic phase (sustained contraction of skeletal muscles; abnormal postures, such as opisthotonos; and absence of respirations, during which the person becomes cyanotic) and the clonic phase (rapid rhythmic and symmetric jerking movements of the body).
4. People with minimal symptoms do not require treatment but should be encouraged to maintain a healthy lifestyle. Those with more extensive symptoms should try to avoid emotional stress, extremes of environmental temperature, and infections.
5. Skeletal muscle relaxants are used primarily as adjuncts to other treatment measures such as physical therapy. Occasionally, parenteral agents are given to facilitate orthopedic procedures and examinations. In spastic disorders, skeletal muscle relaxants are indicated when spasticity causes severe pain or for inability to tolerate physical therapy, sit in a wheelchair, or participate in self-care activities of daily living (e.g., eating, dressing). The drugs should not be given if they cause excessive muscle weakness and impair rather than facilitate mobility and function.

SECTION II: APPLYING YOUR KNOWLEDGE
Activity D CASE STUDIES

Case Study 1
1. Status epilepticus is a life-threatening emergency characterized by generalized tonic–clonic convulsions lasting for several minutes or occurring at close intervals during which the patient does not regain consciousness. Hypotension, hypoxia, and cardiac dysrhythmias may also occur.
2. In a person taking medications for a diagnosed seizure disorder, the most common cause of status epilepticus is abruptly stopping AEDs.

Case Study 2
1. Physical therapy may help maintain muscle tone, and occupational therapy may help maintain ability to perform activities of daily living.
2. Oral baclofen begins to act in 1 hour, peaks in 2 hours, and lasts 4 to 8 hours. It is metabolized in the liver and excreted in urine; its half-life is 3 to 4 hours. Dosage must be reduced in patients with impaired renal function.
3. When oral baclofen is discontinued, dosage should be tapered and the drug withdrawn over 1 to 2 weeks.

SECTION III: PRACTICING FOR NCLEX

Activity E

1. **Answer: b, c, and e**
   RATIONALE: Seizures are classified as idiopathic or secondary. In infants, secondary causes include metabolic disorders, birth injury, and fever.

2. **Answer: a**
   RATIONALE: The home care nurse must work with patients and family members to implement and monitor AED therapy. When an AED is started, a few weeks may be required to titrate the dosage and determine whether the chosen drug is effective in controlling seizures. The nurse can play an important role in clinical assessment of the patient by interviewing the family about the occurrence of seizures (using a log of date, time, duration, and characteristics of seizures).

3. **Answer: c**
   RATIONALE: The community health nurse may assist the physician to titrate drug doses by ensuring that the patient keeps appointments for serum drug level testing and follow-up care.

4. **Answer: b**
   RATIONALE: The use of continuous nasogastric enteral feedings may decrease the absorption of phenytoin administered through the same route, predisposing the patient to the risk of seizure activity.

5. **Answer: d**
   RATIONALE: The occurrence of nystagmus (abnormal movements of the eyeball) indicates phenytoin toxicity; the drug should be reduced in dosage or discontinued until serum levels decrease.

6. **Answer: a**
   RATIONALE: Oral drugs are absorbed slowly and inefficiently in newborns. If an antiseizure drug is necessary during the first 7 to 10 days of life, IM phenobarbital is effective.

7. **Answer: c**
   RATIONALE: AEDs must be used cautiously to avoid excessive sedation and interference with learning and social development.

8. **Answer: a**
   RATIONALE: In older adults, decreased elimination by the liver and kidneys may lead to drug accumulation, with subsequent risks of dizziness, impaired coordination, and injuries due to falls.

9. **Answer: d**
   RATIONALE: An IV benzodiazepine (e.g., lorazepam 0.1 mg/kg at 2 mg/min) is the drug of choice for rapid control of tonic–clonic seizures.

10. **Answer: d**
    RATIONALE: Oxcarbazepine decreases effectiveness of felodipine and oral contraceptives, and a barrier type of contraception is recommended during oxcarbazepine therapy.

11. **Answer: b**
    RATIONALE: Sexually active adolescent girls and women of childbearing potential who require an AED must be evaluated and monitored very closely, because all of the AEDs are considered teratogenic. In general, infants exposed to one AED have a significantly higher risk of birth defects than those who are not exposed, and infants exposed to two or more AEDs have a significantly higher risk than those exposed to one AED.

12. **Answer: b**
    RATIONALE: Valproic acid preparations (Depakene, Depakote, and Depacon) are chemically unrelated to other AEDs. They are thought to enhance the effects of GABA in the brain and are also used to treat manic reactions in bipolar disorder and to prevent migraine headache.

13. **Answer: b**
    RATIONALE: Baclofen is metabolized in the liver and excreted in urine. The patient must be monitored for adverse effects on liver function.

14. **Answer: b, c, and e**
    RATIONALE: Patients should be instructed to avoid alcohol. The medication causes transient drowsiness, dizziness, weakness, fatigue, confusion, headache, insomnia, hypotension, and urinary frequency.

15. **Answer: d**
    RATIONALE: The skeletal muscle relaxants should be used cautiously in patients with renal impairment. Dosage of baclofen must be reduced.

16. **Answer: a**
    RATIONALE: For most of the skeletal muscle relaxants, safety and effectiveness for use in children 12 years of age and younger have not been established. The drugs should be used only when clearly indicated, for short periods, when close supervision is available for monitoring drug effects (especially sedation), and when mobility and alertness are not required.

17. **Answer: c**
    RATIONALE: Tizanidine (Zanaflex) is given orally, and it begins to act within 30 to 60 minutes, peaks in 1 to 2 hours, and lasts 3 to 4 hours.

18. **Answer: d**
    RATIONALE: Common adverse effects with methocarbamol drug include drowsiness, dizziness, nausea, urticaria, fainting, incoordination, and hypotension.

19. **Answer: a**
    RATIONALE: Carisoprodol (Soma) is used to relieve discomfort from acute, painful musculoskeletal disorders. It is not recommended for long-term use. If used long term or in high doses, it can cause physical dependence, and it may cause symptoms of withdrawal if stopped abruptly.

20. **Answer: a**
    RATIONALE: Most skeletal muscle relaxants cause CNS depression and have the same contraindications as other CNS depressants. They should be used cautiously in patients with impaired renal or hepatic function or respiratory depression and in patients who must be alert.

CHAPTER 53

SECTION I: ASSESSING YOUR UNDERSTANDING

Activity A FILL IN THE BLANKS

1. Antianxiety drugs, anxiolytics, sedatives
2. benzodiazepines, nonbenzodiazepine
3. Anxiety
4. Situational anxiety
5. Insomnia

Activity B MATCHING

1. c   2. a   3. e   4. b   5. d

Activity C SHORT ANSWERS

1. The pathophysiology of anxiety disorders is unknown, but there is evidence of a biologic basis and possible imbalances among several neurotransmission systems. A simplistic view involves an excess of excitatory neurotransmitters (e.g., norepinephrine) or a deficiency of inhibitory neurotransmitters (e.g., GABA).
2. The serotonin system, although not as well understood, is also thought to play a role in anxiety. Both selective serotonin reuptake inhibitors (SSRIs) and serotonin receptor agonists are now used to treat anxiety disorders. Research has suggested two possible roles for the serotonin receptor HT1A. During embryonic development, stimulation of HT1A receptors by serotonin is thought to play a role in development of normal brain circuitry necessary for normal anxiety responses. However, during adulthood, SSRIs act through HT1A receptors to reduce anxiety responses.
3. Activities that occur during the various sleep stages include increased tissue repair, synthesis of skeletal muscle protein, and secretion of growth hormone. At the same time, there are decreased body temperature, metabolic rate, glucose consumption, and production of catabolic hormones. Stage IV is followed by a period of 5 to 20 minutes of REM, dreaming, and increased physiologic activity.
4. Insomnia has many causes, including such stressors as pain, anxiety, illness, changes in lifestyle or environment, and various drugs. Occasional sleeplessness is a normal response to many stimuli and is not usually harmful. Insomnia is said to be chronic when it lasts longer than 1 month. As in anxiety, several neurotransmission systems are apparently involved in regulating sleep–wake cycles and producing insomnia.
5. The noradrenergic system is associated with the hyperarousal state experienced by patients with anxiety (i.e., feelings of panic, restlessness, tremulousness, palpitations, hyperventilation), which is attributed to excessive norepinephrine.

SECTION II: APPLYING YOUR KNOWLEDGE

Activity D CASE STUDY

1. Eszopiclone is rapidly absorbed after oral administration, reaching peak plasma levels 1 hour after administration. Onset of action may be delayed by approximately 1 hour if the drug is taken with a high-fat or heavy meal. Eszopiclone has a half-life of 6 hours.
2. Mr. Petski may be experiencing an adverse reaction to the medication. Adverse reactions include behavior changes such as reduced inhibition, aggression or bizarre behavior, worsening depression and suicidal ideation, hallucinations, and anterograde amnesia (short-term memory loss).
3. Review Mr. Petski's current drug regimen to determine whether he is taking any drugs that inhibit CYP3A4 enzymes (e.g., antidepressants, antifungals, erythromycin, grapefruit, protease inhibitors), which may require the physician to lower the dose of his medication to reduce adverse effects. Eszopiclone should not be taken with alcohol or other CNS depressants, to avoid additive effects.

SECTION III: PRACTICING FOR NCLEX

Activity E

1. **Answer: b**
   RATIONALE: Eszopiclone (Lunesta) is the first oral nonbenzodiazepine hypnotic to be approved for long-term use (up to 12 months). During drug testing, tolerance to the hypnotic benefits of eszopiclone was not observed over a 6-month period.
2. **Answer: c**
   RATIONALE: Eszopiclone is rapidly absorbed after oral administration, reaching peak plasma levels 1 hour after administration. Onset of action may be delayed by approximately 1 hour if the drug is taken with a high-fat or heavy meal. Eszopiclone has a half-life of 6 hours.
3. **Answer: b**
   RATIONALE: Temazepam is the benzodiazepine that is the drug of choice for elderly patients.
4. **Answer: a**
   RATIONALE: Situational anxiety is a normal response to a stressful situation. It may be beneficial when it motivates the person toward constructive, problem-solving, coping activities. Symptoms may be quite severe, but they usually last only 2 to 3 weeks.
5. **Answer: b**
   RATIONALE: Although there is no clear boundary between normal and abnormal anxiety, when anxiety is severe or prolonged and impairs the ability to function in usual activities of daily living, it is called an *anxiety disorder*.

6. Answer: d
RATIONALE: Benzodiazepines are widely used for anxiety and insomnia and are also used for several other indications. They have a wide margin of safety between therapeutic and toxic doses and are rarely fatal, even in overdose, unless combined with other CNS depressant drugs, such as alcohol. They are schedule IV drugs under the Controlled Substances Act. They are drugs of abuse and may cause physiologic dependence; therefore, withdrawal symptoms occur if the drugs are stopped abruptly.

7. Answer: b
RATIONALE: Diazepam (Valium) is the prototype benzodiazepine. High-potency benzodiazepines such as alprazolam (Xanax), lorazepam (Ativan), and clonazepam (Klonopin) may be more commonly prescribed due to their greater therapeutic effects and rapid onset of action.

8. Answer: c
RATIONALE: Eszopiclone (Lunesta): Adverse reactions include behavior changes such as reduced inhibition, aggression or bizarre behavior, worsening depression and suicidal ideation, hallucinations, and anterograde amnesia (short-term memory loss).

9. Answer: d
RATIONALE: Ramelteon does not cause physical dependence.

10. Answer: b
RATIONALE: Ramelteon is rapidly absorbed orally, reaching peak plasma levels in about 45 minutes.

11. Answer: a
RATIONALE: Zaleplon is well absorbed, but bioavailability is only about 30% because of extensive presystemic or "first-pass" hepatic metabolism. Action onset is rapid and peaks in 1 hour. A high-fat, heavy meal slows absorption and may reduce the drug's effectiveness in inducing sleep.

12. Answer: b
RATIONALE: Zaleplon should not be taken concurrently with alcohol or other CNS depressant drugs because of the increased risk of excessive sedation and respiratory depression.

13. Answer: b
RATIONALE: Cimetidine inhibits both the aldehyde oxidase and the cytochrome P450 CYP3A4 enzymes that metabolize zaleplon. If cimetidine is taken, zaleplon dosage should be reduced to 5 mg. It is very important that patients taking zaleplon be taught about this interaction, because cimetidine is available without prescription, and the patient may not inform the health care provider who prescribes zaleplon about taking cimetidine.

14. Answer: d
RATIONALE: A newer controlled-release form of zolpidem (Ambien CR) contains a rapid-releasing layer of medication, which aids a person in falling asleep, and a second layer, which is released more slowly to promote sleep all night.

15. Answer: c
RATIONALE: Adverse effects of zolpidem include daytime drowsiness, dizziness, nausea, diarrhea, and anterograde amnesia. Rebound insomnia may occur for a night or two after stopping the drug, and withdrawal symptoms may occur if it is stopped abruptly after approximately 1 week of regular use.

16. Answer: a
RATIONALE: Alprazolam is the most commonly prescribed benzodiazepine; its dose should be reduced by 50% if it is given concurrently with the antidepressant fluvoxamine.

17. Answer: b
RATIONALE: In older adults, most benzodiazepines are metabolized more slowly, and half-lives are longer than in younger adults. Exceptions are lorazepam and oxazepam, whose half-lives and dosages are the same for older adults as for younger ones. The recommended initial dose of zaleplon or zolpidem is 5 mg, one half of the initial dose recommended for younger adults. Dosages of eszopiclone should also be reduced for older adults, beginning with 1 mg initially, not to exceed 2 mg at bedtime.

18. Answer: b
RATIONALE: When benzodiazepines are used with opioid analgesics, the analgesic dose should be reduced initially and increased gradually to avoid excessive CNS depression.

19. Answer: c
RATIONALE: The antianxiety benzodiazepines are often given in three or four daily doses. This is necessary for the short-acting agents, but there is no pharmacologic basis for multiple daily doses of the long-acting drugs. Because of their prolonged actions, all or most of the daily dose can be given at bedtime. This schedule promotes sleep, and there is usually enough residual sedation to maintain antianxiety effects throughout the next day.

20. Answer: c
RATIONALE: Kava is the nutritional/herbal supplement that is recommended for the treatment of anxiety. Caffeine may possibly increase symptoms of anxiety. Melatonin is used to reestablish sleep–wake cycles, and whey is used to build muscle mass.

CHAPTER 54

SECTION I: ASSESSING YOUR UNDERSTANDING

Activity A FILL IN THE BLANKS

1. Postnatal depression
2. Major depression
3. Bipolar disorder type I
4. Bipolar disorder type II
5. antidepressant discontinuation syndrome

Activity B MATCHING

1. e   **2.** b   **3.** a   **4.** c   **5.** d

Activity C SHORT ANSWERS

1. Toxicity is most likely to occur in depressed patients who intentionally ingest large amounts of drug in suicide attempts and in young children who accidentally gain access to medication containers. Measures to prevent acute poisoning from drug overdose include dispensing only a few days' supply (i.e., 5 to 7 days) to patients with suicidal tendencies and storing the drugs in places that are inaccessible to young children. General measures to treat acute poisoning include early detection of signs and symptoms, stopping the drug, and instituting treatment if indicated.

2. For patients with certain concurrent medical conditions, antidepressants may have adverse effects. For patients with cardiovascular disorders, most antidepressants can cause hypotension, but the SSRIs, bupropion, and venlafaxine are rarely associated with cardiac dysrhythmias. Duloxetine, venlafaxine, and MAOIs can increase blood pressure. For patients with seizure disorders, bupropion, clomipramine, and duloxetine should be avoided. SSRIs, MAOIs, and desipramine are less likely to cause seizures. For patients with diabetes mellitus, SSRIs may have a hypoglycemic effect. Duloxetine may slightly increase fasting glucose levels, and bupropion and venlafaxine have little effect on blood sugar levels. Duloxetine can cause mydriasis, increasing intraocular pressure in patients with narrow-angle glaucoma.

3. Lithium is the drug of choice for patients with bipolar disorder. When used therapeutically, lithium is effective in controlling mania in 65% to 80% of patients. When used prophylactically, the drug decreases the frequency and intensity of manic cycles.

4. With SSRIs and venlafaxine, therapy is begun with once-daily oral administration of the manufacturer's recommended dosage. Dosage may be increased after 3 or 4 weeks if depression is not relieved. As with most other drugs, smaller doses may be indicated in older adults and in patients taking multiple medications. Duloxetine is initiated with twice-a-day oral administration without regard to food.

5. Serotonin syndrome, a serious and sometimes fatal reaction characterized by hypertensive crisis, hyperpyrexia, extreme agitation progressing to delirium and coma, muscle rigidity, and seizures, may occur due to combined therapy with an SSRI and an MAOI or other drugs that potentiate serotonin neurotransmission. An SSRI or SNRI and an MAOI should not be given concurrently or within 2 weeks of each other. In most cases, if a patient taking an SSRI is to be transferred to an MAOI, the SSRI should be discontinued at least 14 days before starting the MAOI. However, because of its prolonged half-life, fluoxetine should be discontinued at least 5 weeks before starting an MAOI.

SECTION II: APPLYING YOUR KNOWLEDGE

Activity D CASE STUDIES

Case Study 1

1. If an antidepressant medication was recently started, the nurse may need to remind the patient that it usually takes 2 to 4 weeks to take effect. The nurse should encourage the patient to continue taking the medication.

2. The family should be taught to report any change in the patient's behavior, especially anxiety, agitation, panic attacks, insomnia, irritability, hostility, impulsivity, akathisia, hypomania, or mania. A patient who has one or more of these symptoms may be at greater risk for worsening depression or suicidality.

Case Study 2

1. Adverse effects include a high incidence of gastrointestinal (GI) symptoms (e.g., nausea, diarrhea, weight loss) and sexual dysfunction (e.g., delayed ejaculation in men, impaired orgasmic ability in women). Most SSRIs also cause some degree of CNS stimulation (e.g., anxiety, nervousness, insomnia), which is most prominent with fluoxetine.

2. Fluoxetine also forms an active metabolite with a half-life of 7 to 9 days. Therefore, steady-state blood levels are achieved slowly, over several weeks, and drug effects decrease slowly (over 2 to 3 months) when fluoxetine is discontinued.

SECTION III: PRACTICING FOR NCLEX

Activity E

1. Answer a
   RATIONALE: Third-trimester intrauterine exposure to fluoxetine or other SSRIs may result in a *neonatal withdrawal syndrome*, which shares some similarity to a mild serotonin syndrome. Common symptoms include irritability, prolonged crying, respiratory distress, rigidity, and possibly seizures. Care for an infant with neonatal withdrawal syndrome is supportive; symptoms usually abate within a few days.

2. Answer c
   RATIONALE: Weight loss is a common side effect of SSRIs and is particularly undesirable in older adults.

3. Answer b
   RATIONALE: A black box warning alerts health care providers to the increased risk of suicidal ideation in children, adolescents, and young adults 18 to 24 years of age when taking antidepressant medications.

4. Answer c
   RATIONALE: Bipolar disorder type II is characterized by episodes of major depression plus hypomanic episodes and occurs more frequently in women.

5. Answer d
RATIONALE: Critically ill patients may be receiving an antidepressant when the critical illness develops, or they may need a drug to combat the depression that often develops with major illness. The decision to continue or start an antidepressant should be based on a thorough assessment of the patient's condition, other drugs being given, potential adverse drug effects, and other factors. If an antidepressant is given, its use must be cautious and slow, and the patient's responses must be carefully monitored, because critically ill patients are often frail and unstable, with multiple organ dysfunctions.

6. Answer b
RATIONALE: Hepatic impairment leads to reduced first-pass metabolism of most antidepressant drugs, resulting in higher plasma levels. The drugs should be used cautiously in patients with severe liver impairment. Cautious use means lower doses, longer intervals between doses, and slower dose increases than usual.

7. Answer a
RATIONALE: SSRIs are the drugs of choice in older adults, as in younger ones, because they produce fewer sedative, anticholinergic, cardiotoxic, and psychomotor adverse effects than the TCAs and related antidepressants.

8. Answer b
RATIONALE: A TCA probably is not a drug of first choice for adolescents, because TCAs are more toxic in overdose than other antidepressants, and suicide is a leading cause of death in adolescents.

9. Answer d
RATIONALE: Amitriptyline, desipramine, imipramine, and nortriptyline are the TCAs most commonly prescribed to treat depression in children older than 12 years of age. Because of potentially serious adverse effects, blood pressure, ECG, and plasma drug levels should be monitored.

10. Answer b
RATIONALE: For most children and adolescents, it is probably best to reserve drug therapy for those who do not respond to nonpharmacologic treatments such as cognitive behavioral therapy.

11. Answer a
RATIONALE: African Americans tend to have higher plasma drug levels for a given dose, respond more rapidly, experience a higher incidence of adverse effects, and metabolize TCAs more slowly than whites. To decrease adverse effects, initial doses may need to be lower than those given to whites, and later doses should be titrated according to clinical response and serum drug levels.

12. Answer c
RATIONALE: Lithium should be stopped 1 to 2 days before surgery and resumed when full oral intake of food and fluids is allowed. Lithium may prolong the effects of anesthetics and neuromuscular blocking drugs.

13. Answer a, b, d, and e
RATIONALE: The most clearly defined withdrawal syndromes are associated with SSRIs and TCAs. With SSRIs, withdrawal symptoms include dizziness, gastrointestinal upset, lethargy or anxiety/hyperarousal, dysphoria, sleep problems, and headache. Symptoms can last from several days to several weeks.

14. Answer a, b, and e
RATIONALE: Patients who are taking phenelzine must avoid certain foods to prevent serious complications. The patient must avoid game meats, soy products, sesame seeds, brewers yeast, sauerkraut, seafood, aged cheeses and meats, and fava beans.

15. Answer d
RATIONALE: When lithium therapy is being initiated, the serum drug concentration should be measured two or three times weekly in the morning, 12 hours after the last dose of lithium.

16. Answer b
RATIONALE: Fluoxetine may cause hypoglycemia in patients who have diabetes mellitus.

17. Answer b
RATIONALE: Bupropion does not cause orthostatic hypotension or sexual dysfunction.

18. Answer a, b, d, and e
RATIONALE: Because the available drugs have similar efficacy in treating depression, the choice of an antidepressant depends on the patient's age; medical conditions; previous history of drug response, if any; and the specific drug's adverse effects. Cost also needs to be considered.

19. Answer a
RATIONALE: St. John's wort may reduce the effectiveness of cyclosporine, HIV protease inhibitors, oral contraceptives, digoxin, warfarin, and theophylline through interactions mediated by CYP3A4, CYP2C9, CYP1A2, and CYP2C19 enzyme systems as well as other mechanisms.

20. Answer b
RATIONALE: The patient must stop taking imipramine a few days prior to surgery and will not be able to resume it for a few days after surgery.

CHAPTER 55

SECTION I: ASSESSING YOUR UNDERSTANDING
Activity A FILL IN THE BLANKS
1. psychosis
2. Hallucinations
3. Delusions
4. paranoia
5. neuroleptics

Activity B   MATCHING

1. b   **2.** e   **3.** a   **4.** c   **5.** d

Activity C   SHORT ANSWERS

1. Psychosis is a severe mental disorder characterized by disordered thought processes (disorganized and often bizarre thinking); blunted or inappropriate emotional responses; bizarre behavior ranging from hypoactivity to hyperactivity with agitation, aggressiveness, hostility, and combativeness; social withdrawal, in which a person pays less than normal attention to the environment and other people; deterioration from previous levels of occupational and social functioning (poor self-care and interpersonal skills); hallucinations; and paranoid delusions.

2. Acute psychotic episodes, also called confusion or delirium, have a sudden onset over hours to days and may be precipitated by physical disorders (e.g., brain damage related to cerebrovascular disease or head injury, metabolic disorders, infections); drug intoxication (e.g., adrenergics, antidepressants, some anticonvulsants, amphetamines, cocaine); or drug withdrawal after chronic use (e.g., alcohol; benzodiazepine antianxiety or sedative–hypnotic agents).

3. The neurodevelopmental model proposes that schizophrenia results when abnormal brain synapses are formed in response to an intrauterine insult during the second trimester of pregnancy, when neuronal migration is normally taking place. Intrauterine events such as upper respiratory tract infection, obstetric complications, and neonatal hypoxia have been associated with schizophrenia. The emergence of psychosis in response to the formation of these abnormal circuits in adolescence or early adulthood corresponds to the time period of neuronal maturation.

4. Genetics is strongly suspected to play a role in the development of schizophrenia. Family studies identify increased risk if a first-degree relative has the illness (10%), if a second-degree relative has the illness (3%), if both parents have the illness (40%), and if a monozygotic twin has the illness (48%). Adoption studies of twins suggest that heredity, rather than environment, is a key factor in the development of schizophrenia. Many genetic studies are under way to identify the gene or genes responsible for schizophrenia. Possible genes linked to schizophrenia include *WKL1* on chromosome 22, which is thought to play a role in catatonic schizophrenia; *DISC1*, mutations of which cause delays in migration of brain neurons in mouse models; and the gene responsible for the glutamate receptor, which regulates the amount of glutamine in synapses.

5. Negative symptoms of schizophrenia include lack of pleasure (anhedonia), lack of motivation, blunted affect, poor grooming and hygiene, poor social skills, poverty of speech, and social withdrawal.

SECTION II: APPLYING YOUR KNOWLEDGE

Activity D   CASE STUDIES

Case Study 1

1. Advantages of clozapine include improvement of negative symptoms without the extrapyramidal side effects associated with older antipsychotic drugs. However, despite these advantages, it is a second-line drug, recommended only for patients who have not responded to treatment with at least two other antipsychotic drugs or who exhibit recurrent suicidal behavior.

2. Clozapine is associated with agranulocytosis, a life-threatening decrease in white blood cells (WBCs) that usually occurs during the first 3 months of therapy. A black box warning alerts health practitioners to this dangerous side effect. Weekly WBC counts are required during the first 6 months of therapy; if acceptable WBC counts are maintained, then WBC counts can be monitored every 2 weeks thereafter.

3. Black box warnings for clozapine (especially in the first months of treatment) include increased risk for fatal myocarditis, orthostatic hypotension with or without syncope, and, rarely, cardiopulmonary arrest. Clozapine is also more likely to cause constipation, drowsiness, and weight gain than other atypical drugs. Clozapine is metabolized primarily by CYP1A2 enzymes and, to a lesser degree, by CYP2D6 and CYP3A4 enzymes.

Case Study 2

1. For patients who are unable or unwilling to take the oral drug as prescribed, a slowly absorbed, long-acting formulation (haloperidol decanoate) may be given IM, once monthly.

2. The signs and symptoms of extrapyramidal side effects include twisting and rhythmic movements (acute dystonia), tremors (parkinsonism), and inability to sit or remain still (akathisia).

SECTION III: PRACTICING FOR NCLEX

Activity E

1. Answer b, d, and e
   RATIONALE: Symptoms of neuroleptic malignant syndrome include severe hyperthermia, confusion, tachycardia, agitation, delirium, dyspnea, respiratory failure, and acute renal failure.

2. Answer d
   RATIONALE: Tardive dyskinesia, a late extrapyramidal effect, may occur with all phenothiazine and typical nonphenothiazine drugs and is generally

considered to be irreversible. It may be treated by reducing the dosage or switching to a second-generation antipsychotic. Prevention through early detection is key.

3. Answer c
RATIONALE: Early extrapyramidal effects are treated by reducing dosage, changing to a second-generation antipsychotic, or using anticholinergic medications. Akathisia may also be treated with benzodiazepines and beta-blockers to reduce the urge to move.

4. Answer a
RATIONALE: Antipsychotics may take several weeks to achieve maximum therapeutic effect.

5. Answer b
RATIONALE: The home care nurse must assist and support caregivers' efforts to maintain medications and manage adverse drug effects, other aspects of daily care, and follow-up psychiatric care. In addition, the home care nurse may need to coordinate the efforts of several health and social service agencies or providers.

6. Answer d
RATIONALE: If haloperidol is used in adolescents who have Tourette's, the usual initial dose is 1.5 mg to 6 mg PO.

7. Answer c
RATIONALE: Some patients become acutely agitated or delirious and need sedation to prevent their injuring themselves by thrashing about, removing tubes and intravenous (IV) catheters, and so forth. Some physicians prefer a benzodiazepine-type sedative, whereas others may use haloperidol. Before giving either drug, causes of delirium (e.g., drug intoxication or withdrawal) should be identified and eliminated if possible.

8. Answer c
RATIONALE: Antipsychotic drugs undergo extensive hepatic metabolism and then elimination in urine. In the presence of liver disease (e.g., cirrhosis, hepatitis), metabolism may be slowed and drug elimination half-lives prolonged, with resultant accumulation and increased risk of adverse effects. Therefore, these drugs should be used cautiously in patients with hepatic impairment.

9. Answer a
RATIONALE: Because most antipsychotic drugs are extensively metabolized in the liver and the metabolites are excreted through the kidneys, the drugs should be used cautiously in patients with impaired renal function. Renal function should be monitored periodically during long-term therapy. If renal function test results (e.g., blood urea nitrogen) become abnormal, the drug may need to be lowered in dosage or discontinued.

10. Answer b
RATIONALE: Jaundice has been associated with phenothiazines, usually after 2 to 4 weeks of therapy. It is considered a hypersensitivity reaction, and patients should not be reexposed to a phenothiazine.

11. Answer c
RATIONALE: African Americans tend to respond more rapidly; experience a higher incidence of adverse effects, including tardive dyskinesia; and metabolize antipsychotic drugs more slowly than whites. When compared with haloperidol, olanzapine has been associated with fewer extrapyramidal reactions in African Americans.

12. Answer d
RATIONALE: Patients with dementia may become agitated because of environmental or medical problems. Alleviating such causes, when possible, is safer and more effective than administering antipsychotic drugs. Inappropriate use of antipsychotic drugs exposes patients to adverse drug effects and does not resolve underlying problems.

13. Answer d
RATIONALE: If antipsychotic drugs are used to control acute agitation in older adults, they should be used in the lowest effective dose for the shortest effective duration. If the drugs are used to treat dementia, they may relieve some symptoms (e.g., agitation, hallucinations, hostility, suspiciousness, uncooperativeness), but they do not improve memory loss and may further impair cognitive functioning.

14. Answer d
RATIONALE: Children usually have a faster metabolic rate than adults and may therefore require relatively high doses of antipsychotics for their size and weight.

15. Answer a
RATIONALE: A major concern about giving traditional antipsychotic drugs perioperatively is their potential for adverse interactions with other drugs. For example, antipsychotic drugs potentiate the effects of general anesthetics and other CNS depressants that are often used before, during, and after surgery. As a result, risks of hypotension and excessive sedation are increased unless doses of other drugs are reduced.

16. Answer a, b, and c
RATIONALE: Acute dystonia (manifested by severe spasms of muscles of the face, neck, tongue, or back) typically occurs early in treatment and constitutes an emergency. Severe manifestations of acute dystonia include oculogyric crisis (severe involuntary upward rotation of the eyes) and opisthotonus (severe spasm of back muscles causing head and heels to bend backward with the body bowed forward).

17. Answer b
RATIONALE: Acute dystonia is treated with intramuscular or intravenous administration of anticholinergic medications such as benztropine or diphenhydramine.

18. Answer b
RATIONALE: Olanzapine takes approximately 1 week to reach a steady state of concentration.

19. Answer a
RATIONALE: The nurse would be most concerned about a patient's temperature of 102 because clozapine can cause agranulocytosis.

20. Answer b
RATIONALE: Clinically significant drug interactions may occur with drugs that induce or inhibit the liver enzymes, and dosage of quetiapine (Seroquel) may need to be increased in patients who are taking enzyme inducers (e.g., carbamazepine, phenytoin, rifampin) or decreased in patients who are taking enzyme inhibitors (e.g., cimetidine, erythromycin).

CHAPTER 56

SECTION I: ASSESSING YOUR UNDERSTANDING

Activity A FILL IN THE BLANKS

1. ADHD
2. Narcolepsy
3. ADHD, narcolepsy
4. ADHD
5. learning disabilities

Activity B MATCHING

1. b   **2.** a   **3.** d   **4.** e   **5.** c

Activity C SHORT ANSWERS

1. ADHD is the most common psychiatric or neurobehavioral disorder in children. It is usually diagnosed between 3 and 7 years of age and may affect as many as 6% or 7% of school-age children. It is characterized by persistent hyperactivity, short attention span, difficulty completing assigned tasks or schoolwork, restlessness, and impulsiveness. Such behaviors make it difficult for the child to get along with others (e.g., family members, peer groups, teachers) and to function in situations requiring controlled behavior (e.g., classrooms).
2. Narcolepsy is a sleep disorder characterized by daytime "sleep attacks" in which the person goes to sleep at any place or at any time. Signs and symptoms also include excessive daytime drowsiness, fatigue, muscle weakness and hallucinations at onset of sleep, and disturbances of nighttime sleep patterns.
3. In addition to drug therapy, prevention of sleep deprivation, regular sleeping and waking times, avoiding shift work, and short naps may be helpful in reducing daytime sleepiness.

4. CNS stimulants act by facilitating initiation and transmission of nerve impulses that excite other cells. The drugs are somewhat selective in their actions at lower doses but tend to involve the entire CNS at higher doses. In ADHD, the drugs improve academic performance, behavior, and interpersonal relationships.
5. Amphetamines increase the amounts of norepinephrine, dopamine, and possibly serotonin in the brain, thereby producing mood elevation or euphoria, increasing mental alertness and capacity for work, decreasing fatigue and drowsiness, and prolonging wakefulness.

SECTION II: APPLYING YOUR KNOWLEDGE

Activity D CASE STUDIES

Case Study 1
1. Acceptable nursing diagnoses are
   - Sleep Pattern Disturbance related to hyperactivity, nervousness, insomnia
   - Risk for Injury: Adverse drug effects (excessive cardiac and CNS stimulation, drug dependence)
   - Deficient Knowledge: Drug effects on children and adults
2. Try to identify potentially significant sources of caffeine intake.
3. The patient will take CNS stimulants safely and accurately.

Case Study 2
1. This statement by Jane's mother indicates that she requires further education regarding the administration of stimulants to her child. You should include in your education of the patient's parents the following points:
   - Stimulant drugs should be taken only as prescribed.
   - These drugs have a high potential for abuse.
   - The risks of serious health problems and drug dependence are lessened if they are taken correctly.
   - The likelihood of medical problems is greatly increased when ADHD medication is used improperly or in combination with other drugs.
2. Jane's weight should be recorded at least weekly, and excessive losses should be reported. The drugs may cause weight loss; caloric intake (of nutritional foods) may need to be increased, especially in children. Alterations in attention span and task performance should be noted.
3. Monitor for symptoms of drug dependence and stunted growth. You should assist parents in scheduling drug administration to increase beneficial effects and help prevent drug dependence and stunted growth. In addition, ask parents to control drug distribution and monitor the number of pills or capsules available and the number prescribed. The goals are to prevent overuse by the child for whom the drug is prescribed and to prevent the

child from sharing the medication with other children who wish to take the drug for nonmedical purposes.

SECTION III: PRACTICING FOR NCLEX
Activity E

1. **Answer a**
   RATIONALE: All of the CNS stimulants, including caffeine, can cause life-threatening health problems with excessive intake.

2. **Answer b, d, and e**
   RATIONALE: Narcolepsy is characterized by daytime drowsiness, unpredictable "sleep attacks," and cataplexy, which is episodic loss of muscle functioning.

3. **Answer c**
   RATIONALE: CNS stimulants improve behavior and attention in patients with ADHD.

4. **Answer d**
   RATIONALE: ADHD usually starts in childhood and may persist through adulthood.

5. **Answer a, c, and d**
   RATIONALE: ADHD is characterized by hyperactivity, impulsivity, and a short attention span. Most often, they do not get along well with other children because of their impulsivity and difficulty maintaining control.

6. **Answer b**
   RATIONALE: Older adults are likely to experience anxiety, confusion, insomnia, and nervousness from excessive CNS stimulation. In addition, older adults often have cardiovascular disorders (e.g., angina, dysrhythmias, hypertension) that may be aggravated by the cardiac-stimulating effects of the drugs, including dietary caffeine. In general, reduced doses are safer in older adults.

7. **Answer b**
   RATIONALE: A drug holiday (i.e., stopping drug therapy) is recommended at least annually to evaluate the child's treatment regimen. Dosage adjustments are usually needed as the child grows and hepatic metabolism slows. Also, drug holidays decrease weight loss and growth suppression.

8. **Answer d**
   RATIONALE: Methylphenidate is commonly prescribed and is usually given daily for the first 3 to 4 weeks of treatment to allow caregivers to assess beneficial and adverse effects.

9. **Answer b, d, and e**
   RATIONALE: Drug therapy is indicated when symptoms are moderate to severe; are present for several months; and interfere in social, academic, or behavioral functioning.

10. **Answer b and d**
    RATIONALE: Treatment is largely symptomatic and supportive. In general, place the patient in a cool room, monitor cardiac function and body temperature, and minimize external stimulation. Activated charcoal (1 g/kg of body weight) may be given.

11. **Answer a**
    RATIONALE: Caffeine is well absorbed from the GI tract and reaches a peak blood level within 30 to 45 minutes after oral ingestion. It easily crosses the blood–brain barrier and has a half-life of 3.5 to 5 hours. It is extensively metabolized, mainly in the liver, and excreted mainly in urine.

12. **Answer d**
    RATIONALE: Caffeine is an ingredient in some nonprescription analgesic preparations and may increase analgesia. It is combined with an ergot alkaloid to treat migraine headaches (e.g., Cafergot).

13. **Answer a.**
    RATIONALE: Brewed coffee may have up to 180 mg of caffeine. Instant coffee has a maximum of 120 mg. The maximum of caffeine in an energy drink is 160 mg, and brewed tea has a maximum of 80 mg.

14. **Answer b**
    RATIONALE: Modafinil is not recommended for patients with a history of left ventricular hypertrophy or ischemic changes on electrocardiograms.

15. **Answer a**
    RATIONALE: In general, the caffeine content of a guarana product is unknown, and guarana may not be listed as an ingredient. As a result, consumers may not know how much caffeine they are ingesting in products containing guarana.

16. **Answer c**
    RATIONALE: The main goal of therapy with CNS stimulants is to relieve symptoms of the disorders for which they are given. A secondary goal is to have patients use the drugs appropriately.

17. **Answer a, c, and e**
    RATIONALE: CNS stimulants are contraindicated for those who drive long distances, those with cardiac dysrhythmias, and those with peptic ulcer disease.

18. **Answer b**
    RATIONALE: When a CNS stimulant is prescribed, it is started with a low dose that is then increased as necessary, usually at weekly intervals, until an effective dose (i.e., decreased symptoms) or the maximum daily dose is reached. In addition, the number of doses that can be obtained with one prescription should be limited. This action reduces the likelihood of drug dependence or diversion (use by people for whom the drug is not prescribed).

19. **Answer d**
    RATIONALE: CNS stimulants are not recommended for ADHD in children younger than 3 years of age.

20. **Answer d**
    RATIONALE: Caffeine withdrawal symptoms may begin approximately 18 to 24 hours after the last drink of coffee.

CHAPTER 57

SECTION I: ASSESSING YOUR UNDERSTANDING

Activity A FILL IN THE BLANKS

1. Substance abuse
2. CNS
3. tolerance
4. pleasure (or reward)
5. dependence

Activity B MATCHING

1. b **2.** d **3.** a **4.** c **5.** e

Activity C SHORT ANSWERS

1. Substance abuse is defined as self-administration of a drug for prolonged periods or in excessive amounts to the point of producing physical or psychological dependence, impairing functions of body organs, reducing the ability to function in usual activities of daily living, and decreasing the ability and motivation to function as a productive member of society.
2. Commonly abused drugs include CNS depressants (e.g., alcohol, antianxiety and sedative–hypnotic agents, opioid analgesics), CNS stimulants (e.g., cocaine, methamphetamine, methylphenidate, nicotine), and other mind-altering drugs (e.g., marijuana, "ecstasy").
3. Although these drugs produce different effects, they are associated with feelings of pleasure, positive reinforcement, and compulsive self-administration.
4. Drugs of abuse seem to be readily available. Internet Web sites have become an important source of the drugs. In some instances, instructions for manufacturing particular drugs are available. Although patterns of drug abuse vary in particular populations and geographic areas, continuing trends seem to include increased use of methamphetamine, "club drugs," prescription drugs, and using multiple drugs at the same time.
5. Characteristics of drug dependence include craving a drug, often with unsuccessful attempts to decrease its use; compulsive drug-seeking behavior; physical dependence (withdrawal symptoms if drug use is decreased or stopped); and continuing to take a drug despite adverse consequences (e.g., drug-related illnesses, mental or legal problems, job loss or decreased ability to function in an occupation, impaired family relationships).

SECTION II: APPLYING YOUR KNOWLEDGE

Activity D CASE STUDY

1. Physical dependence involves physiologic adaptation to chronic use of a drug so that unpleasant symptoms occur when the drug is stopped, when its action is antagonized by another drug, or when its dosage is decreased. The withdrawal or abstinence syndrome produces specific manifestations according to the type of drug and does not occur as long as adequate dosage is maintained. Attempts to avoid withdrawal symptoms reinforce psychological dependence and promote continuing drug use and relapses to drug-taking behavior.
2. Psychological dependence involves feelings of satisfaction and pleasure from taking the drug. These feelings, perceived as extremely desirable by the drug-dependent person, contribute to acute intoxication, development and maintenance of drug abuse patterns, and return to drug-taking behavior after periods of abstinence.
3. Tolerance means that the body adjusts to the drugs so that higher doses are needed to achieve feelings of pleasure ("reward") or stave off withdrawal symptoms ("punishment"). Both reward and punishment serve to reinforce continued substance abuse.

SECTION III: PRACTICING FOR NCLEX

Activity E

1. **Answer: a, c, and e**
   RATIONALE: The combination of disulfiram with alcohol may result in headaches, confusion, seizures, chest pain, flushing, palpitations, hypotension, sweating, blurred vision, nausea, vomiting, and a garlic-like aftertaste. More severe effects (with alcohol) include dysrhythmias, cardiovascular collapse, heart failure, myocardial infarction, and death.
2. **Answer: d**
   RATIONALE: With oral anticoagulants (e.g., warfarin), alcohol interactions vary. Acute ingestion increases anticoagulant effects and the risk of bleeding.
3. **Answer: d**
   RATIONALE: Chronic ingestion decreases anticoagulant effects by inducing drug-metabolizing enzymes in the liver and increasing the rate of warfarin metabolism. However, if chronic ingestion has caused liver damage, metabolism of warfarin may be slowed. This increases the risk of excessive anticoagulant effect and bleeding.
4. **Answer: c**
   RATIONALE: With oral antidiabetic drugs that decrease blood sugar, alcohol potentiates hypoglycemic effects. These drugs include acarbose (Precose), exenatide (Byetta), glipizide (Glucotrol), glyburide (DiaBeta), glimepiride (Amaryl), miglitol (Glyset), nateglinide (Starlix), pioglitazone (Actos), pramlintide (Symlin), repaglinide (Prandin), and rosiglitazone (Avandia).
5. **Answer: b**
   RATIONALE: With antihypertensive agents, alcohol potentiates vasodilation and hypotensive effects.
6. **Answer: b**
   RATIONALE: With other CNS depressants (e.g., sedative–hypnotics, opioid analgesics, antianxiety

agents, antipsychotic agents, general anesthetics, tricyclic antidepressants), alcohol potentiates CNS depression and increases risks of excessive sedation, respiratory depression, and impaired mental and physical functioning. Combining alcohol with these drugs may be lethal and should be avoided.

7. Answer: c
RATIONALE: Patients who receive opioid medications such as morphine sulfate do not usually experience addiction once the reason for the pain has gone.

8. Answer: d
RATIONALE: Abusers of alcohol and other drugs are not reliable sources of information about the types or amounts of drugs used. Most abusers understate the amount and frequency of substance use.

9. Answer: a
RATIONALE: Heroin addicts may overstate the amount used in attempts to obtain higher doses of methadone.

10. Answer: c
RATIONALE: The patient is experiencing symptoms of dextromethorphan overdose that include blurred vision, brain damage, confusion, dizziness, drowsiness, excessive sweating, hallucinations, impaired breathing, impaired judgment and mental functioning, loss of consciousness, loss of physical coordination, muscle twitches, nausea and vomiting, paranoia, rapid and irregular heartbeat, seizures, slurred speech, and death.

11. Answer: a
RATIONALE: Health care professionals (e.g., physicians, pharmacists, nurses) are considered to be at high risk for development of substance abuse disorders, at least partly because of easy access.

12. Answer: b
RATIONALE: Psychological rehabilitation efforts should be part of any treatment program for a drug-dependent person.

13. Answer: d
RATIONALE: Inhalants can harm the brain, liver, heart, kidneys, and lungs, and abuse of any drug during adolescence may interfere with brain development. Substances containing gasoline, benzene, or carbon tetrachloride are especially likely to cause serious damage to the liver, kidneys, and bone marrow. Inhalants can also produce psychological dependence, and some produce tolerance.

14. Answer: d
RATIONALE: Usage of GHB has increased in recent years, mainly in the party or dance-club setting, and GHB is increasingly involved in poisonings, overdoses, date rapes, visits to hospital emergency departments, and fatalities.

15. Answer: d
RATIONALE: Phencyclidine (PCP) produces excitement, delirium, hallucinations, and other profound psychological and physiologic effects, including a state of intoxication similar to that produced by alcohol; altered sensory perceptions; impaired thought processes; impaired motor skills; psychotic reactions; sedation and analgesia; nystagmus and diplopia; and pressor effects that can cause hypertensive crisis, cerebral hemorrhage, convulsions, coma, and death. Death from overdose also has occurred as a result of respiratory depression. Bizarre murders, suicides, and self-mutilations have been attributed to the schizophrenic reaction induced by PCP, especially in high doses. The drug also produces flashbacks.

16. Answer: b
RATIONALE: Nicotine is available in transdermal patches, chewing gum, an oral inhaler, and a nasal spray. The gum, inhaler, and spray are used intermittently during the day; the transdermal patch is applied once daily. Transdermal patches produce a steady blood level of nicotine, and patients seem to use them more consistently than they use the other products. The patches and gum are available over the counter; the inhaler and nasal spray require a prescription. The products are contraindicated in people with significant cardiovascular disease (angina pectoris, dysrhythmias, or recent myocardial infarction).

17. Answer: a, b, and c
RATIONALE: Drug therapy for cocaine dependence is largely symptomatic. Agitation and hyperactivity may be treated with a benzodiazepine antianxiety agent, psychosis may be treated with haloperidol (Haldol) or another antipsychotic agent, cardiac dysrhythmias may be treated with usual antidysrhythmic drugs, myocardial infarction may be treated by standard methods, and so forth. Initial detoxification and long-term treatment are best accomplished in centers or units that specialize in substance abuse disorders. Long-term treatment of cocaine abuse usually involves psychotherapy, behavioral therapy, and 12-step programs. Caffeine and nicotine are CNS stimulants and would not be used in his treatment.

18. Answer: c
RATIONALE: Heroin may be taken by IV injection, smoking, or nasal application (snorting). IV injection produces intense euphoria, which occurs within seconds, lasts a few minutes, and is followed by a period of sedation. Effects diminish over approximately 4 hours, depending on the dose. Addicts may inject several times daily, cycling between desired effects and symptoms of withdrawal. Tolerance to euphoric effects develops rapidly, leading to dosage escalation and continued use to avoid withdrawal. Like other opioids, heroin causes severe respiratory depression with overdose and produces a characteristic abstinence syndrome.

19. Answer: c

RATIONALE: Convulsions are more likely to occur during the first 48 hours of withdrawal and delirium after 48 to 72 hours for patients with benzodiazepine dependence.

20. Answer: d

RATIONALE: Flumazenil is the antidote for benzodiazepine overdose.

CHAPTER 58

SECTION I: ASSESSING YOUR UNDERSTANDING

Activity A FILL IN THE BLANKS

1. myopia
2. hyperopia
3. presbyopia
4. retina
5. diagnosis

Activity B MATCHING

1. a   **2.** c   **3.** e   **4.** b   **5.** d

Activity C SHORT ANSWERS

1. The eyelids and lacrimal system function to protect the eye. The eyelid is a barrier to the entry of foreign bodies, strong light, dust, and other potential irritants. The conjunctiva is the mucous membrane lining of the eyelids. The canthi (singular, *canthus*) are the angles where the upper and lower eyelids meet. The lacrimal system produces a fluid that constantly moistens and cleanses the anterior surface of the eyeball. The fluid drains through two small openings in the inner canthus and flows through the nasolacrimal duct into the nasal cavity. When the conjunctiva is irritated or certain emotions are experienced (e.g., sadness), the lacrimal gland produces more fluid than the drainage system can accommodate. The excess fluid overflows the eyelids and becomes tears.

2. Pupil constriction is called miosis; dilation is called mydriasis.

3. The eyeball is a spherical structure composed of the sclera, cornea, choroid, and retina, plus special refractive tissues. The sclera is a white, opaque, fibrous tissue that covers the posterior five sixths of the eyeball. The cornea is a transparent, special connective tissue that covers the anterior sixth of the eyeball. The cornea contains no blood vessels. The choroid, composed of blood vessels and connective tissue, continues forward to form the iris. The iris is composed of pigmented cells, the opening called the pupil, and muscles that control the size of the pupil by contracting or dilating in response to stimuli.

4. For vision to occur, light rays must enter the eye through the cornea; travel through the pupil, lens, and vitreous body; and be focused on the retina.

5. Light rays do not travel directly to the retina. Instead, they are deflected in various directions according to the density of the ocular structures through which they pass. This process, called *refraction*, is controlled by the aqueous humor, lens, and vitreous body.

SECTION II: APPLYING YOUR KNOWLEDGE

Activity D CASE STUDY

1. Diagnosis of glaucoma is based on the results of a number of tests. Tests for glaucoma include ophthalmoscopic examination of the optic disk, measurement of intraocular pressure (IOP; tonometry), and testing of visual fields. Glaucoma is often characterized by increased IOP (greater than 22 mm Hg) but may also occur with normal IOP (less than 21 mm Hg); the average IOP is 15 to 16 mm Hg.

2. Mrs. Lincoln has most common type of glaucoma, primary open-angle glaucoma. Its cause is unknown, but contributing factors include advanced age, a family history of glaucoma and elevated IOP, diabetes mellitus, hypertension, myopia, long-term use of corticosteroid drugs, and previous eye injury, inflammation, or infection. Her hypertension put her at risk for this condition. In addition, the incidence of glaucoma in African Americans is about three times higher than in non–African Americans. Glaucoma is one of the leading causes of blindness in the United States and the most common cause of blindness in African Americans.

3. Glaucoma is a group of diseases characterized by optic nerve damage and changes in visual fields.

4. These are signs of closed-angle glaucoma, which is usually an acute situation requiring emergency surgery. It may occur when pupils are dilated and the outflow of aqueous humor is blocked. Darkness and drugs with anticholinergic effects (e.g., atropine, antihistamines, tricyclic antidepressants) may dilate the pupil, reduce outflow of aqueous humor, and precipitate acute glaucoma.

SECTION III: PRACTICING FOR NCLEX

Activity E

1. Answer: b

RATIONALE: Local eye medications may cause systemic effects; systemic drugs may affect eye function.

2. Answer: b

RATIONALE: Eye medications should be kept sterile, to avoid infection.

3. Answer: d

RATIONALE: Therapeutic effects of eye drops depend on accurate administration.

4. Answer: a, b, c, and e

RATIONALE: Drug therapy of eye disorders is unique because of the location, structure, and function of the eye and the blood–eye barrier.

5. **Answer: a, b, and c**
   RATIONALE: The home care nurse may be involved in the care of patients with acute or chronic eye disorders. As with other drug therapies, the nurse may need to teach patients and caregivers reasons for use, accurate administration, and assessment of therapeutic and adverse responses to eye medications. The nurse would not be responsible for the administration of all medications.

6. **Answer: c**
   RATIONALE: Accurate dosage and occlusion of the nasolacrimal duct in the inner canthus of the eye are needed to prevent adverse drug effects such as hypertension, tachycardia, or dysrhythmias with adrenergic drugs and bradycardia, heart block, or bronchoconstriction with beta-blockers.

7. **Answer: a and d**
   RATIONALE: Acetazolamide is administered both orally and intravenously.

8. **Answer: b**
   RATIONALE: When treating children, the short-acting mydriatics and cycloplegics (e.g., cyclopentolate, tropicamide) are preferred because they cause fewer systemic adverse effects than atropine or scopolamine.

9. **Answer: b**
   RATIONALE: For chronic glaucoma, the goal of drug therapy is to slow disease progression by reducing IOP. Topical beta-blockers are first-line drugs and are commonly used.

10. **Answer: c**
    RATIONALE: Patients who wear contact lenses are at higher risk of developing abrasions that become infected and ulcerate. For these patients, an antipseudomonal antibiotic (such as gentamicin or a fluoroquinolone) should be used. In addition, the patient should avoid wearing contact lenses until the abrasion is healed and antibiotic therapy is completed.

11. **Answer: a**
    RATIONALE: Brimonidine is an alpha$_2$-adrenergic agonist that is used to treat open-angle glaucoma and ocular hypertension. It reduces aqueous humor production.

12. **Answer: b**
    RATIONALE: Natamycin (Natacyn) is the drug of choice in fungal eye infections. It has a broad spectrum of antifungal activity and is nonirritating and nontoxic.

13. **Answer: b**
    RATIONALE: In severe infections, antibacterial drugs may be given both topically and systemically. Because systemic antibiotics penetrate the eye poorly, large doses are required to attain therapeutic drug concentrations in ocular structures. Drugs that reach therapeutic levels in the eye when given in proper dosage include ampicillin and dicloxacillin.

14. **Answer: a, d, and e**
    RATIONALE: Timolol maleate is a beta-blocker used for the treatment of open-angle glaucoma and is contraindicated in patients with asthma, COPD, cardiogenic shock, heart failure, and left ventricular dysfunction.

15. **Answer: d**
    RATIONALE: Drug therapy is usually initiated as soon as culture material (eye secretions) has been obtained and often includes a broad-spectrum antibacterial agent or a combination of two or more antibiotics.

16. **Answer: a**
    RATIONALE: Some eye drops contain benzalkonium hydrochloride, a preservative, that is absorbed by soft contact lenses. The medications should not be applied while wearing soft contacts; they should be instilled 15 minutes or longer before soft contacts are inserted.

17. **Answer: c and d**
    RATIONALE: Phenylephrine eye drops are contraindicated in patients who have hypertension, ventricular tachycardia, and narrow-angle glaucoma.

18. **Answer: a, b, and c**
    RATIONALE: Topical ophthalmic medications should not be used after the expiration date; cloudy, discolored solutions should be discarded. Stinging upon administration is a common side effect of instillation of eye drops and does not signify the need for the medication to be discarded.

19. **Answer: a**
    RATIONALE: Ointments are administered less frequently than drops and often produce higher concentrations of drug in target tissues.

20. **Answer: a and d**
    RATIONALE: Atropine sulfate (ophthalmic) produces mydriasis and pupillary dilation. It prevents the accommodation of near vision.

CHAPTER 59

SECTION I: ASSESSING YOUR UNDERSTANDING

Activity A FILL IN THE BLANKS

1. Otitis externa
2. Otitis media
3. eustachian
4. otalgia, otorrhea
5. otic

Activity B MATCHING

1. b   2. e   3. a   4. d   5. c

Activity C SHORT ANSWERS

1. Otitis externa involves the presence of moisture in the external ear canal, leading to the development of inflammation of the pinna and canal. The canal becomes itchy, red, and tender, and increased swelling makes it narrower. Ear pain occurs with movement because of the inflammation. There may be watery or purulent drainage, and intermittent hearing loss may result.

2. In acute otitis externa, the patient complains of ear pain and discharge from the external auditory canal. The discharge may be yellow or green, possessing a foul odor. The patient may also report a feeling of "fullness" in the ear, decreased hearing, and pruritus.

   In necrotizing otitis externa, the presenting symptoms are *otalgia*, or ear pain, and *otorrhea*, or purulent drainage. The pain is primarily experienced at night and may extend to the temporomandibular joint when chewing.

3. In acute otitis media, marked fluid and inflammation in the mucosa lining the middle ear space are present. Otalgia and diminished hearing occur. Fever may or may not be present. An upper respiratory tract infection or seasonal allergic rhinitis commonly precedes acute otitis media. Changes in equilibrium may occur. If the tympanic membrane ruptures, patients report a reduction or relief of ear pain.

4. Neomycin and polymyxin B are antibiotics, which combat bacterial infections. Hydrocortisone is a steroid, which reduces the actions of chemicals in the body that cause inflammation, redness, and swelling.

5. The proper administration of ear drops requires tilting the head toward the opposite shoulder, pulling the superior aspect of the auricle upward, and instilling the ear drops into the ear canal. The patient should then lie on the side opposite the side of administration for 20 minutes. To maximize medication absorption, the patient should have a cotton ball placed in the ear canal.

SECTION II: APPLYING YOUR KNOWLEDGE

Activity D CASE STUDY

1. The nurse anticipates that the physician will order Cortisporin Otic. Administration of Cortisporin Otic is directly in the external ear canal. Prior to administering the otic suspension, it is necessary to shake the medication well. In addition, if cerumen is present, cleaning of the ear canal with a cotton swab is important.

2. The nurse will instruct the mother to dry the ear carefully whenever it is wet because of swimming or bathing. The ear may be dried with a hair dryer set to the cool setting. Also, the child should wear earplugs to prevent water from entering the ear when swimming.

3. In otitis externa, the infection is in the external canal. The patient may experience some decrease in hearing due to swelling of the external canal, but it does not permanently damage the ear. Otitis media is an infection of the middle ear, and chronic infections can cause permanent loss of hearing.

SECTION III: PRACTICING FOR NCLEX

Activity E

1. **Answer: c**
   RATIONALE: Amoxicillin should be administered around the clock.

2. **Answer: c**
   RATIONALE: Ofloxacin is the only otic topical preparation that can be administered if the patient has a perforated ear drum.

3. **Answer: a**
   RATIONALE: Coly-Mycin is contraindicated in patient with known hypersensitivity to aminoglycosides as well as the presence of herpes simplex, vaccinia, or varicella.

4. **Answer: b**
   RATIONALE: Patients who are taking ciprofloxacin should avoid dairy products within 2 hours of taking the medication.

5. **Answer: a**
   RATIONALE: Patients who are 60 years of age and older are at higher risk for tendon rupture.

6. **Answer: b, c, and d**
   RATIONALE: Symptoms of necrotizing otitis externa include otalgia, otorrhea, and pain while chewing.

7. **Answer: c**
   RATIONALE: A vaginal infection in a patient who is taking amoxicillin is an example of a superinfection. The nausea and abdominal pain are adverse effects of the medication, and swelling and itching of the throat are an example of possible allergy to the drug.

8. **Answer: c**
   RATIONALE: In the event of a penicillin allergy without urticaria or anaphylaxis, the patient is prescribed cefdinir, cefpodoxime, or cefuroxime

9. **Answer: b, d, and e**
   RATIONALE: Indications of a resolution of otitis media include the absence of otalgia and otorrhea; improved hearing; a gray, dull tympanic membrane with a cone of light; no bulging of the tympanic membrane; and normal body temperature.

10. **Answer: b**
    RATIONALE: Alternating acetaminophen and ibuprofen has proven to control elevated body temperature in children better than monotherapy. Aspirin is never administered for control of fever to a child.

11. **Answer: b**
    RATIONALE: A patient with otitis media would demonstrate an absence of a cone of light on the ear drum when the ear is examined with an otoscope.

12. **Answer: c**
RATIONALE: Impaired skin integrity related to an auricle lesion is the most appropriate nursing diagnosis for a patient with necrotizing otitis externa. The other nursing diagnoses are not related to otitis externa.

13. **Answer: d**
RATIONALE: The most important thing the patient can do to prevent the development of otitis externa is to wear ear plugs when swimming and to dry the ear thoroughly if the ear gets wet.

14. **Answer: a**
RATIONALE: A baby should never be allowed to sleep while drinking a bottle because of the short, straight eustachian tube of the infant, which allows fluid to enter the ear when the child is lying down.

15. **Answer: d**
RATIONALE: *Pseudomonas aeruginosa* is the most common bacteria that causes otitis externa.

16. **Answer: b**
RATIONALE: Evidence has proven that the occurrence of otitis externa can be reduced if public swimming pools enforce swimmers to bathe prior to entering the pool.

17. **Answer: b**
RATIONALE: Cortisporin Otic is used for 10 days.

18. **Answer: c**
RATIONALE: Ciprofloxacin can cause tendon rupture, especially in patients younger than 18 and older than 60.

19. **Answer: a**
RATIONALE: Tetracycline, if taken with amoxicillin, inhibits the action of amoxicillin.

20. **Answer: c**
RATIONALE: The patient with renal impairment will need to have reduced dose of ciprofloxacin.

CHAPTER 60

SECTION I: ASSESSING YOUR UNDERSTANDING

Activity A FILL IN THE BLANKS

1. erythema, pruritus
2. Contact dermatitis
3. urticaria
4. Rosacea
5. staphylococci, streptococci

Activity B MATCHING

1. c   2. a   3. e   4. b   5. d

Activity C SHORT ANSWERS

1. Tinea infections (ringworm) are caused by fungi (dermatophytes). These infections may involve the scalp (tinea capitis), the body (tinea corporis), the foot (tinea pedis), and other areas of the body. Tinea pedis, commonly called athlete's foot, is a type of ringworm infection.

2. At least four pathologic events take place within acne-infected hair follicles: (1) androgen-mediated stimulation of sebaceous gland activity, (2) abnormal keratinization leading to follicular plugging (comedone formation), (3) proliferation of the bacterium *Propionibacterium acnes* within the follicle, and (4) inflammation.

3. General treatment goals for many skin disorders are to relieve symptoms (e.g., dryness, pruritus, inflammation, infection), eradicate or improve lesions, promote healing and repair, restore skin integrity, and prevent recurrence. Specific goals often depend on the condition being treated.

4. Oral antimicrobials are first-line treatment for patients with moderate to severe inflammatory acne. These drugs have both antimicrobial and anti-inflammatory effects. They reduce *Propionibacterium acnes* organisms and thereby inhibit production of *P. acnes*–induced inflammatory cytokines.

5. The FDA has issued a black box warning stating that isotretinoin, in pregnancy category X, causes both spontaneous abortions and severe life-threatening congenital malformations. In addition, women of childbearing potential should not take isotretinoin unless they have had two negative pregnancy test results before beginning therapy, will begin drug therapy on the second or third day of the next menstrual period, and will comply with stringent contraceptive measures for 1 month before therapy, during therapy, and for 1 month after therapy (iPLEDGE program).

SECTION II: APPLYING YOUR KNOWLEDGE

Activity D CASE STUDY

1. "No, the treatment is for a secondary infection on your forearm." Scratching damages the skin and increases the risk of secondary infection, which may be treated by the use of an oral antibiotic.

2. Dermatitis, also called eczema, is not a contagious disease. It is caused by an inflammatory response of the skin to injuries from irritants, allergens, or trauma.

3. Atopic dermatitis is a common disorder characterized by dry skin, pruritus, and lesions that vary according to the extent of inflammation, stages of healing, and scratching. Acute lesions are reddened skin areas containing papules and vesicles; chronic lesions are often thick, fibrotic, and nodular. The cause of atopic dermatitis is uncertain but may involve allergic, hereditary, or psychological elements. Approximately 50% to 80% of patients have asthma or allergic rhinitis; some have a family history of these disorders.

4. Significant stress associated with her profession could be an exacerbating factor in Mrs. Benjamin's condition. Other exacerbating factors are allergens, irritating chemicals, and certain foods, and these should be avoided if possible.

5. Mrs. Benjamin should bring her child to the pediatrician for an assessment. The development of atopic dermatitis may have a hereditary component, so, if she has it, it may be that her child has it too. Furthermore, although atopic dermatitis may occur in all age groups, it is more common in children.

SECTION III: PRACTICING FOR NCLEX

Activity E

1. **Answer: c**
   RATIONALE: Systemic adverse effects may occur with topical drug therapy; skin disorders may occur with systemic drugs.
2. **Answer: d**
   RATIONALE: Special precautions are needed for safe use of oral retinoids in female patients of childbearing potential.
3. **Answer: c**
   RATIONALE: Special precautions are needed for safe use of topical corticosteroids, especially in children.
4. **Answer: a**
   RATIONALE: Topical drugs are used to treat most skin disorders; accurate application is essential to maximize therapeutic effects.
5. **Answer: a, c, and e**
   RATIONALE: Careful assessment of types, color, and locations of lesions can aid diagnosis and treatment of many skin disorders.
6. **Answer: a and d**
   RATIONALE: Staphylococci and streptococci are the most common bacterial causes of skin infection, and methicillin-resistant *Staphylococcus aureus* (MRSA) infections are increasing.
7. **Answer: c**
   RATIONALE: Two topical agents for which there is some support of safety and effectiveness are aloe and oat preparations.
8. **Answer: b**
   RATIONALE: Older adults often have thin, dry skin and are at risk of pressure ulcers if mobility, nutrition, or elimination is impaired. Principles of topical drug therapy are generally the same as for younger adults. In addition, topical corticosteroids should be used with caution on thinned or atrophic skin.
9. **Answer: b**
   RATIONALE: With topical agents, cautious use is recommended. Infants, and perhaps older children, have more permeable skin and are more likely than adults to absorb topical drugs.
10. **Answer: c**
    RATIONALE: Tacrolimus ointment carries a black box warning that this medication carries with it an increased risk of skin cancer.

11. **Answer: d**
    RATIONALE: Because children are at high risk for development of systemic adverse effects with topical corticosteroids, these drugs should be used only if clearly indicated, in the smallest effective dose, for the shortest effective time, and usually without occlusive dressings.
12. **Answer: c**
    RATIONALE: With chronic urticaria, the goal of treatment is symptom relief. Antihistamines are most effective when given before histamine-induced urticaria occurs and should be given around the clock, not just when lesions appear.
13. **Answer: b**
    RATIONALE: Glycolic acid is the agent that is added to decrease skin wrinkles and is used to make cosmetics antiaging.
14. **Answer: a, d, and e**
    RATIONALE: Older adults are more prone to skin cancer, actinic keratoses, and dry skin.
15. **Answer: a**
    RATIONALE: Sedating, systemic antihistamines such as diphenhydramine or hydroxyzine are often used to relieve itching related to dermatitis and promote rest and sleep.
16. **Answer: b**
    RATIONALE: Oral antiandrogens may be given to female patients with high blood levels of androgens (e.g., testosterone). Combination oral contraceptive pills decrease the amount of free testosterone circulating in the bloodstream and therefore may improve acne. Norgestimate/ethinyl estradiol (Ortho Tri-Cyclen) and norethindrone acetate/ethinyl estradiol (Estrostep) are FDA approved for treatment of acne.
17. **Answer: d**
    RATIONALE: Retinoids, in both systemic and topical forms, may be used for moderate to severe acne. All topical retinoids (tretinoin, adapalene, tazarotene) reduce acne lesions, usually within 12 weeks.
18. **Answer: a, c, d, and e**
    RATIONALE: Rosacea symptoms are made worse by spicy food, alcohol, embarrassment, and becoming hot.
19. **Answer: d**
    RATIONALE: Combination products of topical clindamycin or erythromycin and benzoyl peroxide are more effective than antibiotics alone.
20. **Answer: b**
    RATIONALE: The most common adverse effects related to isotretinoin are dermatologic.